Current practice in gerontological nursing

VOLUME ONE

Current practice in gerontological nursing

Edited by

ADINA M. REINHARDT, Ph.D.

Associate, Rocky Mountain Gerontology Center,
University of Utah; Health Care Coordinator,
Office of Health Care Financing,
Utah State Department of Social Services,
Salt Lake City, Utah

MILDRED D. QUINN, R.N., M.S.

Professor Emeritus and Dean Emeritus,
College of Nursing, University of Utah,
Salt Lake City, Utah

The C. V. Mosby Company

ST. LOUIS • TORONTO • LONDON   1979

Copyright © 1979 by The C. V. Mosby Company

All rights reserved. No part of this book may be reproduced
in any manner without written permission of the publisher.

Printed in the United States of America

The C. V. Mosby Company
11830 Westline Industrial Drive, St. Louis, Missouri 63141

Library of Congress Cataloging in Publication Data

Main entry under title:

Current practice in gerontological nursing.

    Bibliography: p.
    1. Geriatric nursing. I. Reinhardt, Adina M.
II. Quinn, Mildred D.
[DNLM: 1. Geriatric nursing — Essays. WY152 C976]
RC954.C87   610.73'65   78-31424
ISBN 0-8016-4113-6 (Paperback)   02/B/216
ISBN 0-8016-4122-5 (Hardbound)   02/C/216

GW/CB/B 9 8 7 6 5 4 3 2 1

NATHANIEL N. WAGNER
1930-1978

Nathaniel N. Wagner was born on January 31, 1930, in Brooklyn, New York, obtained his Ph.D. in 1956 from Columbia University, and joined the faculty of the University of Washington in 1962, where he obtained the Distinguished Teacher Award in May of 1978.

A clinical psychologist, Nathaniel Wagner strongly believed that human suffering could be greatly alleviated via a candid effort to explore the human condition, despite social taboos. In conjunction with others, he contributed over 75 journal and book articles on minority affairs, human sexuality, aging, and cardiac rehabilitation. In his writings he sought to offer comfort and hope to the victims of hatred, prejudice, agism, and illness.

Nathaniel Wagner understood the plight and struggle of the afflicted, as he himself was afflicted by a heart attack at the age of 35, followed by two others in later years. Nevertheless, with a reverence for life, he responded by refusing to become a "cardiac cripple," and he led as full a life as possible. It is perhaps fitting that this present work on the Chicano aged, in life and death, should have been among his final contributions. His ideals live on in the many individuals he managed to touch — students, advisees, colleagues, and others.

Nathaniel N. Wagner died suddenly of coronary arrhythmias in Cleveland, Ohio, on June 14, 1978; he was a man who touched many lives.

Felipe G. Castro

Contributors

ALICE M. AKAN, A.M., R.N.

Instructor, Department of Nursing,
Herbert H. Lehman College of the City University of New York,
Bronx, New York

FELIPE G. CASTRO, M.S.W.

Department of Psychology, University of Washington,
Seattle, Washington

ALAN CHEUNG, Pharm.D., M.P.H., F.C.P.

Associate Clinical Professor, School of Pharmacy,
University of Southern California,
Los Angeles, California

SHERMAN R. DICKMAN, Ph.D.

Department of Biochemistry, University of Utah,
Salt Lake City, Utah

CHARLOTTE ELIOPOULOS, R.N., M.P.H.

Consultant in Gerontological Nursing, Division of Nursing,
State of Maryland, Department of Health and Mental Hygiene,
Baltimore, Maryland

PAUL A. L. HABER, M.D.

Assistant Chief Medical Director for Professional Services,
Department of Medicine and Surgery,
Veterans Administration,
Washington, D.C.

EDWARD O. MOE, Ph.D.

Principal Sociologist and Coordinator for Rural Development,
United States Department of Agriculture,
Cooperative State Research Service,
Washington, D.C.

DOROTHY V. MOSES, R.N.

Professor of Nursing, School of Nursing,
San Diego State University,
San Diego, California

ROSEMARY MURRAY, M.A., R.N.

Director, The Mount Sinai Hospital,
School of Continuing Education in Nursing,
New York, New York

MARTHA C. PRIMEAUX, R.N., M.S.

Associate Professor of Nursing, The University of Oklahoma
Health Sciences Center, College of Nursing,
Oklahoma City, Oklahoma

MILDRED D. QUINN, R.N., M.S.

Professor Emeritus and Dean Emeritus,
College of Nursing, University of Utah,
Salt Lake City, Utah

ADINA M. REINHARDT, Ph.D.

Associate, Rocky Mountain Gerontology Center,
University of Utah; Health Care Coordinator,
Office of Health Care Financing,
Utah State Department of Social Services,
Salt Lake City, Utah

KATHRYN L. RIFFLE, R.N., Ph.D.

Associate Professor, School of Nursing,
Duke University Medical Center,
Durham, North Carolina

PAULETTE ROBISCHON, R.N., Ph.D.

Professor and Coordinator, Community Health Nursing,
Department of Nursing, Herbert H. Lehman College of the
City University of New York,
Bronx, New York

E. PERCIL STANFORD, Ph.D.

Professor and Director, Center on Aging,
San Diego, California

LILLIAN G. STOKES, R.N., M.Sc.N., Ph.D.

Associate Professor of Nursing,
Indiana University School of Nursing,
Indianapolis, Indiana

THERESE SULLIVAN, R.N., Ph.D.

Head, Department of Nursing;
Chairman, Division of Health Sciences, Carroll College,
Helena, Montana

JACK L. TEDROW, M.D., J.D.

Clinical Associate Professor, Department of Psychiatry,
University of Utah College of Medicine;
Member, Utah State Bar Association;
Member, State Board of Mental Health,
Salt Lake City, Utah

NATHANIEL N. WAGNER, Ph.D.†

Professor of Psychology, Director of Clinical
Psychology Training, University of Washington,
Seattle, Washington

THELMA J. WELLS, R.N., Ph.D.

Assistant Professor of Nursing (Gerontology),
School of Nursing, University of Rochester,
Rochester, New York

NANCY FUGATE WOODS, R.N., Ph.D.

Associate Professor of Physiological Nursing,
University of Washington,
Seattle, Washington

---

†Deceased.

Foreword

Nurses have taken the leadership in the care of older Americans, both as community health nurses and in nursing homes, doing so under very adverse conditions. Little wonder that a small number — only 50,000 of our nearly 1 million nurses — work in nursing homes, although there are more older patients in nursing homes than there are in hospitals.

The United States has a new, growing minority group: the aged. Four percent of the population in 1900 was over 65 years of age, almost 11% was in 1976, and by the year 2030 a projected 17% to 20% will be in that age group. In fact, those people over 85 years of age are the fastest growing age group in the country. This is indeed a remarkable scientific and social achievement, but one with extensive consequences for our country.

Some effects of these demographic changes are already being experienced, especially in the health field. Few medical personnel are trained to improve the longer lives of the elderly. To work effectively with members of this minority, today's gerontological nurse must be many things, including a health practitioner, sociologist, psychologist, and politician.

Gerontological nursing is advancing despite the adverse conditions under which a good many of these nurses must often work: run-down or dangerous neighborhoods where some elderly are forced to live, scandalous conditions in some nursing homes, inadequate pay, and poor advancement opportunities. Thus, it is not surprising that a determined effort is needed to attract more qualified nurses to the field. This is especially true since the Department of Health, Education, and Welfare estimated that broadening nurses' roles, such as the increased use of nurse practitioners, will create a shortage of 220,000 American nurses by 1980.

Nurses are the medical profession's primary contact with the elderly, whether in the clinic, the private physician's office, the nursing home, or the aged person's own residence. The nurse may conduct a detailed screening before a visit with a doctor, administer needed medication, or instruct the older person in its use; or the nurse may visit the elderly at home to monitor their condition or to determine ways to improve their general health and life-style. A nurse may perform the many routine tasks involved in the daily care of a chronically ill patient in a nursing home. The knowledge, time, and understanding these professionals display greatly affects the elderly's view of medicine and its ability to improve their lives.

Nursing's commitment to the care of older Americans extends to educational programs, and specialized texts such as this one are essential educational tools in an emerging field. There are approximately 100 baccalaureate nursing programs that include the subject of geriatrics, but these are still not sufficient. Gerontological care needs to be further complemented by the teaching of geriatric medicine in American medical schools. Few such schools provide any special emphasis on the subject.

As new people enter the nursing profession, they will learn, from books on gerontological nursing, the range of career possibilities and rewards to be found in this field. Our older citizens are extremely diverse because of the many experiences they have had during their long lives. Contrary to popular belief, the elderly do not need only routine chronic care; rather, one fourth of all doctor contacts with older patients relate to acute infectious diseases. There are also special challenges for minority group nurses in caring for the elderly members of their minorities.

Current Practice in Gerontological Nursing specifically addresses the diverse needs of the geriatric patient. The state of our knowledge on the physiological changes associated with aging, pharmacology for the elderly, nutrition, psychological aspects of aging, the unique needs of minority group aged, health programs for older Americans, and legal aspects of aging is detailed by experts in each field.

The elderly have been described as a subculture of society, people brought together by a feeling that their age excludes them from the rest of the population. With training in geriatrics, our nurses may be able to change this feeling. They will gain a clearer understanding of the elderly and their special needs and, in turn, may be able to integrate these people back into the society they helped to create.

Robert N. Butler, M.D.

Director, National Institute on Aging

Preface

Today is a "new age for old age"; the sudden and dramatic increase in the number and relative proportion of elderly in our society has been referred to as a demographic revolution.[1] Now exceeding 23.5 million persons, the number of senior citizens in the United States represents more than 10% of our population. This expansion in the size of the older age group will demand from our country adaptations in regard to economic, social, and, in particular, *health* realities. For example, increasing Social Security taxes have been mandated by growing numbers of recipients. Likewise, the movement to abolish mandatory retirement, initially and most prominently supported by the Gray Panthers, will soon become law.[2] Stronger lobbying efforts by organized senior groups such as the Gray Panthers, the American Association of Retired Persons/National Retired Teachers' Association, and other senior citizens' coalitions are highly visible and effective aspects of today's political scene.

Most important, however, health care providers and health care delivery systems are being pressed to reorient themselves to the ever-increasing needs for providing preventive and supportive services, home health care services, treatment of chronic degenerative diseases, and improvement in long-term care facilities.[3]

In its attempt to respond to the needs of the elderly for comprehensive, coordinated, and continuing quality health care, including preventive and supportive ambulatory care as well as institutional care, the nursing profession has recently accepted an expanded responsibility for preparing nurses in gerontological nursing. Nursing must now meet the challenge of caring for the aged who have a wide variety of needs in diverse settings, while utilizing a sophisticated blend of knowledge and skills from the sciences of gerontology and geriatrics. New concepts of gerontology and geriatrics are being incorporated into baccalaureate and continuing education programs. Growing numbers of schools of nursing are now offering a specialty in gerontological nursing at the master's and doctoral levels.

New and more humane concepts concerning supportive care for the terminally ill are being proposed. For example, the nurse thanatologist, a gerontological nurse skilled in working with the terminally ill and their families, is a new development, as are the emerging proposals concerning pain medication for the terminally ill that will necessitate changes in narcotics laws in this country.[4] Also new in the United States is the notion of hospice, an attitude of supportive care for terminally ill patients enabling them to live as comfortably, fully, and effectively as possible until death does occur.[5] Clearly, gerontological nurses must become advocates for the health and mental health needs of the elderly and for the improvement and coordination of health delivery services and programs for this group. In their caring and counseling roles with patient-clients and their families, these nurses need to assume responsibility for providing information and guidance that may lead to changes in health care habits, attitudes, and life-styles from infancy (through parental education) through adulthood, maturity, aging, and dying.

Caring for the health needs of older people requires a unique blend of multidisciplinary knowledge and skills in identifying and assessing normal and abnormal physiological, pharmacological, nutritional, and other biopsychosocial reactions in the aging individual. For example, illnesses may manifest themselves quite differently in older persons than in younger people. Gerontological health care providers must be carefully trained in the complex tasks of assessing, planning, and implementing care for older patients and in evaluating the outcome of such care.

With the increasing activity in development of curricula in gerontological nursing education, there is a pressing need for a text written primarily by gerontological nurses for nursing students and practitioners who care for the elderly. All material in this text is original and has been specifically designed and developed for this book.

The purpose of this book is to bring together material of a multidisciplinary nature that will aid the health care provider to understand in greater depth the physiological, cultural, psychosocial, pharmacological, nutritional, and other aspects of providing effective care and service for seniors, including information concerning legal issues affecting the elderly. This book will be of value to undergraduate and graduate nursing students, practitioners in gerontological health care, and practitioners in the areas of community health, psychosocial, and medical-surgical nursing. It is hoped that the resource material included will provide a broader base of understanding for students in allied health fields such as health education and social work.

Current Practice in Gerontological Nursing is divided into seven parts. Part I provides an overview of physical and mental health care for the elderly and of the politics of providing health care for the elderly in the United States.

Part II deals with the physiological bases of advancing age. The three chapters comprising Part II are devoted to the physiological, pharmacological, and nutritional aspects of aging. Chapter 3 is a comprehensive, detailed study of the physiology of bodily changes in aging and the nurse's assessment of these changes. Chapter 4, "Drugs for the Aging: Use and Abuse," discusses altered physiological absorption of drugs by the elderly, negative drug interactions, and other important aspects of drug use, abuse, and prescription methods. Nutritional needs and the effects of poor nutrition are the topics of concern in Chapter 5. The author concludes by stating, "If only one physician, nurse, or attendant recognizes that the irrational, irascible behavior of one older person may be due to nutritional factors and acts accordingly, it will have been worthwhile writing this chapter."

Part III presents four chapters that deal with the social and cultural implications of advanced maturity. These chapters focus on the historical aspects of aging in four diverse cultures: black, Chicano, American Indian, and Anglo. Customs and rituals concerning chronic care, illness, death, and burial practices in the above cultures can, in many instances, be compared and contrasted in these unique chapters.

The chapters in Part IV are devoted to the psychosocial needs of the aged. In Chapter 10, Rosemary Murray addresses psychosocial aspects of aging from a more general orientation; the following two chapters focus on more specific topics. For example, in Chapter 11, Nancy Fugate Woods explores some of the pertinent research findings regarding sexual potential among aging persons, the need for such expression, and the barriers, social, rather than biological, instituted by our society. Paulette Robischon and Alice M.

Akan (Chapter 12) perceptively discuss, and illustrate with a case vignette, the role of the family with an elderly parent.

Part V is entitled "Action and Service for the Elderly: Nursing Education and Agency Collaboration." The emerging network concerning agency collaboration in health care planning and service for the elderly is the topic addressed by Edward O. Moe, a nationally prominent health care planner and sociologist. In Chapter 14, Thelma J. Wells discusses activity on the educational front in gerontological nursing. Charlotte Eliopoulos describes the specific role and functioning of the gerontological nurse specialist in Chapter 15.

Part VI, "Understanding the Law and the Nurse's Role as Health Advocate with the Elderly," contains two chapters unique for a gerontological nursing text. In Chapter 16, "The Law and the Elderly," Jack L. Tedrow focuses his writing on pertinent and specific legal information that can be of great value to gerontological nurses in their counseling and supportive roles with elderly clients and their families. Dorothy V. Moses, a pioneering gerontological nurse, discusses in Chapter 17 the timely issue of advocacy for and with the elderly. A psychiatric nurse who has devoted 20 years or more to working with the aged, she issues a challenge to nurses to function as health advocates.

In Part VII, "Looking to the Future," a prominent national authority in gerontological nursing and health care for the elderly anticipates future directions in this field. A physician long active and involved in improved health care delivery for the elderly, Paul A. L. Haber, presents a discursive overview regarding future trends and issues in the field of gerontology. This paper points to the problems of aging and expansion of the care-giving role. This role offers much promise for nursing.

We wish to express our appreciation to Dr. Robert N. Butler, Director, National Institute on Aging, for his support of this project from its inception and particularly for his support of nursing, medical, and all professional and paraprofessional health care providers who work patiently and supportively with the elderly. As editors of a multiauthored text, we are in debt to each author who has generously provided his or her concepts, ideas, insights, and experiences concerning health care issues for the elderly. All of them are recognized leaders in the areas of gerontological and geriatric care.

We also owe thanks to our teachers — the elderly patients and clients we have served in care and counseling roles. In addition, a personal note of appreciation goes to L. L. C., whose encouragement and support have been of immeasurable assistance in the task of completing this manuscript. Finally, we sincerely hope that nurses and other practitioners serving the aged may profit from the concepts and insights expressed by our contributors and, indeed, may "catch attitudes" of humane caring, warmth, and acceptance of the elderly. May they strive to become competent and effective health care providers for and with the elderly. In due course, we shall all join that growing group.

Adina M. Reinhardt
Mildred D. Quinn

REFERENCES

1. Butler, R. N.: Statement before the Special Committee on Aging of the United States Senate on "International Perspectives on Aging," Nov. 10, 1977.
2. When retirement takes hold at age 70—, U.S. News and World Report, **84**(10):82-83, March 13, 1978.
3. Horn, L., and Griesel, E.: Nursing homes: a citizens' action guide, Boston, 1977, Beacon Press.
4. Butler, R. N.: A humanistic approach to our last days, March, 1978, Personal communication.
5. Butler, R. N., and Toufexis, A.: Hospice: putting more living into dying, Medical News and International Report **1**:7, March 20, 1978.

Contents

Part I

HEALTH CARE FOR THE ELDERLY: AN OVERVIEW

1 The elderly: health and mental health care — a nursing challenge, 3
ADINA M. REINHARDT
MILDRED D. QUINN

2 The politics of providing health and mental health care for the aged, 18
E. PERCIL STANFORD

Part II

PHYSIOLOGICAL BASIS OF ADVANCED MATURITY

3 Physiological changes of aging and nursing assessment, 39
KATHRYN L. RIFFLE

4 Drugs for the aging: use and abuse, 64
ALAN CHEUNG

5 Nutritional needs and effects of poor nutrition in elderly persons, 74
SHERMAN R. DICKMAN

Part III

SOCIOCULTURAL IMPLICATIONS OF ADVANCED MATURITY

6 The subculture of the aging and its implications for health and nursing care to the elderly, 91
THERESE SULLIVAN

7   Growing old in the black community, 105
       LILLIAN G. STOKES

8   The Chicano community and its aged, 115
       FELIPE G. CASTRO
       NATHANIEL N. WAGNER

9   Health care and the aging American Indian, 130
       MARTHA C. PRIMEAUX

Part IV

PSYCHOSOCIAL NEEDS OF THE AGING

10 Psychosocial aspects of aging, 141
       ROSEMARY MURRAY

11 Sexuality and aging, 151
       NANCY FUGATE WOODS

12 The family and its role with the elderly parent, 161
       PAULETTE ROBISCHON
       ALICE M. AKAN

Part V

ACTION AND SERVICE FOR THE ELDERLY: NURSING EDUCATION AND AGENCY COLLABORATION

13 Agency collaboration in planning and service:
       the emerging network on aging, 173
       EDWARD O. MOE

14 Nursing committed to the elderly, 187
       THELMA J. WELLS

15 The gerontological nurse specialist, 197
       CHARLOTTE ELIOPOULOS

Part VI

UNDERSTANDING THE LAW AND THE NURSE'S ROLE AS HEALTH ADVOCATE FOR THE ELDERLY

16 The law and the elderly, 207
JACK L. TEDROW

17 The nurse's role as advocate with the elderly, 221
DOROTHY V. MOSES

Part VII

LOOKING TO THE FUTURE

18 Issues and trends in gerontology, 229
PAUL A. L. HABER

part I
HEALTH CARE FOR THE ELDERLY: AN OVERVIEW

The first two chapters of this book provide an overview and discussion of the current concerns, issues, and politics related to health care and mental health care for the elderly in this country.

In Chapter 1, the authors have described the problems associated with the economic, physical, and social changes that occur during the later years of life. The article points out the relationship between the changes in society (historical changes) and the economic circumstances that affect the elderly. The pros and cons of the Social Security Act and a brief discussion of mandatory retirement are included. A number of issues and challenges for health care providers are described and documented in this chapter.

Four key issues that are identified, along with some recommendations for desirable social action, include the following. First, the loss of a productive role and the associated economic deprivation as a result of heretofore mandatory retirement at age 65 years, combined with inflationary pressures, is discussed. Second, such economic deprivation frequently results in a perception of lessened self-worth, a contributory factor to mental and physical health problems. The third issue is the need for education of nurses and physicians and associated health care providers in geriatrics and gerontology in order that they may be made more aware of the multiple problems that are unique to this age group.

The fourth issue concerns the need for a more humanistic approach in caring for the terminally ill. Frequently, the dying patient elicits a response of frustration from both physicians and nurses as they are unable to effect a cure or alter the sequence of events made final by death. The terminally ill also produce a response of acute awareness of one's own mortality in those involved in providing care. The normal response engendered by this stress is one of avoidance, if possible. The concept of hospice is an attitude of supportive care for the terminally ill to effect a better quality of remaining life and to assist the patient and family in coping with the problems associated with the terminal illness, including their own acceptance of the inevitable event of death.

The politics of providing health and mental health care for the elderly is dealt with comprehensively by Dr. E. Percil Stanford in Chapter 2. Dr. Stanford points out that there currently exist adequate federal, state, and local legislation, authorities, and programs to ensure better health for older persons. However, Dr. Stanford implies that there is some question as to whether the federal financing mechanisms could be more effectively implemented at the various levels of government. A national focal point for implementing a sound program to monitor and enhance the quality of care for the elderly is needed. A number of additional issues and implied challenges for health care providers are described and documented in this comprehensive article.

Gerontological nursing students and practitioners can gain greater awareness of the political issues surrounding the delivery of health and mental health care for the aged by close scrutiny of the wealth of information contained in this chapter.

1 The elderly: health and mental health care—a nursing challenge

ADINA M. REINHARDT
MILDRED D. QUINN

Life is a continuing process from birth until death and it seems strange that it so seldom occurs to us to study life as a whole.[1]

Aging is a natural phenomenon that, as far as is known, affects all higher forms of life and perhaps all living things. No matter how aging is defined, its implications for the individual and for society are profound. Twenty-two million Americans, 10% of our population, are now over 65 years old. In 50 more years, 40 million persons may be that old. Two thirds of the federal money spent on health in this country is directed toward care of the aged. One million people over 65 years of age live in institutions, and a significant proportion of them are incapacitated by a variety of diseases and degenerative conditions. Thus, it is everyone's responsibility to study the phenomenon of aging throughout the life span.

Most particularly, such a study of aging is a major responsibility of health care providers, both nurses and physicians. Most physicians are trained more extensively in the treatment of acute diseases, however, than in the treatment of chronic diseases of the elderly. As a consequence, nurses must become more interested in and involved in providing care for the aged. They can have a significant impact on suffering resulting from chronic diseases among the elderly, since their basic philosophy is one of caring, teaching and educating clients on health problems, and health promotion and maintenance.[2] Furthermore, they are the largest group of health care providers in the United States today.

In 1973 we noted that "the public views health as a fundamental right to which all people are entitled regardless of their ability to pay," and that consumers "are demanding an increased quantity and an improved quality of health care services."[3] Since that time, the provision of health care has become a major issue in the United States.[4] Watkin has recently pointed out:

> The cost of appropriate health care . . . has brought the issue to prominence. With health costs rising at an unprecedented rate, outstripping the increments attributable solely to inflation, American society is searching desperately for solutions which will satisfy public demand for quality health care and at the same time contain costs not only to the individual but also to society as a whole. Among proposed solutions, one in particular is rational and of proven effectiveness: individuals' *acceptance of life-long personal responsibility for their health.*[5]

Continuing life crises help develop coping mechanisms throughout childhood, adolescence, young adulthood, middlescence, older adulthood, and most particularly, during the aging years. Increased awareness on the part of each individual regarding how to successfully cope with critical life events and how to accept personal responsibility for health would add to the richness of "life experienced and lived deeply and fully" in optimum health, and would result in greater productivity, more and better longevity, and less misery and suffering for most elderly in our society.[6] Parents and the individual adolescent's responsibility for learning, practicing, and adopting healthful life-styles such as good nutritional habits and avoidance of gluttony, smoking, drinking, and other destructive lifestyle habits,[7] would lead more and more people to grow to a healthful and good old age.[8]

To provide an overview to this text, the discussion in this chapter will consider the following, in sequence: (1) some demographic aspects of the elderly population explosion, (2) changes — physical, economic, and social — associated with aging and often experienced as losses and deprivation by the elderly, (3) the changing social environment of today's elderly, (4) social forces propelling the federal government's concern for the elderly since 1935 to the present and the development of gerontological nursing, (5) some issues and recommendations for social action by, and in behalf of, the elderly.

THE ELDERLY POPULATION EXPLOSION: DEMOGRAPHIC ASPECTS

During this century, there has been a striking increase in the age group 65 years and older in the United States. Butler has noted that "a population explosion of older people has been under way for a number of decades, and the elderly are now the fastest growing group in the United States. Between 1960 and 1970 the aging increased by 21% compared with an 18% increase among those under 65."[9] Before 1900, relatively few people attained that age and "in 1900 only three million or 4% of the population, were 65 and older."[10] At the turn of the century, the average life span was 47 years; now it is 70.4 years. It is predicted that "by the year 2000, just over twenty years from now, 1 out of every 3 Americans will be sixty five or over. That is a large segment of society even if the proportions are overstated. If you are over forty, you are going to be in that segment. Nearly half of the United States' population is going to be age fifty and over by the year 2000."[11]

Dr. Robert N. Butler, Director, National Institute on Aging, has noted, "Paradoxically, (this) extended average life expectancy . . . has reduced that already limited social status of the old."[12] Furthermore, anticipated discoveries and breakthroughs in medical science, an improved health-care delivery system and the presently declining birth rate, make it possible that the age group 65 and over will comprise one quarter of the total population by the year 2000. It is not the number of elderly persons that has produced this contemporary social problem. Rather, it is the lack of adequate preparation by our society for the population increase among the elderly.[13,14] Most perceptively, Dr. Butler states, "the truth is that we cannot promise a decent existence for those elderly now alive."[15] On a more positive note, Butler adds, "What is clear is that the presence of so many elderly in the United States will result in enormous change in every part of society."[16] For example, we believe that in the next two decades, changes will occur in our society's definition of the aging process itself, in current retirement practices, and, it is hoped, in improvement in the physical health of the majority of tomorrow's elderly and in their social and economic statuses.

Elsewhere, Butler has pointed out, "The biggest single major issue we have to face is that of looking realistically at aging and not trying to pretend that it does not occur. Clearly, unless we understand it, research it, do everything we can to control it, we open ourselves up to problems when we grow older."[17]

Demographically, there are 68.7 men per 100 women for the white group, and 72.9

men per 100 women for the black group. More than 70% of the men in this age group are living with their wives. The rest are widowed, divorced, or single. Only 37.6% of the women in this age group are living with their husbands. Of the rest, more than half are widowed. The living arrangements of this age category are that over 95% of the men live in households (either with their wives or with someone else). About 5% do not live in a household. About 94% of the women live in a household (either with their husbands or with someone else). About 5.6% do not live in a household.[18,19]

ECONOMIC, PHYSICAL, AND SOCIAL CHANGES IN LATER LIFE

Aging inevitably brings economic, physical, and social changes that test the coping skills of the elderly individual; the person's inner resources can assist the elderly individual to experience old age as a time of fulfillment, a "time of integrity,"[20] a vegetative state of disengagement from living, or as some other state along that continuum. These economic, physical, and social changes may be reacted to by the aging individual either as challenges to be overcome or as overwhelming problems. The facts would appear to indicate that 85% of the elderly in the United States today are coping realistically with the economic, physical, and social problems to which they must adjust. Although economic, physical, and social changes that affect the elderly are complex and interwoven, a brief discussion of each factor follows.

Economic changes and problems in later life

The majority of elderly in our society are economically deprived. It has been noted that "to live in retirement in the 1960's . . . was to suffer an income gap separating the old from the young—a gap that did not narrow during the decade."[21] Nor did this economic gap narrow a great deal in the 1970s. Kreps notes that "the incomes of older people have improved during recent years, but they remain low both in absolute amount and in relation to the incomes of younger families."[22] In summary:

1. Median income of families with heads age 65 and over was just under $7,300 in 1974; the median for families with heads of all ages was approximately $13,000.
2. For persons aged 65 years or over, the median income was about $3,000 compared with a median of approximately $4,500 for unrelated individuals of all ages.
3. About 16% of all the elderly were at or below the poverty level.
4. Among very old persons, incomes were particularly low: $2,700 for men and $2,200 for women aged 73 years and over who are living with relatives.

Kreps has recently pointed out:

Low incomes, now the number one problem of the aged, are likely to persist. Particular study should be made of the income problems of aged widows, health needs and rising medical costs, problems associated with home ownership and taxation, and the implications of early retirement from the labor force. In view of these difficulties and unless positive action is taken, the future elderly may suffer the deprivation characteristic of today's old people.[22]

Physical changes and health problems in later life

Physical changes and health problems of aging affect every aspect of the older person's life. As previously noted, these are interwoven with other problems—cultural, environmental, economic, and social. For example, Goldfarb has pointed out that in determining the degree of physical disability of the older person, the professional must consider numerous factors, including (1) personality (way of life, emotional, psychological, and cultural factors), (2) any possible organic brain syndrome, (3) environmental factors including danger, physical challenges, absence of aids and supports (physical and social supports), and (4) financial and social factors, including helpful or troublesome family, friends, or neighbors.[23] (The reader is here referred to Chapters 3, 4, and 5 for material relating to the physical changes and health problems of the elderly.)

Social changes in later life

One major distinguishing social characteristic of the elderly is their social isolation or social marginality, which entails the absence of meaningful social roles. Social isolation may be thought of as socially induced sensory or stimulus deprivation. Research has demonstrated that there is a significant relationship between social isolation, morale, and key mental health variables such as social adjustment, mental status, and cognitive functioning in the aging person.[24]

Such social isolation and social marginality are results of a multiplicity of factors, including (1) mandatory retirement rules with meager financial resources, (2) reduced mobility caused by physical infirmity, (3) loss of spouse, relatives, friends, and other peers through death, (4) social and geographic mobility of offspring, and (5) widespread prejudice against the aged in our society, which has aptly been termed "ageism" by Butler and Lewis.[25]

A vital concept of wide currency among gerontologists, "ageism" has been defined by Butler and Lewis as:

> a systematic stereotyping of and discrimination against people because they are old, just as racism and sexism accomplish this in relation to skin color and gender. Elderly people are categorized as senile, rigid in thought and manner, garrulous, and old-fashioned in morality and skills; and a multitude of other labels are applied. Ageism allows the younger generations to see older people as different from themselves; thus they subtly cease to identify with their elders as human beings. Mental and physical health problems can be more easily ignored, as can the frequently poor social and economic plight of older people.[26]

Ageism as a stereotype applied to people over 65 years of age is basically a myth because statistically, as Butler has pointed out, the physical health of the greatest proportion of the elderly is better than generally believed. "Eighty-one percent of those over sixty-five are fully ambulatory and move about independently on their own. Ninety-five percent live in the community; at any one time only 5 percent are in nursing homes, chronic-disease hospitals and other institutions—a startling fact when one thinks of the popular image of the old "dumped" en masse into institutions by their families because they have become enfeebled."[27]

Stereotypes and myths become discriminatory thought barriers, shaping attitudes between specific groups of people. Just as ageism shapes the attitudes of the younger generations towards the elderly, numerous additional stereotypic myths abound in our society today. The following myths or social fictions about the elderly are the most frequently encountered:

1. Intellectual deterioration is inevitable.
2. Mental and emotional deterioration are inevitable.
3. Most older people are institutionalized.
4. People die of old age.

5. Older people should not live alone.
6. Sexual activities and interest decline sharply with age.
7. Most marriages in later life are a mistake.
8. The problems of older people are best solved by agencies and professionals.

We strongly believe that the attitudes of the general public, professionals, youth, and the elderly themselves need to be modified based on facts rather than on these social fictions. It seems to us that professional health care providers have been influenced (as has the general public) by what Kuhn describes as the "Detroit syndrome," which builds obsolescence into all our thinking and production. Kuhn states, "Only the new model is desirable, marketable, profitable. The 'Detroit' mentality has taken us over as a society."[28] In this view, the elderly are seen as people who cannot produce, as surplus, as scrap, and as dependent "nonpeople."

Instead, professional health care providers need to view the elderly as experienced, mature people, and as growing adults who have a great responsibility for the continued survival of our society. Thus, to decrease morbidity and increase effective longevity among the elderly, we endorse Watkin's perceptive observation: "Attacking the *Carpe diem* philosophies in youth-oriented societies requires building a new image for the latter half of life. The joys of late maturity and old age need reinforcement based on real achievements by the natural, biologic, clinical, social, economic and political sciences. No one will strive to be alive in the latter half of life if that epoch holds forth only an image of illness, disability, loneliness, poverty, and indifference by family, society, and government."[29]

THE CHANGING SOCIETY: HISTORICAL LIFE CIRCUMSTANCES OF TODAY'S ELDERLY

At the turn of the century, the United States was still predominantly rural, with the majority of the population living on or near the country's farms. By 1920, however, a striking change had occurred. America had become an urbanized nation with the bulk of its people now concentrated in towns of populations of at least 2,500. Because younger segments of the population were more willing and able to relocate, the population movement for younger people was to the cities where more varied and numerous employment opportunities existed.

Because today's elderly began their lives during the first decade and a half of this century, these individuals experienced the following historical life circumstances or phenomena during their life spans: (1) lack of indoor plumbing facilities, (2) no electric lights or appliances, (3) horses used for transportation because few families owned automobiles, (4) none or few residential telephones, (5) lack of exposure to mass media, that is, few newspapers in rural areas, few families having radios and none having television. In short, the elderly experienced none of the conveniences of the automated, "electrified" society of today. Most important, these individuals have lived through more technological changes than any other group of human beings in history.

Often, as Maggie Kuhn has pointed out, the value of this experience is not appreciated due to society's foolishness, attitudes, and lack of insight as to what makes human beings really human. Kuhn states, "Old people ought to have a sense of history. They must be encouraged to review their own history, valuing their origins and past experiences. With rapid technological change, we are made to feel that our experience is useless."[30]

The life review technique illustrates the extent of technological changes experienced by today's elderly and also serves as a therapeutic aid in helping older people favor successful aging. Developed and implemented by Butler, the life review technique integrates persons ranging from the age of 15 years to over age 80 into age-integrated psychotherapy groups.[31] This helping technique brings out the importance of personal and social interactions that aid the individual in recalling the social and historical events and forces that have been influential in helping him to cope and survive in his dramatically changing society. As Butler points out, "Such life review therapy can be conducted in a variety of settings ranging from outpatient individual psychotherapy to counseling in senior centers to skilled listening in nursing homes. Even nonprofessionals can function as therapists by becoming trained listeners as older persons recount their lives."[32] Conducting age-integrated groups prevents younger people from losing important social roots contained in the life stories and autobiographies of the elderly. Maggie Kuhn notes, "If we could stimulate a life review, we would see what we have lived through, the ways in which we have coped and survived, the changes we have seen—all of this is the history of the race." Also, Kuhn would agree with Butler in that life review is helpful in a personal way by giving old people emotional reinforcement. By recalling past accomplishments and half-forgotten skills, memories can motivate and give new energy.[33]

A similar technique to the Butler life review is one developed by Roy Fairchild entitled Your Life Line[34] and used in Kuhn's consciousness-raising groups. Personal history and events are written above a vertical line and major societal events, such as the Depression, below the line. This technique connects an individual's personal history with the social history that has had a major influence on the individual's life.

THE AMERICAN DEPRESSION AND FEDERAL CONCERN FOR THE ELDERLY

What finally propelled the Federal government into action on behalf of the elderly was in a large part the result of the depression of the 1930's. The traditional American dream of an ever brighter tomorrow met with the stark reality of widespread economic blight that cut across all social classes. Butler notes, "Americans born in the 1900's found themselves, in the prime of their earning years, trapped in the massive depression of the 1930's. Many lost jobs, homes, savings and their morale. . . . By the 1960's when they were retiring, inflation eroded their fixed incomes to an alarming degree. Economic forces, not improvidence, have placed today's elderly in their predicament."[35]

Even rugged individualists were convinced by the depression that forces beyond the control of the individual could bring widespread devastation and poverty. A legislative landmark of the Roosevelt Administration was the passage of the Social Security Act in 1935, a collective insurance policy form of income maintenance for the retired and disabled. The Social Security Act has had vast impact on the society and since its passage, has undergone numerous modifications and additions for health benefits, among which are Title 18 (Medicare) and Title 19 (Medicaid). At present, 85 cents of every federal dollar now expended annually for programs for the elderly are derived from Social Security trust funds. Although Social Security, Medicare, and federal housing programs have helped to gain *some* income security, *some* health care, and *some* housing for the elderly, the efforts do not match the needs. (For a comprehensive discussion of Medicare, see Chapter 7, pp. 174 to 224, of Butler's *Why Survive? Being Old in America.*)

SOCIAL SECURITY ACT AND MANDATORY RETIREMENT

The Social Security Act defined age 65 as the beginning of old age through the concept of mandatory retirement, which has become a controversial policy as most of the arguments for it are based on false or exaggerated assumptions.[36] (A detailed discussion of the pros and cons regarding abolition of mandatory retirement is found in Chapter 17.) Less than a century ago in 1890, workers over 65 years old made up 68% of the labor force. In 1960 they comprised only 30.5%.[37] Mandatory retirement labels workers as worthless. The retiree often suffers a substantial loss of income. The average retiree can expect to have only half of his annual pre-retirement income. In fact, more than half of all retirees have no private pensions to supplement Social Security. One out of every six retirees lives at or below the poverty level. There has been an increase in both the number and proportion of aged poor (although a decrease in other age groups) and the elderly are the fastest growing poverty group.[38]

There are no scientific data to support mandatory retirement on the basis of chronological age. As Kanin has written, ''Working men and women should retire for two reasons only: if they want to retire or if they are unable to function. These conditions may occur at age forty-two, or twenty-six, or thirty-eight or eighty-seven.''[39] Also, the individual who is a product of a society that values the work role as a necessary function of the healthy adult finds himself in a complicated and often stressful situation at retirement. Mandatory retirement gradually enforces poverty and induces stress. Basically, it is a nonproductive role in and for society. Butler puts the issue succinctly: ''Each year as thousands of people are encouraged or forced to retire, their skills, knowledge and wisdom are lost and their opportunities to instruct, teach, consult or advise, listen and reflect, as well as to work, are cut off.''[40] According to a Harris and Associates survey, ''almost half of all retirees report a very keen feeling of loss of identity and self-worth. For those who want to work, mandatory retirement means enforced idleness, a social stigma.''[41]

Even the American Medical Association has opposed forced retirement and offered empirical evidence of the negative physiological and psychological effects on retired persons. The American Medical Association's Committee on Aging has found that mandatory retirement inflicts ''a disease — or disability-producing condition upon working men and women that is no less devastating than cancer, tuberculosis, or heart disease. This condition — enforced idleness — robs those affected of the will to live full, well-rounded lives, deprives them of opportunities for compelling physical and mental activity, and encourages atrophy and decay. . . . It robs the worker of his initiative and independence. It narrows physical and mental horizons.''[42]

Recent legislation ending mandatory retirement heralds a new era of freedom of choice for the individual. In the future, personal interest, ability, health, and economic circumstances rather than chronological age will determine work eligibility for continued employment. A review of the legal history of mandatory retirement is given by Botelho and Associates.[43]

THE OLDER AMERICANS ACT AND COMMUNITY SERVICES
FOR THE ELDERLY

The passage of the Older Americans Act in 1965 was another significant turning point in the role of the federal government in providing leadership and services for the elderly.

This act created the Administration on Aging (AOA) and put into law ten objectives of Title I that cut across all areas of federal programming and created three operating programs in AOA: grants to the states for community services projects (Title III), research and demonstration projects (Title IV), and training programs (Title V).

The 1969 amendments gave AOA authority under Title III to fund, on a project-grant basis, area-wide model projects to test a variety of approaches to achieving coordination between existing public and private service providers that serve the elderly, and that set priorities for filling service gaps and drawing in new monies to fund these projects.

For the first time, these 1969 amendments expressly provided that the state agencies on aging were to have responsibility for statewide planning, coordination, and evaluation of programs for the aging at the state level. Another addition of the 1969 amendments was a new Title VI, the National Older Americans Volunteer Program, that included the Foster Grandparent Program and the Retired Senior Volunteer Program (RSVP). In 1972, Title VII established the nutrition programs for the elderly.

The second White House Conference on Aging, held in 1971, focused on a wide range of problems facing older people, developed numerous recommendations that resulted in the 1973 amendments to the Older American Act. The 1973 amendments called for a network of state and area agencies on aging (AAA) that would be charged with working to establish a comprehensive coordinated system of services to meet needs of older Americans at the community level. Numerous other changes in the law to date are covered in *Aging* (Volume 247, May, 1975).

ESTABLISHMENT OF THE NATIONAL INSTITUTE ON AGING

The Research on Aging Act (P.L. 93-296, May 31, 1974) authorized the establishment of the National Institute on Aging within the National Institutes of Health for the support and conduct of biomedical, social and behavioral research and training related to the aging process, and also diseases and other special problems and needs of the aged. Dr. Robert N. Butler, internationally noted psychiatrist and gerontologist, was appointed Director of the Institute, and assumed the leadership position on May 1, 1976. Butler states that the broad mandate of the Institute presents an exciting opportunity to support studies on physiological, psychological, social, educational, and economic aspects of aging in order to effectively understand the whole aging process. Discussing the early direction and goals of the Institute, Butler writes:

> Our concern about program balance reflects the fact that it is not the extension of life per se, but the improvement in the quality of life that deeply interests the NIA . . . basic research is not only biological research in molecular or cellular aging and immune biology, but fundamental investigations of the interpersonal and social aspects of human experience. In this regard, we are very interested in preventive medicine, individual and family life styles, personal, social and physical fitness — including exercise, dietary habits and the adverse effects of so-called recreational drugs like tobacco, alcohol, and caffeine.[44]

Another goal is ". . . to improve the quality of life by lengthening the vigorous and productive middle years."[44]

At the new Institute, aging is no longer defined as a disease process, but simply as the organism's progressive loss of ability, after maturity, to function optimally within its environment. As a consequence, NIA's research extends into many special fields of inquiry: cellular biochemistry, molecular biology, enzymology, behavioral sciences, sociology, and other disciplines. For example, sociologists working on problems of the relationships between health and social stresses, such as relocation and loss of friends and spouse, think that their study will furnish a basis for helping aged persons adjust better to new circumstances.

A recent meeting of the Directors of National Institutes with Programs in the Field of Aging pointed out, ''In the future, there should be expanded investigation of 'aging' individuals, perhaps 40 to 50 years, which are as essential to understanding gerontology as are studies of 'aged' people, those over 65.''[45]

DEVELOPMENT OF GERONTOLOGICAL NURSING

Geriatric nurses, although traditionally involved in providing care for the elderly in general hospitals, were often seen as incompetent or inferior to nurses working in acute settings; often this was true as nursing education included little content on physiological and psychosociocultural aspects of caring for the elderly. Only recently has nursing education accepted responsibility for providing the multidisciplinary blend of education and experience in the knowledge and skills required to provide effective, competent care for elderly patients. For example, Eliopoulos has noted:

> To elevate their status, a small group of geriatric nurses appealed to the ANA for assistance. In 1961 . . . the ANA recommended that a specialty group of geriatric nurses be formed; the following year this group held its first national meeting. Full recognition as a nursing specialty came in 1966 when this group became known as the Division on Geriatric Nursing. The development of standards for geriatric nursing practice came in 1969 and certification for excellence in geriatric nursing practice and publication of the Journal of Gerontological Nursing in 1975. Only as late as the early 1970's did interest grow in changing the name of the Division on Geriatric Nursing to the Gerontological Nursing Division in an effort to reflect the broader scope of nursing's involvement with the aging population; this change came as late as 1976.[46]

New concepts of gerontological education for nursing practice are now being presented to nurses in basic baccalaureate, master's, some doctoral programs, and most widely in continuing education courses. (See Chapter 17.) However, the effort is still vastly short of what is needed in terms of the increasing demand.

Clearly, nurses must become involved in advocacy groups and in the political process at the local level for planning health care delivery programs. (See Chapters 2 and 16.) Nurses in care-giving and counseling roles with patients and clients must assume responsibility for providing information that will lead to changing health care habits and life-styles of clients from infancy (through the parents' education) through adulthood, aging, and dying.

HOME HEALTH CARE AND INSTITUTIONAL CARE

Nurses can help more elderly persons to maintain their independence and remain in their own homes by providing more information for the elderly on how to use whatever preventive services exist on the local level. In *Aging and Mental Health,* Butler and Lewis devote an entire chapter to ''How to keep people at home'' and it is required reading for all gerontological nurses.[47,48] A growing number of studies demonstrates that many elderly patients, often with severe chronic conditions, can be maintained at home at roughly one third the cost of institutional care, *if* supportive home care services are used.[49,50]

"In the U.S., 80% of home health care for older people is performed by families, primarily the middle-aged daughters of older men and women. As these women become increasingly employed outside the home, . . . more supplemental care will be needed."[51] Because of the current lack of adequate home health care services, large numbers of the elderly are forced into nursing homes, at a high cost to Medicare and Medicaid, simply because public programs could not give attention to alternative ways to meet their needs. The average age of nursing home residents is 78 years. "Some 85% to 90% of persons who enter nursing homes do not leave them alive."[52]

A proprietary industry with strong profit motives,[52,53,54] nursing homes in the United States have been labeled a failure in public policy.[55] The United States is one of the few countries in the world in which care of the sick elderly has become "big business" run primarily for commercial gain. Ninety percent of the 23,000 nursing homes in the United States are profit making, some owned by large chains with publicly sold stock, which is a glamour investment, according to financial experts. Even physicians, despite an obvious conflict of interest, often invest in and own nursing homes.

National attention has recently been focused on the welfare of the millions of nursing home patients supported through Medicare and Medicaid. One study revealed that mentally ill patients in nursing homes received an increase in prescribed psychoactive medication and showed a decrease in activity levels, both negative consequences of placing these patients in nursing home facilities.[56]

Although a great deal of emphasis is placed on alternatives to institutionalization, there will always be a necessary role for long-term care facilities. Our social responsibility is to see that these institutions meet approved standards of care and safety. We believe that nurses must become involved as reformers and, as Maggie Kuhn has written, "they cannot be sissies. . . . Nursing homes reflect our society's attitude toward old age and dependency."[57]

Required reading for the gerontological nurse is *Nursing Homes: A Citizens' Action Guide,*[58] by Horn and Griesel. This book is an outstanding guide concerning the ways in which citizens' action groups can organize, plan, and achieve nursing home reform in their communities. Griesel,[58] a co-author of this book, is the informal leader of an important volunteer group, The National Citizens Coalition for Nursing Home Reform. The effective advocacy pressure of this group, along with a recent federal general accounting office study and a substantial documentation concerning the inadequacy of present nursing home care, has resulted in the introduction (by Representative Claude Pepper D. Fla.), of several bills that we hope will become laws. Pepper's proposed legislation is aimed at expanding home health care alternatives for the elderly.[59]

Horn and Griesel point out forcefully that "as a society, we have entrusted the care of the ill elderly to nursing homes, to our government and to health professionals." These two authors emphatically state that all these groups, in addition to our educational institutions, have perpetuated a negative image of old people and of caring for old people by failing to recognize their health needs and failing to provide education in geriatrics and gerontology (see Horn and Griesel,[58] pp. 17 and 18). They challenge the present state of affairs by stating, "A lesson learned from existing citizen action groups is that anyone and everyone has the potential for being an organizer."[60] However, it does require commitment of time and energy to change the existing negative stereotypes.

A "NEW AGE FOR OLD AGE": ISSUES AND RECOMMENDATIONS FOR ACTION

In this introductory chapter, we have attempted to provide an overview of some of the major issues related to health and mental health care for the elderly in this country. However, consideration of issues requires the identification of problems. We have attempted to identify the major problems of the elderly in regard to their health and mental health care needs. In this section we will summarize what we consider to be four major issues and set forth some alternative solutions or recommendations for social action that may help toward the resolution of problems affecting the well-being of the elderly in our society.

The first issue is that of economic deprivation, a basic problem of aging. Too many of America's elderly are living below the poverty level, despite a lifetime of productive work and carefully thought out savings and retirement plans that are being eroded by the continuing inflationary increases in the costs of basic necessities of living, for example, housing, utilities, and food. In addition, costs of medical, dental, and other health care are skyrocketing. Through mandatory retirement, too many of the well, productive, and able elderly have been forced into loss of their productive roles in society, resulting in loss of self-esteem as well as income.

With the new federal legislation abolishing mandatory retirement at age 65, those elderly who are healthy and productive on the job will have the right to continue working until the age of 70. We view this new law as a significant step in federal legislation.

Whether they continue their employment after age 65 or elect to retire from a full-time work role, activity and involvement is increasingly being viewed by health experts as an essential aspect of successful aging. On a simplistic level, "you lose what you don't use," physically and mentally. Both mental and physical health are improved through involvement in productive volunteer and advocacy roles that are so essential to the improvement of conditions for the physically disabled and homebound elderly. Certainly, seniors today want to be in the mainstream of living and we need to be reminded that approximately 95% of the elderly are living and coping in the community, meeting head-on the daily problems and challenges of living.

We recommend that gerontological nurses review the journal of The American Association of Retired Persons, entitled *Modern Maturity,* which reflects the thinking of the association, their political lobbying efforts, and their philosophy and motto: "To serve and not to be served."[61] This organization is undergoing phenomenal growth and undoubtedly will continue to grow in the future. Also the News Bulletin of the AARP will assist the gerontological nurse in staying abreast of current legislative developments regarding health care for the elderly. In addition, gerontological nurses should be aware of any local chapters of the Gray Panther organization, which lobby for reforms in nursing home care and home health care alternatives.

In our communities, we need also to provide meaningful part-time paid employment for seniors. Programs such as the Foster Grandparent program have been highly productive and successful. In summary, we believe that productive involvement adds to the quality of life by providing additional income for and enhancing self-esteem of the elderly.

The second issue is that of physical and mental health of the elderly. A comprehensive review of the normal physiological declines of aging is contained in Chapter 3 of the text, whereas Chapter 4 addresses the problems associated with poor nutrition among the elderly. Because of lack of adequate income and lack of knowledge of good nutritional principles, in addition to loneliness and lack of motivation to prepare meals, the elderly often experience physiological problems caused by poor nutrition. Health counseling of seniors by gerontological nurses and other health care providers, in addition to re-education of the public in the principles of good nutrition, could go far in helping to correct this problem. Although some senior nutritional programs are excellent, many need to be improved. Research and experience have shown repeatedly that social isolation, poverty, loss of productive social roles, and loss of spouse and friends through death all test in a profoundly significant manner the coping skills of the elderly.

We also recommend that gerontological nurses review the special issue of *Innovations** entitled "The Greening of Old Age."[62] This particular issue of *Innovations* reviews the problems and issues our society faces in dealing with the health and mental health care needs of the elderly, pointing out that much more needs to be done in terms of changing the attitudes of professionals and developing innovative programs. The issue highlights several innovative programs developed by community agencies in California, Texas, and Minnesota that can serve as models for care providers in developing activities to involve the elderly in growth experiences, such as programs that stress exercise, physical vigor, yoga, meditation, dance therapy, and other activities.[62]

The third issue we have selected to consider briefly is the need for a general and extensive reeducation of health care professionals serving the elderly, especially in regard to medical education and nursing education. In respect to the care of the elderly, nursing education is now beginning to meet this challenge by developing basic and graduate level programs in gerontological nursing. In regard to medical education, we believe that geriatric content must be incorporated into the education of all future physicians. Doctors need to be exposed not only to the chronically ill elderly, but to healthy, vigorous older people as well, in the same way they are exposed to healthy babies in nurseries. In the very near future, we foresee that medical schools will be prodded by the federal government to include geriatric content in their curricula. Recently, a bill was introduced in the Senate that would help schools of medicine establish geriatric programs.

The attitudes of the public need to be changed in regard to the general negative image of aging held by the current generation of adults and youth. However, we see some changes emerging. For example, the public television program "Over Easy" is an outstanding example of a positive view of aging. This program includes absorbing interviews with community leaders and elderly citizens that can significantly work toward changing attitudes of viewers.

Public attitudes can also be changed by increasing publicity concerning the lobbying efforts of organizations such as the AARP and the Gray Panthers. New organizations, such as the National Coalition for Nursing Home Reform, will have an impact on the nursing home reform movement in this country. As more and more publicity is focused on the problems of the elderly in communities and nursing homes, and on the advocacy groups pressuring for reform, changes in attitudes will undoubtedly come about.

The fourth issue we choose to address is that of society's attitude toward the terminally ill. Specifically, health care professionals, particularly physicians and many nurses, need to develop a more humanistic approach to the dying.

The concept of hospice, whose original definition was a place dedicated to providing

---

Innovations is an experimental magazine published by the American Institutes for Research in collaboration with the National Institute of Mental Health, Mental Health Services Development Branch.

comfort, support, and dignity for those who were dying, is an idea whose time has come. It need not be a separate specific place, but an attitude or awareness toward the dying, an attitude of acceptance of death as a part of life, an attitude of support and caring, the opposite of abandonment, which is often the case in nursing homes and hospitals. Nurses and physicians need to learn to provide the dying patient with continuity of care whether this be in the home, hospital or nursing home environment.

Nurses, as well as physicians and all other health care providers, need reeducation in the process of death and dying. A growing volume of literature is available in this area. Some of the most recent and revealing works are those of Dr. E. Kubler-Ross on death as a final growth process and the work of Dr. Raymond Moody.[63-66]

A more humanistic approach to dying needs to be learned and practiced by gerontological nurses in their care for terminally ill patients and in their counseling roles with the patients' families. In the future it appears that changes will be made in federal narcotics laws to allow the administration of more effective medication to the terminally ill, particularly those suffering from severe pain.[67-69] The challenge is not only to help patients die better but to help them live better until they die.

SUMMARY

The demographic revolution among the elderly in America, referred to as the "graying of America," is a phenomenon that will have profound social, economic, and political consequences for our social systems.

The challenge for gerontological nursing and for all health professionals is to respond to the many problems evident that have been described in this chapter, and to utilize to the fullest extent the multiple resources available in bringing about a more independent, healthy, and contributory elderly population.

REFERENCES

1. Butler, R. N.: Why survive? Being old in America, New York, 1975, Harper & Row, Publishers, Inc.
2. Kinlein, L.: Point of view: on the front: nursing and family and community health, Family Community Health 1(1):57-58, April, 1978.
3. Reinhardt, A. M., and Quinn, M. D.: Community health nursing: new directions for practice. In Reinhardt, A. M., and Quinn, M. D., editors: Family-centered community nursing: a sociocultural framework, St. Louis, 1973, The C. V. Mosby Co., p. 5.
4. Medicine in America: life, death and dollars, National Broadcasting Co., New York, Jan. 3, 1978. (Television documentary.)
5. Watkin, D. M.: Personal responsibility—key to effective and cost-effective health, Family Community Health 1(1):1-7, April, 1978.
6. Watkin, D. M.: Aging, nutrition, and the continuum of health care, Ann. N.Y. Acad. Sci. **300:** 290-297, Nov., 1977.
7. Belloc, N. B., and Breslow, L.: Relationship of physical health status and health practices, Prev. Med. **1:**409-421, 1972.
8. Kubler-Ross, E.: Death: the final stage of growth, Englewood Cliffs, N.J., 1975, Prentice-Hall, Inc.
9. Butler, p. 16.
10. Ibid.
11. Hessell, D. T., editor: Maggie Kuhn on aging: a dialogue, Philadelphia, 1977, The Westminster Press, p. 16.
12. Butler, p. xi.
13. Neugarten, D.: The aged in American society. In Becker, H. S., editor: Social problems: a modern approach, Chicago, 1968, The University of Chicago Press.
14. Rose, A. M.: Future developments in aging perspectives. In Hoffman, A. M., editor: The daily needs and interests of older people, Springfield, Ill., 1970, Charles C Thomas, Publisher.
15. Butler, p. xi.
16. Ibid., p. 17.
17. Butler, R. N.: Address, National Institute on Aging open house, Washington, D.C., May 1, 1976, U.S. Department of Health, Education, and Welfare.
18. U.S. Department of Commerce, Bureau of the

Census: Demographic aspects of aging and the older population in the United States, current population reports, Special Studies Series, P-23, No. 56, May, 1976.

19. Hessell, p. 16.
20. Erikson, E. H.: Childhood and society, New York, 1950, W. W. Norton & Co., Inc., ed. 2, 1963.
21. Kreps, J. M.: Economics of retirement. In Busse, E. W., and Pfeiffer, E., editors: Behavior and adaptation in late life, ed. 2, Boston, 1977, Little, Brown & Co., pp. 59-77.
22. Ibid. pp. 59-60.
23. Goldfarb, A. I.: Integrated psychiatric services for the aged, Bull. N.Y. Acad. Med. **49:**1070-1083, Dec., 1973.
24. Bennett, R.: Social isolation and isolation-reducing programs, Bull. N.Y. Acad. Med. **49:** 1143-1163, Dec., 1973.
25. Butler, R. N., and Lewis, M. I.: Aging and mental health: positive psychosocial approaches, ed. 2, St. Louis, 1977, The C. V. Mosby Co., p. ix.
26. Ibid.
27. Butler, Why survive? p. 17.
28. Hessell, p. 16.
29. Watkin, D. M.: Aging, nutrition, and the continuum of health care, Ann. N.Y. Acad. Sci. **300:**293, 1977.
30. Hessell, p. 30.
31. Butler, R. N.: Successful aging and the role of the life review, J. Am. Geriatr. Soc. **22:**529-535, 1974.
32. Ibid.
33. Hessell, pp. 30-31.
34. Fairchild, R.: Life-story conversations: dimensions in a ministry of evangelistic calling, New York, 1977, United Presbyterian Program Area on Evangelism.
35. Butler, Why survive? p. 17.
36. U.S. News & World Report, March 13, 1978, pp. 82-83.
37. Clague, E., Palli, B., and Kramer, L.: The aging worker and the union, New York, 1971, Praeger Publishers, Inc.
38. Butler, Why survive? p. 24.
39. Kanin, G.: It takes a long time to become young, Garden City, N.Y., 1978, Doubleday & Co., Inc., p. 4.
40. Butler, Why survive? p. 24.
41. Harris, L., and Associates, Inc.: The myth and reality of aging in America, Washington, D.C., 1975, National Council on Aging.
42. Retirement: A medical philosphy and approach, Chicago, 1972, American Medical Association.
43. Botelho, B. M., Cain, L. D., and Friedman, S. M.: Mandatory retirement: the law, the courts,

and the broader social context, Willamette Law J. **2:**398-416, Summer, 1976.
44. Butler, R. N.: Guest editorial: early directions for the National Institute on Aging, Gerontologist **16:**293-294, 1976.
45. Summary of second meeting of directors of national institutes with programs in the field of aging, sponsored by National Institute on Aging, Fogarty International Center, and World Health Organization, Washington, D.C., November 9-12, 1977.
46. Eliopoulos, C.: Assessment and action in gerontological nursing, Family Community Health **1**(1):81-90, April, 1978.
47. Butler, R. N., and Lewis, M. I., pp. 211-235.
48. U.S. House of Representatives Subcommittee on Health and Long Term Care: Comprehensive home health care: recommendations for action, Washington, D.C., 1976, U.S. Government Printing Office.
49. Colt, A. M., Anderson, N., Scott, H. D., and Zimmerman, H.: Home health care is good economics, Nursing Outlook **25**(10):632-636, 1977.
50. Davis, E.: "Funding rural nurse practitioner care," Nursing Outlook **25**(10):628-631, 1977.
51. Butler and Lewis, p. 214.
52. Butler and Lewis, p. 245.
53. Mendelson, M. A.: Tender loving greed, New York, 1974, Alfred A. Knopf, Inc.
54. Moss, F. E., and Halamandaris, V. J.: Too old, too sick, too bad, Germantown, Md., 1977, Aspen Systems Corp.
55. Nursing home care in the United States: failure in public policy, hearings before the Senate Subcommittee on Long-Term Care of the Special Committee on Aging, U.S. Senate, ninety-third Congress, Second Session, Dec. 19, 1974.
56. Schmidt, L. J., Reinhardt, A. M., Kane, R. L., and Olsen, D. M.: The mentally ill in nursing homes: new back wards in the community, Archives of Gen. Psych. **34**(6):687-691, June, 1977.
57. Kuhn, M.: Introduction. In Horn, L., and Griesel, E., editors: Nursing homes: a citizens' action guide. Boston, 1977, Beacon Press, pp. x-xii.
58. Horn, L., and Griesel, E.: Nursing homes: a citizens' action guide, Boston, 1977, Beacon Press.
59. News: GAO study confirms home care for elderly cuts costs and affects quality of life, Am. J. N. **78**(3):347, March, 1978.
60. Horn and Griesel, p. 19.
61. VanLandingham, A.: The joy of serving, Modern Maturity **21**(1):7, Feb.-March, 1978.
62. The greening of old age, Innovations **4**(1), 1977. (Entire issue.)

63. Kubler-Ross, E.: Death: the final stage of growth, Englewood Cliffs, N.J., 1975, Prentice-Hall, Inc.

64. Moody, R. A.: Life after life, New York, 1975, Bantam Books.

65. Kastenbaum, R. J.: Death, society & human experience, St. Louis, 1977, The C. V. Mosby Co.

66. Davis, R. H., editor: Dealing with death, Los Angeles, 1973, University of Southern California Ethel Percy Andrus Gerontology Center.

67. Butler, R. N.: "A humanistic approach to our last days," National Institute on Aging, Washington, D.C., 1977, Department of Health, Education, and Welfare.

68. McCorkle, R.: Hospices: a British reality and an American dream. In Kellog, C. J., and Sullivan, B. P., editors: Current practice in oncologic nursing, St. Louis, 1978, The C. V. Mosby Co.

69. Nowlis, E. A.: "Odyssey to Mare street: lessons learned at St. Joseph's hospice." In Kellog, C. J., and Sullivan, B. P., editors: Current practice in oncologic nursing, St. Louis, 1978, The C. V. Mosby Co.

2 The politics of providing health and mental health care for the aged

E. PERCIL STANFORD

Health affects every aspect of the older person's life: financial status, personal welfare, participation in society, use of time, and expectations for the future. Millions of older people are reasonably healthy and others suffer from diseases and disabilities of various sorts. The increasing incidence of chronic conditions with advancing age contributes to the problem of health care and the financing of medical costs. National Health Survey data show that three fourths of all aged persons not in institutions have one or more chronic conditions. Two out of every five have chronic conditions that prevent or limit normal activity. About one out of every five older persons is either confined to the house or has trouble getting about alone. The health outlook for most older people becomes worse with advancing age. Among those 75 years old or older, almost every third person is confined to the house or needs help getting around outside the home.

Older persons have a higher rate of physician visits, spend much more time in hospitals, and their drug bills are likely to be much higher. An indication of their greater use of health services is the fact that almost 20% of public health expenditures or medical services are in behalf of aged persons, although this group comprises less than 10% of the population. Private expenditures for medical care are much higher per person for the aged than for those under 65 years old. Relatively little of the aged person's total medical bill generally is covered by insurance.

The greater than average health needs of older persons are accompanied by decreased financial ability to meet the soaring costs. Public programs now assure older persons of some regular income even though it is a very small amount. The fact is that as earnings decline or cease altogether, most persons 65 years and older must make do on relatively low incomes. Exactly how many are in low-income groups depends not only on what is meant by "low," but also on the survey instrument used. No matter what survey is used, it is likely to show that some 50% to 60% of the aged have less than $1,000 cash income of their own to live on for a year. For many of the aged, current cash income does not represent the total amount of resources available to them. Older persons are more likely than younger persons to have savings to draw on. Many also own homes, usually mortgage free, which can mean they do not have to spend as much for housing. Some, particularly in rural areas, can reduce grocery bills by raising food. However, the aged with incomes on the high side, not the low, more often have the advantage of additional resources. No budget standards can be applied across the board to all the different circumstances in which the elderly find themselves.

HEALTH AND POLITICS

Contrary to common belief, health and politics are not uncommonly related. Health care and health services have long been the focal point for debate among politicians.

There are many schools of thought and ideologies that are debated vigorously for purposes of gaining political clout as well as for establishing a means for providing much needed services. Jerry L. Weaver stated it succinctly when he indicated that in the arena of national health policymaking, in the operation of health care delivery industries, and in the provider-consumer relationship, we witness a ritualized struggle for dominance and advantage among industries, classes, age cohorts, men and women, and ethnic and racial communities. Health is viewed as a major personal concern, in addition to being such a massive economic sector that political decisions related to it are not socially trivial or commercially insignificant. In essence, national health policy provides a primary opportunity to observe the responses of the political elite to the needs and preferences of the greater part of our society.[1]

The decade of 1960 to 1970 was one of upheaval in both the public and private sector with respect to the provision and delivery of medical and related health services. At the beginning of the decade, a major effort, supported by federal funds, for the development of innovative programs for providing health services to the elderly, along with action leading toward the passage of a program to finance health insurance for the aged through Social Security mechanisms, was initiated. About halfway through the decade, enactment of this legislation came about, followed by an intensive gearing-up period, increasing demands for services aggravated by shortages in personnel and programs, skyrocketing costs, and a mushrooming of long-term care facilities, especially those operated for profit. Near the end of the decade the grim reality of the enormous cost involved, caused at least in part by abuses, lead to a tightening of controls. It was obvious that remedial measures and innovative delivery systems were necessary. In 1970 congressional committees and the Department of Health, Education, and Welfare intensified their efforts in the search for effective solutions to the long-standing problems in health care for the aged and to the more recent problems raised by the activities and events of the past decade.

Politics of providing health care

There is little doubt that health care is a political issue of particular importance to the elderly. One consideration is that the cost of personal health care services is one of the major blocks to a reasonable life-style for many older people. Most health literature regarding older people shows that as many as one third or more older Americans are afflicted by at least one chronic disease or health-related impairment causing them to limit their activity.[2] It has been shown that the older population tends to seek hospital and other medical care more often and tends to receive it for longer periods of time than any other population group. Medicare was originally brought about to eradicate much of the health cost burden from the lives of older persons; in fact, it only covers about 40% of the total health bill. The facts and circumstances surrounding health costs and the ways in which they are controlled provide the basis for political action on the part of older persons. Research data have shown that many older people react to the rising costs by expecting the federal government to help provide relief for them. Contrary to many reports, a significant number of older people do not react with disfavor toward receiving public assistance.[3]

Home health care has been defined by the National Council for Homemaker–Home Health Aide Services, Inc., in the following manner. Home health service is that component of comprehensive health care whereby services are provided to individuals and families in their places of residence for the purpose of promoting, maintaining, or restoring health or minimizing the effects of illness and disability. Services appropriate to the needs of the individual patient and family are planned, coordinated, and made available by an agency or institution, or a unit of an agency or institution, that is organized for the delivery of health care through the use of employed staff, contractual arrangements, or a combination of administrative patterns. These services are provided under a plan of care that includes, but is not limited to, service components such as, medical care, dental care, nursing, physical therapy, speech therapy, occupational therapy, social work, nutrition, homemaker–home health aid, transportation, laboratory service, medical equipment, and supplies.

The home environment plays an important role in promoting health and facilitating the healing process. Properly coordinated and delivered home health care provides meaningful health services, speech recovery, and rehabilitation for the ill older person, particularly for those with acute or chronic health problems. It also assists in the prevention of disease and disability. Appropriate health care services to older patients in their home benefit not only the patient but the family and community alike. Therefore it is essential that quality health services in the home be a basic component of our health care system. Home health services can contribute to the health and well-being of the patient and his or her family, restore the patient to health and maximum functioning, prevent costly and inappropriate admission to institutions, reduce readmission to institutions, and enable earlier discharge from hospitals, extended or intermediate care facilities, or nursing homes.

Controversy has surrounded the quality and image of home care services. It has been noted that health services at home have been characterized by provision of high quality care to patients, professional coordination of the services being delivered to individuals and families, and appropriate administrative controls and proper evaluative measures to insure the appropriateness and quality of care provided. Levels of care of varying degrees are available to meet the individual needs of patients at home. It is now up to many local governments and state governments to ensure that these services can be delivered. As patients' needs change, there must be adequate mechanisms for movement of patients within levels of home care, as well as for transfer to other care settings. Another factor to consider is the reality of cost of services to individuals, families, and communities. It is therefore imperative that health services at home be included in all present and future health care delivery systems. If that is to come about, it is then mandatory that present and future funding mechanisms, governmental and nongovernmental, adequately finance all levels and service components of health care on a continuing basis. Availability and accessibility of home health services for all populations must be assured. In addition, developmental funds must be an integral part of all financing for the expansion of existing services and initiation of new programs.

One only has to examine the changing age composition of our society and the proportionate increase in long-term illness and disabilities to immediately recognize the need for improving and re-examining traditional methods of health care services. During the past 50 years, the increase in chronic diseases such as hypertensive and arteriosclerotic heart disease, cerebrovascular disease, arthritis, neurological disorders, malignancies, and pulmonary disorders has expanded demands for a long-term medical and supportive care. Many diseases, after a dramatic acute phase, are followed by long periods of convalescent rehabilitation that are often punctuated by additional acute episodes. Other medical problems have a less acute onset phase that requires definitive diagnosis followed by a long course of definitive therapy. Congenital defects and disabilities resulting from accidents also contribute their share to long-term care problems.

Home care services are delivered at a variety of levels and in many different ways.

They may be provided through single service agencies, such as a homemaker–home health aid services program or a Meals-On-Wheels program; a multiple service agency that arranges for two or more types of services, such as nursing care, physical therapy, and home health aid; or a coordinated home care program that arranges for a wide range of home services designated to meet the patient's individual needs through one centralized administration. The coordinated home care program is also responsible for the planning, evaluation, and follow-up procedures that provide physician-directed medical, nursing, social, and related services to selected patients at home. Home care is generally considered to be categorized into three levels: concentrated or intensive care, intermediate services, and basic services.

The most concentrated or intensive service is for patients who would ordinarily require admission to inpatient institutions. Some patients require complex professional services on a coordinated and continuing basis for a brief period of time. However, they do not require full-time resources and can benefit from intensive home health care services. Intermediate services are those needed on a less intensive basis. Patients who require intermediate services may have long-term problems or may have been recently discharged from an acute care facility. Basic services are those that provide an effective level of health care for an individual within that person's home. These services should be sufficient to sustain patients adequately so they can remain relatively independent. Assuming they have stabilized physical conditions, they do not have to return to an inpatient facility for more intensive care.

Home health services, including follow-ups, can be provided by many different kinds of private and public agencies, including visiting nurse associations (VNA), departments of public health, and hospital-based programs. Visiting nurse associations are voluntary non-profit groups that deliver nursing service in the home. The public health departments are governmental units that have the capability to provide, in addition, a variety of services such as case finding, preventive services, observation, and follow-up. Hospital-based home care programs serve as an extension of hospital services and can provide nursing care plus a variety of other supportive services to noninstitutionalized and posthospital patients.

After the enactment of the Medicare law, programs that were previously providing nursing care of the sick at home expanded their functions to include other services such as physical therapy, home health aide services, and social services. Whether a visiting nurse association, a public health department, or a hospital-based program, a home health agency certified under Medicare must receive referrals from physicians. It provides services for both noninstitutionalized and posthospital patients. Whatever the organizational mechanism, home care services at any level should be viewed as an alternative to hospitals, nursing homes, or other institutional care and as part of a total medical care program. As such, home care can enable the patient to remain in, or return to, a home environment that may be psychologically therapeutic and will probably result in a cost savings. The patient must want to receive care in the home environment, and family relationships should be conducive to care.

Training is an essential element in home care. Training of the patient in self-care and instruction of family members are of prime importance in achieving maximum effective utilization of available professional health personnel. For example, institutional efforts devoted to careful instruction of a diabetic or a postcoronary patient and his or her family before the patient goes home provides for better continuity of care and reinforcement of the educational process in the setting of the patient's home. Home care will be enhanced by having instruction start in the hospital because it will then be reinforced once the patient returns home.[4]

HISTORICAL PERSPECTIVE

The history of mental and physical health in the United States from a policy perspective is relatively brief but complex. It was as recently as 1961 that the Division of Chronic Diseases was organized in the Bureau of State Services of the United States Public Health Service, reflecting a growing concern about the need for positive action to better the health situation of the elderly. Shortly afterward, the passage of the Community Health Service and Facilities Act of 1961 provided supporting funds for demonstrations of community-based programs of preventive and therapeutic services for the aged and the chronically ill. It was about 1962 that a greater emphasis was placed on the development of positive action programs to meet the health and mental health needs of the elderly. This awareness led to the creation of the Gerontology Branch within the Division of Chronic Diseases. This was no doubt an outstanding year for the passage of legislation related to the health needs of the aged.

In 1965 the Social Security Amendments added two titles, XVIII and XIX, to the Social Security Act. Medicare, or Title XVIII, is for people 65 years of age and older. Title XVIII is comprised of two sections known as Part A and Part B. Part A, hospital insurance, pays cost of covered inpatient service in the hospital and also pays for posthospital service in an extended care facility or in the home if such services are provided by a certified home health agency. Part B, medical insurance, provides for partial payment for doctors' services and other medical and health services. Medicaid, Title XIX, is not necessarily age related and is a federal and state medical public assistance program that, at the option of the states, makes vendor payments to providers of health services on behalf of recipients of cash maintenance payments in certain public assistance categories.

It was also during 1965 that the Division of Medical Care Administration was created and given public health services responsibility for the professional health aspects of Medicare. The overall administrative responsibility of the Medicare program was given to the Social Security Administration. In 1967, after an expansion of function and a change in name from the Gerontology Branch to the Adult Health Protection and Aging Branch, the Adult Health Protection and Aging Branch was transferred to the Division of Medical Care Administration.

Many of the regional medical programs initially created by legislation in the mid-1960s and subsequently amended, provide grants to assist health institutions and professionals in putting into general practice the most recent and effective advances of scientific medicine in the prevention, diagnosis, treatment, and rehabilitation of heart disease, cancer, stroke, and related diseases such as emphysema, diabetes, and nutritional disorders. Regional medical programs have traditionally been administered by the Regional Medical Program Service in the Health Services and Mental Health Administration. The program stimulates and provides support to voluntary regional cooperative arrangements among medical schools, hospitals, practitioners, and other health resources. The partnership for a health program was created in 1966 to enable governmental and nongovernmental health and health-related agencies and groups to develop a cooperative and coordinated approach toward the goal of achieving and maintaining good health for every individual. The partnership for health amendments of 1967 strengthened the program by increasing authorizations, and 1970 legislation was enacted to extend the program to 1973.

The expressed advantages of merging the activities of the Division of Medical Care Administration and the Office of Comprehensive Health Planning led to the formation of the Community Health Service in 1968. The service had a significant program commitment to the health needs of the aged, because of its Medicare responsibility and the functions of the Adult Health Protection and Aging Branch that were retained in the Community Health Service. The responsibility for serving as a focal point for information for the aged and about health services remained with the Community Health Service, which then created the role of Coordinator of Health of the Aging to carry out the prescribed function.[5]

PUBLIC POLICY AND ITS IMPACT ON HEALTH CARE

The past decade has shown many changes in both the definition of needs and the implementation of services in health care programs throughout the United States. Programs have been developed in the belief that they would demonstrate, through reduced mortality and morbidity, improved health status. However, priorities have varied as national attention has been focused on particular health care problems. The mid-1960s showed an emphasis on increased consumer participation, use of indigenous personnel, the clinically dependent, and abuse and neglect. Federal attention has been directed, although somewhat unsuccessfully, toward developing a form of national health insurance with concomitant concerns for providing a national health strategy.

The somewhat unplanned approach to solving the nation's health care problem is attributable, to some degree, to an insistence that needs can be established and priorities set intuitively. There has been a refusal to document the existence and extent of the needs to be met by specific programs. In the zeal to bring about change, program administrators and commissions have frequently failed to measure and document programs' successes and failures. As a result, while presumably meeting clients' and patients' needs, practitioners have failed to build even a minimal data base that is essential and convincing for sustaining the trust of programs.

It has been aptly pointed out that the a priori approach to health care by health care providers is detrimental to the role of health care providers and those who support their mission. Increasingly, legislators and governmental program heads are no longer willing to accept "professional belief" as a justification for funding new programs or continuing existing ones. Instead there should be a more concrete and substantive data base to justify the use of resources. Some recent legislation incorporates provisions regarding the appropriateness, feasibility, effectiveness, and efficiency of whatever programmatic activities are being funded.

The emergence of health care issues at the political level has sensitized many legislators to the fact that making right decisions on health matters is important. The increased politicization of health matters in this country has brought about considerable attention from health care professionals and professionals in related areas. A growing body of literature describes the political impact of specific health-related legislative and executive transactions.[6-9]

Legislative proposals

Proposals for federal programs for health care related to the aged brought about increasing congressional concern in the late 1950s and early 1960s beginning particularly with the eighty-sixth Congress (1959-1960). Proposals generally fell into three major categories pertaining to the provision of health care for the elderly: (1) benefits through the Social Security program (old age and survivors insurance), (2) federal grants out of general revenues to states to provide health care to the aged with limited income, and (3) credit against income tax for payment to private insurance carriers. Bills in the first two categories appear throughout the period, whereas those tax related bills proposed in the third appeared in the second session of the Eighty-seventh Congress (1961-1962).

During the early part of the 86th Congress, the debate centered around the Forand Bill (H.R. 4700). This bill would have provided hospital, surgical, and nursing home benefits for old age and survivors insurance eligibles using the Social Security Administrative mechanism. The program could be financed by an increase in the Social Security tax. A number of alternative proposals were subsequently introduced in both the House and the Senate.

On May 4, 1960, Secretary of Health, Education, and Welfare, Arthur S. Flemming, presented the Eisenhower Administration's proposal. The proposal would have instituted a federal-state program to provide low-income individuals 65 years of age and older with protection against the cost of long-term and expensive illness. State and individual participation would have been optional, and income taxes would have shared in financing the cost of a broad range of medical benefits. During the Senate debate, a modified proposal similar to the Forand Bill (the Kennedy-Anderson Amendment would have authorized hospital, nursing home, visiting nursing, and outpatient diagnostic services for old age and survivors insurance eligibles age 68 and older) was defeated, as was an amendment introduced by Senator Javits and others, combining elements of the administration's proposal with his earlier bills that had emphasized federal assistance to voluntary payment health plans for the low-income aged.

The Kerr-Mills proposal, its implementation by the Senate and its enactment as the Social Security Amendments of 1960 (P.L. 86-778) increased the amount of federal grant aid available to States for their medical care programs for aged persons on Old Age Assistance. The increase was spent on vendor medical payments, that is, payments made directly to providers of medical services, to authorize new programs of Medical Assistance for the Aged (MAA) to establish a vendor medical care program for aged persons not receiving Old Age Assistance but with income and resources insufficient to meet the cost of necessary medical service. States participating in the program had wide latitude to determine the standards of eligibility and the medical benefits that they would offer. Federal assistance provided by both programs was derived from general revenue.

Old Age Assistance. The 11 states that did not have programs prior to the effective date of the Kerr-Mills Law adopted them in 1960, 1961, and 1962. Thus Old Age Assistance vendor medical care programs were in effect in 54 states and territories. As of the end of 1962, 24 states had improved the extent of coverage or content of services since the 1960 enactment. Fourteen states had made substantive change in the scope of state Old Age Assistance medical care plans.

Medical assistance for the aged. As of the beginning of March 1963, MAA programs were in effect in 28 jurisdictions. The District of Columbia had submitted its plan; it had not yet been approved by the department. The New Jersey and Wyoming plans were effective in July of 1963 and Virginia's was effective on January 1, 1964. Georgia, Iowa, and New Mexico had authority for programs but no funds had been made available. Appropriate bills were pending in Iowa and New Mexico. Also in 1964, enabling legislation was pending in South Dakota, Indiana, Arizona, Colorado, Kansas, Minnesota, Missouri, Montana, Nebraska, Nevada, North Carolina, Ohio, and Texas, and a bill was being drafted in Rhode Island.

On February 9, 1961, President Kennedy sent his special message on health and hospital care to the Congress urging enactment of a medical care bill under the Social Security system. On February 13, 1961, the administration's proposal was introduced in the House of Representatives by Representative Cecile R. King of California and in the Senate by Senator Clendon P. Anderson of New Mexico. These bills would, in brief, have provided any or all of the following benefits to persons aged 65 and over who were eligible to receive Social Security or Railroad Retirement benefits: (1) inpatient hospital care, 90 days per benefit, subject to a deductible of $10 per day for the first 9 days, but no deductible less than $20 (2) a skilled nursing home care after transfer from a hospital, 120 days per benefit period plus an extra 2 days of nursing home care for each unused day of hospital care, but total nursing care for each benefit period not to exceed 180 days, (3) home health services, 240 visits per calendar year, and (4) outpatient diagnostic services, no durational limit but subject to a deductible of $20 per diagnostic study.

This program would have been financed by: (1) an increase in the Social Security payroll tax rate of ¼ of 1% each for employers and employees and ⅜ of 1% for self-employed persons, and (2) an increase in the amount of annual earnings subject to the payroll tax from $4,800 to $5,000 (later revised to $5,200).

President Kennedy, on February 21, 1963, in a special message on aiding our senior citizens, called for a hospital insurance program for the aged under the Social Security system. The same day Senator Anderson, other senators, and Representative King introduced the administration bill (S. 880 and H.R. 3920). The administration bill was essentially the same as the Anderson-Javits Amendment of the eighty seventh Congress. The principal differences were as follows:

1. The Administration Bill offered individuals the option to elect different types of hospitalization plans as follows:
   a. Payments of all costs on inpatient hospital services up to 90 days, the patient paying $10 a day for the first 9 days with a minimum deductible of $20.
   b. All hospital costs for up to 45 days, no deductible.
   c. All hospital costs up to 180 days with the patient paying the first 2½ days of average cost (set at $92.50 initially).
2. The administration bill provided 180 days of nursing home care after transfer from a hospital without requiring unused hospital days to reach the maximum.
3. The Javits option to purchase private insurance was eliminated.

The private insurance option, however, was included in a Bill (S. 849) introduced by Senator Javits, and the other four Republican Senators who sponsored the Anderson-Javits Amendment, on February 19, 1963, two days prior to the special message of the President. This bill was almost identical to the Anderson-Javits Amendment as voted on by the Senate in 1962. Prior to the introduction of both these bills, Senator McNamara introduced a bill (S. 86) basically similar to the administration bill but differing in several aspects:

1. There would be only one hospital plan of 45 days without a deductible, skilled nursing home care of up to 90 days, and 135 home health visits; combination of the previous options could not exceed 46 units with 1 unit equal to 1 day of hospitalization or 2 days of nursing home care or 3 home health visits.

2. There would be a "retirement test" for both the Social Security and the uninsured groups.
3. The provision for the uninsured elderly would not be a transitional program as provided for in the Administration Bill, that is, S. 86 would apply to uninsured aged at the present time and in the future.
4. Initially (the first 3 years) the skilled nursing homes need not be hospital affiliated.
5. -There would be included certain services provided in the outpatient departments of hospitals within home health benefits.[10]

GENERAL CONCERNS

One of the primary problems leading to the hindrance of adequate provision of health care for the elderly is the negative attitude manifest in our society toward aged persons. Health needs of the elderly can not be overlooked in deference to younger age groups composed of individuals in their productive years. Within the society, there is a negative climate toward the health needs of the elderly. There are many indications that the elderly are victims of more frequent and costly illnesses and are more prone to chronic conditions than their younger cohorts. The high cost of care for the elderly continues to be documented by the fact that a high percentage of the nation's personal health care dollar is spent for services to persons 65 years old and older, although they comprise only 10% of the population. There are those who believe that expenditures by individuals aged 65 years old and older for health services are three times the amount spent by younger individuals.

One factor contributing to the high cost of care for the elderly is the lack of a systematic organization and sufficient alternatives to provide a full range of appropriate levels of service. Very few approaches to programs and services for the elderly have considered the heterogenous characteristics of our population. Rather than providing a continuum of services, prevention and routine health maintenance, home health service, crisis and day care centers, residential facilities and total health care institutions, majority efforts have been directed toward acute episodic conditions using the types of facilities previously mentioned.

Limited fixed incomes of older persons compound the problem of adequate health care by diminishing the effectiveness of preventive measures such as adequate housing, nutrition, and transportation. Further, as individuals grow older and health needs become more acute, the rise in the cost of living becomes a more substantial impediment to the individual's ability to afford adequate health care.

There is a need to consider integration of appropriate health services for the aged with those of other groups, but not without taking a substantial look at the special requirements of the aging. Specialized health care for aged requires professional training, treatment methodology, and facilities unique to the client population.

Preventive programs for the health and mental health needs of the aged cannot be overemphasized. Because of the special social and health needs of the aged, programs must emphasize a number of matters not traditionally considered health concerns, such as adequate retirement plans and programs to reduce social isolation and inactivity. It is important to take these matters into consideration if we are to deal realistically with problems of prolonging life and not merely maintaining existence over a long period of time. Institutionalization is quite often costly and inappropriate.

Carl Eisdorfer has indicated that national health policy and program issues have had a profound effect on state and local planning of services and facilities by both the public and private sectors. Issues such as economics of health services, prevention versus care, bureaucratic gaps and overlaps, quality assurance, training, education with other services and facilities, make apparent that health, malpractice, and health research cannot be ignored when discussing the ramifications of a national health policy. The issue of health planning is not new. It is complex and quite often confusing to the extent that two or more discussants might asume they are debating a common concern when in fact they are not.[11]

Health planners have suggested several strategies for maintaining the health status of our society. They have also realized that there is no more significant group in our society that uses health services than the older population. As individuals age, there are more chronic diseases and therefore more need for health maintenance and health prevention, as well as long-term health care. To date, many of our health maintenance and prevention strategies have not been adequate for the older person. There are many reasons, some of which include the lack of income and inadequate means for individuals to avail themselves of the existing services.

There are those who advocate a better relationship between the socioenvironmental and health issues. It is becoming more common to view health services and health support programs in the same light that social service programs are viewed. A significant trend has been identified that indicates that in health services, money tends to be linked to health care. The economics of health care are somewhat different in that the costs are not mediated by the consumer. Costs have continued to be controlled by the individual provider. The provider recommends and often decides on the need for specific health care expenditures. Providers also get a large share of the health care dollar in return. Some of this is being modified by the increasingly visible role of third party carriers, such as insurance companies or governments, and currently there is a series of readjustments in the economic pattern of health care payment.

In the case of the elderly, the prevention versus care conflict is obviously an issue. There is considerable illness that exists among the late middle-aged and older American population. The Department of Health, Education, and Welfare shows that about 80% of all older Americans suffer from one or more chronic conditions; one out of every four older persons is hospitalized every year, which represents a proportion twice the size of those who are not 65 years old. The hospitalized older individual stays nearly twice as long as his or her younger counterpart. In addition to these situations, nearly 40% of the elderly have some condition that limits their activities of daily living. These figures represent only small portions of the suffering, expense, and frustration that is endured by older persons.[12]

LONG-TERM CARE

The political impact of providing long-term care for the elderly has perhaps been more profound than health care in any other area. Federal support for long-term care for the elderly has climbed from millions of dollars to billions in the last decade. Several scholars who have studied the situation have concluded that public policy has failed to produce either satisfactory institutional care or alternatives for chronically ill elderly. It has been concluded that today's entire population of elderly and their children suffer severe emotional damage because of dread and despair associated with nursing home care in this country today. This policy, or the lack of such policy, may not be entirely responsible for producing such anxiety, but it comes down to the deep-rooted attitudes toward aging and the role or lack of roles of the aged in our society.

Actions of the Congress of the United States and of individual states, as expressed through the Medicare and Medicaid programs, have in many ways intensified existing problems and have been instrumental in developing new ones. Several efforts have been made to deal with more severe problems. Laws have been passed; national commitments have been made; declaration of high purpose has been exposed at national conferences and by representatives of the nursing home industry. Even with all that, long-term care for older Americans stands today as one of the most troubled and troublesome components of our entire health system.

Care of the aged is costly and continues to become more costly. The elderly who need care are increasing in numbers, already demanding more beds than there are beds in general hospitals. There is every reason to believe that many more beds will be needed because the population of old persons in this nation continues to grow faster than any other age group. Nursing home care is associated with scandal and abuse, even though many of the leaders in the field have helped develop vitally needed new methods of care and have shown tremendous concern for elderly clients. Underpaid although compassionate aides in many homes attempt to provide a touch of humanity and understanding care to patients who, though often mute or confused and helpless, feel and appreciate the kindness and skill brought to the job by the aides.

The nursing home industry, which has grown very rapidly in just a few decades and most markedly since 1965 when Medicare and Medicaid were enacted, may take one of three directions: it could continue to grow as it has in the past, spurred on by sheer need but marred by scandal, negativism, and murkiness about its fundamental mission; it could be mandated to transform itself from a predominately proprietary industry into a nonprofit system or into one that takes on the attributes of a quasi-public utility; or it could, with the considered help of government and the general public, move to overcome present difficulties, improve standards of performance, and fit itself more successfully into a comprehensive health care system in which institutionalization is kept to essential minimums. No matter what course is taken, it is certain that the demand for improvement will continue to exist.

In recent years, the Congress has insisted on improvements in the long-term care area. It is also clear that congressional enactments have been thwarted by reluctant administrations or have been completely ignored. With the prospect of action on a national health program for all age groups, Congress will most likely consider a long-term care package as part of the national health programs. If wisely considered, a total health care package could ensure better nursing home care.

Policy makers at the national level have been unresponsive since 1965. At that time there was a congressional mandate to ensure better care for older people in long-term care facilities. There are signs, however, that rising cost and rising public concern have aroused some members of the executive branch over the last few years to see the need for long-term care reform more clearly than ever before. Their actions and initiatives were welcomed, but it is essential that the Department of Health, Education, and Welfare take far more effective, well-paced action than it has in the past. The demand for reform continues to intensify. The general public knows personal care could be a part of everyone's future. There is a tendency at this time to ask why placement in a long-term care facility should be the occasion for such despair and desperation when it could be simply a sensible accommodation. The Subcommittee on Long-Term Care of the Senate Special Committee on Aging has continually asked the same question.

Appropriate care for older persons in need of long-term attention should be one of the most tender and effective services a society can offer to its people. It will be needed more and more as the number of elders increases and as the number of very old among them rises even faster. We are no longer talking about the "young-old"; the "old-old" must be taken very much into consideration. What is needed now is a national health program that offers the opportunity for building good long-term care into a comprehensive program for all Americans. However, the issues related to the care of the chronically ill are far from simple. They are tangled and sometimes obscured. Technical questions related to matters such as reimbursement, establishment of standards, enforcements, and record keeping often attract the attention of policymakers, to the exclusion of other pertinent questions. Other reasonable questions are: Could nursing homes be avoided for some, if other services were available? What assurance is there that the right number of nursing homes are being built where they are most needed? What measures can government take to encourage providers themselves to take action to improve the quality of nursing home care? What can be done to encourage citizen action and patient advocacy at the local level?

MENTAL HEALTH CONSIDERATIONS

It is virtually impossible to discuss health aspects of aging or the political and policy implications of health as it relates to the aged, without being cognizant of the place of mental health in the total matrix. The fact is that personality traits in older persons often change as they grow older. The degree of change no doubt varies among individuals and there is no predictable pattern. It is evident that we are more apt to be critical of observable changes in older people than in most younger people. For example, if an older person tends to be uninvolved or not interested in any particular type of activity or is not close to relatives, he or she is not necessarily in poor mental health. There is a tendency to feel that individuals who do not interact in an aggressive manner are somehow mentally deficient. It is unusual for aging persons to detach themselves from some of the expected obligations held very dear earlier in their lives. The mental health of the individual may depend on the degree to which the person is satisfied and has a positive outlook on life. The problem often becomes the outsider's rather than the older person's.

Forgetfulness or poor judgment may be considered as dire evidence that an older person's mind is beginning to deteriorate. Most persons are on occasion confused about what they want to do or what they have done, or they forget what they were told or possibly do not recall what their assignment was. If an older person, for example, spends or invests foolishly he or she is viewed as being senile or perhaps neurotic. Behavior of elderly persons may reflect the popular image of the aged as helpless, living in the past, cranky, forgetful, long-winded, childish, self-centered, or eccentric. When it helps them get proper care and attention, some folks unconsciously meet all of the aforementioned dismal expectations. In essence, they are made dependent and maladjusted by the stereotypes that are forced upon them.

Many men and women 65 years old and older, and particularly those not bedeviled by poverty, are thought to be more mentally competent. There is little evidence for this conclusion because precise measures of the extent of mental and emotional disorders among the aging do not exist. That only 3% are under care by any kind of institution and that only

1% are in mental hospitals are merely rough indications. No one is really certain of the number who need care in hospitals, nursing homes, or homes for the aged and are not getting it, or of how many now in institutions could, with more community help, be in their own homes. Regardless, the tiny proportion actually receiving institutional care is impressive when contrasted to the widespread notion that when people grow old they inevitably become so irresponsible and befuddled that they must be looked after continuously.

The fact remains that some old people do suffer from mental disorders that range from mild to severe. Although practically all mental illnesses are products of complex, interwoven factors — psychological, physiological, hereditary, social, and economic — for scientific convenience the illnesses are generally classified as ''organic'' or ''functional.'' In organic cases, the primary causes are physical; in functional cases, emotional. The elderly are subject to nearly all the mental disorders that afflict younger people plus some peculiar to themselves. Because of their lowered resistance, older persons can be more vulnerable than their juniors to those organic mental illnesses caused by infections, poisons in the body such as alcohol or barbiturates, severe blows to the head, and so forth. Some of the most devastating organic mental diseases, in which there are actual changes in the brain and its functioning, rarely occur before the individual is 60 years old.[13]

MANPOWER AND TRAINING CONSIDERATIONS

Professional training or training for subprofessionals or paraprofessionals has been lacking for those who desired to either specialize or work with older people in the allied health areas. Few professional groups that serve the health needs of the aged have demonstrated a true awareness of the need for training and a reasonable orientation in applied gerontology for their respective members. It is not sufficient to dwell on the neglect in this area. A positive approach is to consider the direction or multiple directions in which the training process might be moved. Some have suggested a three-pronged approach to enrich the content of the curricula in undergraduate training, to provide programs of continuing education for the health practitioner, and to train new types of paraprofessionals, for example, the geriatric outreach worker. It is recognized that it is much more difficult to motivate the independent private practitioner to participate in training endeavors than it is to bring training to the individual who is working in an institutional setting. An approach that may be considered is one that stimulates both interest and activity. This was the approach followed in the development of gerontological centers at many universities. Several programs were funded by the public health services; however, this type of support was critically reduced because of real or imagined problems.

The Bureau of Health Professions Education and Manpower Training of the National Institutes of Health has historically provided major support for training personnel to meet emerging needs in the health field. The traineeship mechanism within the bureau was responsible for supporting students pursuing full-time graduate training in public health with majors in ''adult health and aging'' and gerontology. Also, support was included for short-term courses relating to geriatric medicine and gerontology. The bureau had been a funded activity in which the Community Health Services and Mental Health Administration worked with several national societies to assist in training health professionals to offer more effective services in long-term care facilities. The American Medical Records Association, the American Pharmaceutical Association, and the American Speech and Hearing Association have been involved in staging national training programs in many regions and states. Other professional societies such as the American Nurses Association, the National Association of Social Workers, and the American Dental Association have agreed to accept some of the training responsibility.

The development of training programs for nursing home administrators was an encouraging factor. The enactment of legislation requiring states to establish programs for the licensing of nursing home administrators and for the development of programs of training for administrators strengthened existing programs and made it possible for potential programs to have specific direction. Regional conferences to strengthen and update training programs for practicing administrators and for those who wished to enter the field were developed by the Community Health Services, working in collaboration with the Medical Services Administration of the Social and Rehabilitation Services. The W. K. Kellogg Foundation provided support for strengthening the capacity of selected university continuing education centers to provide training for long-term care facility administrators. This foundation also supported the extension of programs in continuing education in long-term care administration by the Association of University Programs in hospital administration.[14]

Formal training for nurses in care for the elderly has been slow to develop. Support for geriatric nursing has also been at a minimum. Professor Dorothy T. Moses of San Diego State University makes the point that geriatric nursing education today is about where psychiatric nursing education was about 2½ decades ago. At that time one half of all hospital beds were occupied by mentally ill patients, yet many nursing schools did not include any psychiatric nursing programs in their curricula.

Nurses undoubtedly provide some of the most critical services of any of the health care professionals. It is reasonable to expect that nursing education exists for the purpose of preparing nurses to meet the evolving health needs of our society. It has been pointed out that over a million persons past the age of 65 are institutionalized. It has also been shown that many of those over 65 years old, as a group, require four times more health care than younger individuals. It is significant that nursing school curricula across the country show a differential in developing courses for training nurses to work in geriatric situations. Many of the schools do not have planned clinical experiences so that students can be exposed to older patients. It is recognized that the psychological and mental health of older persons are closely interrelated and in the judgment of many should not be vastly separated. It is for this reason that major problems in geriatric nursing education revolve around attitudes toward older patients. It has been substantiated that many nursing students develop negative attitudes toward older patients from their instructors and from doctors and staff members they observe on a daily basis. We must keep in mind that student nurses, like anyone else, have a tendency to retain more of what they see practiced than what is taught in theory.

Professor Moses makes a very important observation. She indicates that attitudes are caught, not taught, and she believes that education can help modify attitudes. An important factor in improving student attitudes toward geriatric nursing is providing them an opportunity to acquire a positive and pleasant experience. Students should have the chance to observe positive results from their own efforts.

Efforts to improve geriatric nursing education must be focused on the nursing educators themselves. They must examine their own attitudes and feelings about working with the aged and must perceive the challenge that geriatric nursing offers. Gerontological nursing content is admittedly somewhat weak in nursing curricula at the masters as well as the baccalaureate level. Faculty members must take the initiative to inform themselves by attending short-term courses and training programs. The present need for geriatric nurses dictates that more continuing education programs be developed for the nursing population.

There are indications that nurses are beginning to become more involved in care for the elderly in many significant ways. They are more open to understanding the social-psychological aspects of aging that have an impact on the medical and health status of the aged. Nurses, like many other health care professionals, are more comfortable with the team approach to patient care. Therefore they will come in contact with other professionals who are taking seriously their responsibility for the health of older people. This is paramount since most of the curriculum materials developed are interdisciplinary in nature. It also means that the team approach will be taught by individuals from several different disciplines.[15]

There are many positive and innovative approaches to educating and training individuals to work with older persons. Training of employees to provide more than adequate nursing home care is an important and difficult undertaking. Many nurses aides are being paid a bare minimum wage and show a yearly turnover rate of approximately 75%; therefore there may be very little incentive, according to many analyses, to provide proper training. Regardless, there are many nursing homes that fully realize that training not only results in better patient care but helps to develop a stable cadre of employees.[16] There are several good examples of employee training that have been reported:

1. *Employee sensitivity training:* One of the most impressive programs reported has been sensitivity training at the Beaumont Convalescent Hospital in Beaumont, California. The administrator requires each prospective employee in the facility to assume the role of the patient for 24 hours before employment. This experience is expected to give employees a valuable perspective. Employees are groomed by their fellow employees, given baths, fed, and wheeled about in hospital-type gowns opened in the back. They are put to bed about 8 or 9 PM like the other nursing home patients and must remain there until morning. They experience trying to sleep while employees in the hall converse, work, and socialize. There is nothing like being at the mercy of the staff and being wheeled about in a hospital gown with its attendant problems of maintaining modesty and aplomb to help a nurse's aide learn that nursing home patients are dignified human beings, rather than objects incidental to employment.

2. *Accident prevention programs aimed at minimizing possibility of injury to patient or to the nursing staff:* These programs are taking on new importance in view of the Occupational Health and Safety Act, which requires each employer to provide employees with a safe environment in which to work. Employers must comply with a set of safety standards. Employees in nursing homes are accorded the protections of the act. If a nursing home fails to provide a safe living environment, nurses (and other employees) may notify the Department of Labor and ask for an inspection. If the employer is found in violation, a citation and a penalty will be issued. Under the act, nurses are also required to prevent accidents.[17]

3. *In-service training programs:* There are many excellent examples of in-service training programs in the nation's nursing homes. One of the most impressive and important of these programs has been implemented at the Frederick D. Zeman Center for Instruction in New York City. The center has an enrollment of 200 or more volunteers, doctors, and administrators under the direction of the Chief of Medical Services. The cost for

the program is approximately $35 and covers a variety of topics from death and dying to institutional housekeeping and laundry management.[18]

Another unique approach to providing in-service education is the mobile in-service training for nursing homes in Phoenix, Arizona. The prime purpose of the mobile unit is to update training professionals and allied health personnel and to promote better coordination of patient care in nursing homes, extended care facilities, and home health services. Contracts are signed by institutions using the service specifying the hours of training and the programs desired. The facility is usually charged approximately $15 for each hour the unit is actually in the facility. The mobile unit provides direct teaching in formal and informal classes, and at the bedside. In addition, it utilizes closed circuit FM radio broadcasts from the college district radio station.

Another innovation is the Health Employee Learning Program offered by Hoffman-LaRoche, which encompasses 45 programmed audiovisual segments to help nursing homes provide in-service training for employees quickly and inexpensively. Films are provided on a variety of topics such as "How to Move a Patient in Bed." The program is aimed specifically at decreasing the high turnover rate of aides that creates a need for continuing training programs.[19]

4. *Continuing education programs:* Continuing education programs are usually lengthier and more formal than in-facility and in-service education and are focused on an area of concern rather than a specific problem. Continuing education may be offered by a long-term care facility for their employees and outside individuals. For example, the Jewish Home and Hospital for the Aged in New York City conducts several courses and workshops relating to care of the geriatric population. Frequently, however, courses are more suitable in a college or university. The University of Pittsburgh Graduate School of Public Health, Health Services Administration, has established a long-term care education unit. The unit was created to provide courses for long-term care personnel. The courses vary in length from 1 day to 2 weeks, and the registration fee varies accordingly from $30 to $750 per enrollee. The courses are held in various parts of the state and continuing education units are given.[20]

As the health and mental health needs of the elderly have become more acutely evident, so has the lack of knowledge and skills possessed by professional health care workers. Nurses form an important core of the cadre that represents those who are expected to have the skills with which to diagnose, treat, and, if possible, prevent illness in the older individual. It is essential to keep treatment current with research findings and to always be in the process of planning innovative programs to identify those in need and also to consider all possible treatment modalities.

Training programs in health or mental health for the elderly neither exist nor are created in a vacuum. It is necessary to spend thousands of hours with those who are knowledgeable of mental health and health programs. The planners of training programs must continue to ask questions such as (1) What needs to be done? (2) Who knows how to do it? (3) Who pays for it? and (4) What is the content to be included? Educational programs developed in areas such as nursing initially have to be broadly described. There must be consideration for several hours of consultation, in-service training, supervision, seminars, and workshops. The evolution of an educational program for nurses will to some extent continue to evolve as one plans, puts programs into operation, and evaluates.

In developing any training program in an institution of higher education, consideration must be given to where the particular discipline or program area being considered would fit in. It is the intended purpose of each institution that programs and traditional disciplines fill specific needs within the university complex. It is no different with the training of nurses in the gerontological area. Once there is an established fact that geriatric nursing is valuable and will fill obvious gaps, the planners of such programs will have an excellent opportunity to build their case with the appropriate university officials. It is not only essential to build a case with university officials, it is appropriate and necessary to establish collegial understandings and relationships throughout the planning, operational, and evaluation stages.

To develop the best possible program within an institution of higher education, there is a need to involve students, laypersons, and individuals from related health care professional areas. In addition, it is reasonable to develop a program that covers the needs of persons who do not fit the stereotype of an older person. Programs should be developed with the idea that aging is an ongoing process and therefore may include persons who are less than 65 or 55 years old and may include persons who are more than 65 or 70 years old.

CONCLUSIONS

Federal, state, and local legislative authorities and programs currently exist that can adequately be used as resources to ensure better and more stable health for older persons. The major federal programs that provide medical care to specific population groups, including the elderly, are Medicare, Medicaid, Title XX of the Social Security Act, and the Older Americans Act, as well as the programs of the Veterans Administration. There is also federal legislation to build and improve the capacity to deliver health services. Examples include the provisions in the Public Health Services Act for related health laws for the development of community mental health centers and other local health resources, for training in the health and allied health professions, for research on the aging and on the delivery of health services, and for planning and development of health resources at the state and local levels. The Older Americans Act provides for state and area agencies on aging, for training and research, for planning and the development of multipurpose senior centers. There is authorizing legislation for research and experimentation in the delivery of health services, in the Social Security Act, and in the National Health Planning and Resources Development Act of 1974. The Social Security Act gives the federal government authority to recommend standards as to the level, content, and quality of medical care and medical services for which payments are made in behalf of individuals under the Medicare and Medicaid programs.

There are those who believe that existing federal financing mechanisms could be more effectively used to maintain the health and self-sufficiency of the elderly and to meet the needs for care of the mentally ill and chronically disabled elderly. This can only come about if there is a serious move toward a national policy regarding the health and mental health services for the elderly and the development of a central body responsible for implementing a national policy and laying the groundwork for development of a coordinated administrative structure for carrying out existing, modified, and new mental health services mandated by national policy.

A significant aspect of a national policy for meeting the health needs of the elderly that could guide the use of existing resources and the development of new ones is the need to extend the same coverage and benefits for all illnesses that are now available for physical illnesses and to place the providers of health services on an equal basis. However, adequate provisions of funding mechanisms cannot deliver coordinated care to patients in the area of aging. Services and funding sources are so disparate that it is a major undertaking to try to put together even the most modest program for an elderly person in need of care and services. For this reason it is essential to establish a focal point for implementing a sound national health program that will enhance the quality of care to elders.

A policy explicating health care for the elderly would include approaches for coordinating the current fragmented sources of federal funding, for ensuring quality services, and for coordinating the delivery of care to elderly at all levels. Such a policy could provide direction for coordinating the manpower training and research efforts that are appropriate components of several different programs. There is also a need to reorient the long-term care system for a medical approach to a broader health and social service framework. A national policy in the health area for older people could assure that comprehensive services would provide for consistent long-term monitoring and psychosocial support in addition to medical services. Too frequently, elderly persons come into a health care system at the time of catastrophic illness and receive care on a short-term, episodic basis without any provisions for ongoing supportive care. For the frail elderly person who is chronically disabled, there are few, if any, alternatives to institutional care. While recognizing that there are instances in which the individual requires highly specialized services, and institutional care may be the best answer, community and home care should be available as alternatives to institutional care. Planning and developing alternative types of care are essential if they are to be an integral part of a comprehensive and coordinated health delivery and social support system.

There is a need for the development of new health care benefits, such as the assessment of the social and health needs of the individual who requires attention from the health and supports systems in the community. This kind of benefit would be useful for everyone, but is especially needed by mentally ill and frail elderly persons. With a broader array of potential resources available to help the elderly, it seems possible to develop a variety of service packages and to find ways to provide adequate mental health services to the elderly by using existing financial mechanisms. However, there are problems that limit the use and effectiveness of many programs and legislative provisions in ensuring the support of health and mental health services. For several years there have been, and there continue to be, certain limitations of mental health services and exclusions of the mentally ill from basic health care and welfare programs.

It is evident that most of the state and area planning efforts in aging, social services, or health resources do not give high priority or visibility to the problems of the mentally ill elderly or to the mental health services. Operating programs in these same areas seldom provide outreach to persons with mental illness. In fact, ways are often found to exclude them from services. Program policies and regulations frequently express as much hopelessness or stereotyped thinking about the mentally ill and elderly as new program staff members and the community. It is past time for us to recognize that mental illness is as much a part of the health care program for the elderly as are the physical health aspects.

Problems of service coordination are compounded by the closed system approach of many health agencies or staffs and their attempts to directly provide or support complete care within the health facility or program. One of the problems in the development of alternative approaches to institutional care is the difficulty that many community health programs have in directly providing all needed services, from income maintenance to psychotherapy. Community care implies collaboration and multiple source funding, and coordination of resources is not easy to achieve, particularly in the area of health and mental health services.

Many communities do not have an appropriate network of community-based services to meet the needs of those individuals who need help in sustaining themselves in the community. Once it is determined that a person is incapable of living at home without some form of additional support or health care, whether he or she will remain in the community depends on the existence of social support systems and of noninstitutional health and social services. Unfortunately, many of the elderly are poor and have no spouse or relative to assist them with the basic services they need.

REFERENCES

1. Weaver, J.: National health policy and the underserved—ethnic minorities, women, and the elderly, St. Louis, 1976, The C. V. Mosby Co.
2. Marks, H. H.: Prevalence of disease in older persons: nature and interpretation of statistics, Geriatrics **20:**688-690, Aug., 1965.
3. Peters, C. A.: Free medical care, Bronx, New York, 1964, The H. W. Wilson Co.
4. Hearings before the Subcommittee on Health of the Elderly, Special Committee on Aging, United States Senate, Ninety-third Congress, part 5, Washington, D.C., July 11, 1973, U.S. Government Printing Office.
5. Chen, A. B., Colby, E. S., Robbins, E. G., and Simon, A., editors: Physical and mental health background issues. In 1971 White House Conference on Aging, Washington, D.C., March, 1971, U.S. Government Printing Office.
6. Thomas, W. C.: Nursing homes and public health policies: drift and decision in New York state, Ithaca, N.Y., 1969, Cornell University Press.
7. Rosenbaum, W. A.: The politics of environmental concern, New York, 1973, Praeger Publishers, Inc.
8. Marmor, T. R.: The politics of Medicare, Chicago, 1973, Aldine Publishing Co.
9. Fritscher, A. L.: Smoking and politics: policymaking in the federal bureaucracy, New York, 1969, Meredith Corp.
10. Library of Congress Legislative Reference Service: Medical care for the aged: a history of current and past proposals and pro and con arguments, Washington, D.C., March 15, 1963 (rerun Oct. 11, 1963), Education and Public Welfare Division.
11. Eisdorfer, C.: Issues in health planning for the aged, Gerontologist **16**(1):1, Feb., 1976.
12. Ostfeld, A. M.: Frequency and nature of health problems of retired persons. In Carp, F. M., editor: The retirement process, U.S. Public Health Service Publication No. 1788, Washington, D.C., 1968, U.S. Government Printing Office.
13. Department of Health, Education and Welfare, Administration on Aging: Mental disorders of the aged and the aging, Washington, D.C., 1967, U.S. Government Printing Office.
14. Background and issues—physical and mental health. In 1971 White House Conference on Aging, Washington, D.C., March, 1971, U.S. Government Printing Office.
15. Moses, D.: Psychosocial care of the aged: how nurses are going to learn about it, the psychological assessment of aging persons, a Special project funded by California State Board of Trustees Program, San Diego, Calif., 1976, San Diego State University, Campanile Press.
16. Colorado Health Care Association: A team approach training and development, Contract No. HSM-110-72-374, Denver, Dec., 1973.
17. Job safety and health, Washington, D.C., May, 1973, p. 2.
18. New York Times, Feb. 4, 1973.
19. Nursing Homes, Oct., 1972, p. 14.
20. Continuing education courses for long-term care personnel, Winter/Spring Bulletin, Pittsburgh, January-June, 1975, University of Pittsburgh Graduate School of Public Health Services Administration.

part II

PHYSIOLOGICAL BASIS OF ADVANCED MATURITY

The process of aging is continuous from birth until death. As Moss has noted: "Aging is really a subtotal of very many asynchronous, multiple changes that begin with birth and continue throughout the individual's life. . . . Totaling the effects of aging is somewhat like reading a catalogue of losses: physical, social, psychological, sensory losses and many more. Old people are clinically different from other adults."[1] The chapters included in part II address three vitally important areas of knowledge in gerontological nursing: physiological changes in aging, drugs for the elderly (use and abuse), and nutritional needs of the elderly.

In Chapter 3, Kathryn Riffle describes in comprehensive detail the physiological changes associated with the aging of body systems, such as the cardiovascular, nervous, musculoskeletal, and respiratory systems and, in addition, the urinary tract changes, gastrointestinal functioning, alterations in sensory processes, and skin changes. Gerontological nurses must develop skills in assessing these changing bodily functions in their aging patients. Riffle stresses that the nurse needs to view the older person holistically, "taking into consideration behavioral, social and cultural, in addition to physiological data." All of these factors will provide a sound basis for the patient's health care plan.

"It is a known fact that old people are ingesting twenty-five percent of all prescribed medication, even though the elderly comprise only ten percent of the population."[2] Alan Cheung is concerned with drugs for the aging and their use and abuse by the elderly. In Chapter 4, Cheung deals with the problems associated with drug use by the elderly. He focuses on altered physiological responses to drugs, including absorption, metabolism, and excretion. Dr. Cheung describes the clinical use of drugs in the elderly patient in relation to changing physiological processes. A guideline for monitoring and prescribing drugs for the elderly is also included.

As the gerontological nurse is likely to be in closer contact with the patient than any other member of the health care team, the nurse should attempt to coordinate the activities and efforts of these other health professionals by perceptive observation and evaluation of the patient's reaction to prescribed medications and dietary changes and then to provide feedback to the other team members. In addition, the gerontological nurse is in a position to assume the role of teaching the elderly patient the reasons for particular medications prescribed, the methods by which they should be taken, and the results that should be expected. This knowledge results in an improvement of the patient's motivation and compliance in taking prescribed medications appropriately.

In Chapter 5, Sherman R. Dickman assesses the nutritional needs and the effects of poor nutrition in elderly persons. Dickman believes that "good nutrition for the aged does not differ in principle from good nutrition for the young. It does differ in detail." The differences are outlined and the components of a balanced diet are given. The imbalances in many elderly persons' diets are dealt with in detail. The significance of the effects of nutrition on behavior and the effect of drug-induced nutritional deficiencies are examined. A discussion of individual nutritional requirements and of obesity is also included in Chapter 5.

In conclusion, a broad range of relevant material relating to the physiological bases of growing older is discussed in this section. Careful study of this vital, pertinent information will benefit all nurses caring for aging patients.

REFERENCES

1. Moss, B. B.: Effective drug administration as viewed by a physician/administrator. In Davis, R. H., editor: Drugs and the elderly, Los Angeles, 1975, The University of Southern California Press (Publication of the Ethel Percy Andrus Gerontology Center), p. 53.
2. Ibid., p. 55.

3 Physiological changes of aging and nursing assessment

KATHRYN L. RIFFLE

In reviewing the literature on aging, one finds numerous definitions of aging, including the following two:

> . . . a process which occurs with the passage of time in the life of an organism but which progresses more rapidly after maturity. This time-related process is accompanied by changes which decrease the survival potential of the organism and thus increase the probability of death.[1]

> . . . a progressive unfavorable loss of adaptation and a decreasing expectation of life with the passage of time that is expressed in measurement as decreased viability and increased vulnerability to the normal forces of mortality.[2]

A definition of aging that may be particularly useful to the health professional is one embodying a perspective of aging as a series of biopsychosocial changes occurring with the passage of time, resulting in an altered structure and functioning of the organism and an altered relationship of the organism to its environment.

By custom, the age of 65 years denotes the beginning of that period of life known as "old age." Chronological age, however, is a poor criterion by which to determine the beginning of old age, since there are marked intraindividual and interindividual differences in the aging process. Different organ systems age at different rates, manifesting varying degrees of decreases in functioning at any given age after 30 years. The most common pattern of age changes occurs at approximately 30 years of age, when a linear decrease in function begins, continuing thereafter for the remainder of the life span.[3] Some of the more obvious physiological manifestations of aging include a decline in the ability to exercise and do work and in the ability to respond to stress because of a decline in reserve capacity.[4]

Obtaining an adequate data base is requisite to the implementation of a meaningful health care plan at any level of prevention, primary, secondary or teritary. Data for the health assessment of an individual client are obtained through a variety of modalities: interviews, clinical examinations, laboratory reports, and consultations with other persons. In addition, because of the increasing number of persons over 65 years of age in our population, the nurse may also need to engage in health assessment of older persons in a variety of settings — homes, offices, outpatient clinics, apartment complexes for older persons, day care centers, nursing clinics, nursing homes, and hospitals.

In assessing the health status of the older person, the nurse should remember that the older person has a longer life history and thus his health history may be more involved. Because of possible diminished auditory perception and a slower reaction time, the older person may need more time to perceive and respond to a stimulus. Therefore, in conducting both the interview and the clinical examination phases of health assessment, the nurse should evaluate the older person's ability to perceive and to respond to different portions

39

of the health assessment. As an example, for older persons who have difficulty with speech discrimination, speech that is spaced slowly enough to permit better enunciation of syllables will give the older person time to comprehend and process the information. Sometimes, a response may be delayed because the older person does not hear or discriminate and thus has difficulty in processing the information. The slowed reaction time of the older person means that more time is required for him to process information and to respond once he makes a decision.[5] Depending on his state of health, the older person may become fatigued during the examination process. The nurse therefore should allow adequate time for conducting a health assessment of the older person and, if indicated, conduct it in several phases.

The ensuing presentation focuses on the nurse's physical assessment of older persons and examines some of the physiological changes of aging and, in certain instances, selected associated disease processes. In the physical assessment of elderly persons, it is frequently difficult to differentiate between normal aging changes and those associated with a state of disease. Knowledge of pathological processes can assist the nurse in conducting a more detailed assessment when a health problem is suspected or encountered. I also point out relevant modes of intervention by nurses in certain areas.

The type and extent of the physical assessment that the nurse conducts depends on the purposes of the assessment and the setting. The nurse's overall health assessment of the older person is much broader than a physical assessment, of course, and includes both a psychosocial evaluation and a nursing history of the older person's usual patterns of rest, activity, nutritional intake, and responses to stress, as well as his customary health practices and behaviors.

CARDIOVASCULAR SYSTEM

The heart size of older people, in the absence of hypertension, remains about the same as the size of the heart in middle age. In fact, the heart may become slightly smaller because of the reduced physical demands and activities in old age. In the presence of hypertension, however, the heart may enlarge; hypertrophy of the cardiac tissue is caused by the heart muscle having to pump blood against increased peripheral vascular resistance. Under the influence of reduced activity and rest, even hearts that were once enlarged from hypertension or vascular heart disease may shrink.[6]

Age-related endocardial changes include sclerosis and thickening, manifested as thickened whitish patches on the endocardium, the left and right atrium, the papillary muscles, and the apical endocardium of the left ventricle. These endocardial changes develop because of the continuous hemodynamic stress on the endocardium, usually sparing the right ventricle, which is under less pressure.[6]

Continually subjected to hemodynamic stress throughout the life of the individual, the heart valves become thickened and rigid with aging because of sclerosis and fibrosis. The triscupid and pulmonary valves experience slight thickening. The mitral valve is the most severely affected. The aortic valve also demonstrates increased thickness with aging. These changes render the closing of the mitral and aortic valves less accurate, producing murmurs simulating acquired heart disease.

Atherosclerosis

Cardiovascular insufficiency is the major cause of death in the United States and in most of the socioeconomically advanced countries. The physiological alteration accounting for this health problem is associated with arteriosclerosis, a generic term for any vascular degeneration leading to progressive thickening and loss of resiliency of the arterial wall. The most widespread form of arteriosclerosis is atherosclerosis, which refers to certain vascular changes, such as plaques or atheromas, characterized by a combination of fatty accumulation in the intima and an increase in the connective tissue in the subintimal layers of the arterial wall. Atherosclerosis is universal in almost all animal species and in all populations within a species. It is considered to be a general manifestation of aging, a "wearing out" of the arteries. Atherosclerosis, however, is not exclusive to advanced aging, but represents the cumulation of progressive changes in the arterial wall from childhood.

The cardiovascular system diseases most commonly associated with aging are hypertension and myocardial degeneration. Of particular relevance to the development of hypertension in the aged are alterations in peripheral resistance, which are normally governed by circulatory adjustments and affected in turn by chemical and neural mechanisms that alter the caliber of the blood vessels, particularly the arterioles, which are responsible for maintaining peripheral resistance. The walls of the arterioles, compared with the larger arteries, have not only a smaller caliber but contain less elastic tissue and more smooth muscle. Sympathetic nerve fibers, constrictor in function, innervate the arteriolar walls, with small changes in the degree of constriction resulting in changes in the arteriolar caliber, in turn causing large changes in the total peripheral resistance. The arteriosclerotic lesions of the arterioles and arteries, seen in aging, represent one of the causes of hypertension. Many other factors, however, also affect the arteriolar caliber in the elderly: diseased kidneys, disturbances in the neural control of blood pressure at the higher centers of control or the hyperfunction of an endocrine organ, such as the production of abnormally high blood levels of epinephrine and norepinephrine by the adrenal medulla or production of corticoids by the adrenal cortex.[7]

Myocardial degeneration is a term used to denote more of a functional, in contrast to structural, decrement in cardiac efficiency with aging. The decreased reserve capacity of the heart with aging has long been known, although not necessarily well understood. One interpretation holds that the decrease in cardiac reserve is associated with an ischemia that increases with age because of development of diffuse arteriolar disease in the coronary bed. This diffuse arteriolar disease stems from arteriosclerosis, hypertension, or inadequate growth of the capillaries to the myocardial fibers, as would normally occur to compensate for an occlusion of a larger vessel.[7]

With advancing age, the influence of the vagal or parasympathetic branch of the autonomic nervous system increases, resulting in a slower heart rate in old age than earlier in life. An extremely slow heart rate in an older person, however, may indicate pathology of the conduction system of the heart. This slowing of the heart rate with aging may make the assessment of the pulse rate a less useful parameter in detecting the onset of an infection, as contrasted to earlier life periods when an increased pulse rate often signified the onset of an infection.[6]

The aging myocardium exhibits a decrease in the recovery of irritability. When there is an adequate period of rest between beats, the aging myocardium functions satisfactorily. The aging myocardium, however, reacts poorly to tachycardia, such as that caused by fever. Tachycardia in an older person can precipitate heart failure. The aging heart also utilizes oxygen less efficiently.[6] The cardiac output drops at the rate of about 1% per year below the normal value of 5 liters per minute found in a younger person. This reduction in cardiac output results from a decreased stroke volume caused by aging, and a slower heart rate.[6]

The overall effect of these physiological changes in cardiac functioning is a diminished cardiac reserve, the maximum percentage that the cardiac output can increase above normal. Normally, the heart rate can increase its output by four to five times under conditions of stress. Any factor that prevents the heart from pumping blood efficiently decreases the cardiac reserve. Changes in cardiovascular function with aging, such as a slower heart rate and a decreased stroke volume, help to decrease the cardiac reserve of the older person. Therefore the older person's heart has a reduced ability to adapt successfully to those stress situations that call for an increase in the cardiac reserve.[6]

The nurse should be cognizant of the following clinical implications associated with the cardiovascular changes of aging. Knowing that the pulse takes longer to return to normal is significant when taking vital signs. For example, following stressful situations that may lead to an increase in pulse rate, the pulse rate may remain higher than normal for a few hours in older people. Therefore pacing of activity is indicated for the older person since the aging heart has a decreased ability to utilize oxygen. In giving nursing care to the older person, the nurse should plan to provide time for the older person to rest. For example, after the bed bath the older person should be given an opportunity to rest. The nurse should caution older people not to overexert themselves in order to avoid sudden increases in cardiac demand and output.

The nurse, in the assessment of the elderly patient, should be aware of the less common signs of heart disease, such as confusion caused by a reduction in cardiac output and abdominal pain or anorexia, resulting from liver congestion because of right-sided heart failure. The older person may also complain of insomnia because of paroxysmal nocturnal dyspnea.[8]

Breathlessness, a cardinal sign of heart disease, may be modified in the elderly. The nurse should be aware that many older people with heart failure complain of extreme fatigue and inability to walk more than a few steps, rather than breathlessness on exertion. Thus a complaint of fatigue of this severity should lead to a careful assessment of the cardiovascular system. Attacks of breathlessness at night are symptomatic of left-sided heart failure in the older person.

Cerebral symptoms of cardiovascular alterations include mental confusion, unexpected mental changes, vertigo, and syncope. Syncopal symptoms in the elderly may indicate Stokes-Adams' attacks, in which the conduction of impulses from the atria to the ventricles is abnormal. On these occasions when the ventricles fail to beat, the brain receives no blood supply and the afflicted person faints for a few seconds. Digitalis toxicity and fluid and electrolyte imbalance also cause cerebral symptoms such as confusion, vertigo, and syncope.

Cheyne-Stokes respirations may occur in elderly persons, and may be associated with reduced cerebral blood flow caused by cerebral arteriosclerosis and aggravated by heart disease.[6]

In older people, a cough frequently is a symptom of pulmonary congestion and should be distinguished from that of bronchitis.

Changes in blood pressure with aging result from several factors:

1. Loss of elasticity in the walls of the large arteries, which tends to raise systolic blood pressure

2. Increased lability of vasopressor control, which tends to increase both systolic and diastolic blood pressure with aging[6]

There is a steady rise in the average systolic and diastolic blood pressure up to 70 years of age in both sexes. After this age, the average systolic blood pressure tends to be stable for men and to decline for women. The diastolic blood pressure, however, remains stable for both sexes. Normal blood pressure, in extreme old age, usually ranges between 100 to 140 mm Hg systolic and 70 to 90 mg diastolic.[6]

One frequently encounters postural hypertension in the elderly person. Typically, the older person complains of becoming dizzy, weak, or faint on standing, particularly when getting out of bed in the morning. Examination may reveal a systolic blood pressure below 100 mm Hg with the blood pressure returning to normal when the person is placed in the dorsal recumbent position. Among the causes of postural hypertension in older people are the use of drugs, a reduced blood volume such as results from sodium depletion, a reduced cardiac output from heart disease, and a neurological disorder of the reflex mechanisms that usually prevents a fall of blood pressure on standing.[8]

NERVOUS SYSTEM

The brain changes that occur with aging may be a source of great concern and distress to elderly people. Many elderly people show signs such as loss of recent memory, impairment of mental function, and confusion; the realization of this may precipitate depression, irritability or withdrawal.[9]

With aging, the most notable change in the brain is a gradual decrease in its weight. Between 20 and 90 years of age, the brain may lose as much as 10% to 20% of its weight. This loss of neurons reflects both cell loss and individual cell atrophy.[10] Apparently, the brain weight for females peaks at an earlier age and begins to decline sooner.[9]

The brain demonstrates both generalized and regionalized age changes. One of the most consistent of the generalized age changes is the accumulation of the lipofuscin age pigments in the neurons. The cells of the extrapyramidal system seem to accumulate the greatest quantity of these age pigments. At this time the relationships among pigment accumulations, cell functions, and cell death are unclear.[10]

Another generalized aging change affecting the brain is related to the progressive arteriosclerotic changes that affect the cerebral blood vessels.[10] Although some investigations have suggested that changes in the blood vessels represent the basic process that predisposes the brain to physiological impairment, this view has been questioned recently.[10]

The accumulation of abnormal neurofibrils in patch-localized regions of the brain, particularly in the hippocampus, is apparently a universal accompaniment of the aging process. Certain other alterations, such as senile plaques, neurofibrillary tangles, and granulovascular degeneration are found more often in the brains of demented older subjects, as compared with nondemented older subjects.[11]

Examples of regional aging changes in the normal brain include the selective cell loss of the cerebral cortex, with the greatest cell loss occurring in the superior temporal gyrus, the precentral gyrus, and the area striata. Although all cortical layers demonstrate cell loss with aging, the loss of cells in the external and internal granular layers is most notable.[9]

The influence of environmental factors on the aging process may be mediated through the hypothalamus and pituitary gland.[9]

Age and performance of the central nervous system

From a review of the literature, the general picture of the central nervous system function that one receives is one of decreased function in most, but not all, areas of performance.[10]

Memory functions. Decreases may or may not be demonstrated in memory functions, depending on the function being evaluated and how the measurements are made. One often finds a decreased capacity of older people to retrieve items from memory, particularly of recent events. One also may encounter a diminished ability to recall sequences of nonsense symbols or related words. In contrast, the ability to recall complex problems and relationships and to categorize items into associated groups and related tasks is not significantly impaired in the healthy older person. This may be accounted for on the basis of greater practice in performing such tasks caused by greater exposure associated with the normal aging process.[10]

Rigidity. Although it is generally believed that rigidity is common in older people, research data reveal conflicting findings. Rather than a unitary form of rigidity, several forms of rigidity exist. Rigidity may be a consequence of intellectual ability and not of the aging process.[12] Rigidity of reactions may occur because of the need for stability of environmental conditions, since new places and situations may precipitate confusion.[13]

Sleep alterations. When compared to younger adults, older people take longer to fall asleep, awaken more frequently, and spend a greater proportion of their time in bed awake.[13]

Nerve conduction velocity. With aging, nerve conduction velocity declines by about 0.4% per year, which is among the smallest changes shown with aging by any of the physiological parameters. The rate and magnitude of various reflex responses to input stimuli also decrease with aging.[10]

With aging, a progressive alteration, degeneration, and reduction in the number of nerve fibers occurs. As a result, one sees in elderly persons certain physical signs that would be considered abnormal in a younger person, such as loss of tone in the facial, neck, and spinal musculature; loss of position sense in the toes; and diminished tendon reflex responses.[14]

The extrapyramidal system seems particularly sensitive to the aging process. Older people often demonstrate some decrease in movement due to impairment of the extrapyramidal system, such as lessening of spontaneous movements, an impassive facial expression, or an infrequent blinking of the eyes. Tremors are occasionally present.[15,16]

Spontaneous muscular fasciculations may be seen in older people. The major sites of occurrence are the calves, feet, eyelids, and hands. Manifested as flickering movements of the muscle, weakness and wasting are usually evidence of slowly progressive destruction at the anterior horn cells or cranial motor nuclei. In normal persons, muscular fasciculations are shorter in duration and more irregular in rate than those occurring in conjunction with anterior horn cell disease.[7,15]

The nervous system depends on input from other organ systems that, as they decline in effectiveness with aging, send less reliable information to the brain and spinal cord. Therefore the response output to such distorted input may be inappropriate or slow. For the elderly person, a major consequence of altered nervous system function is manifested in a diminished coordination of systems governing human responses, with reactions under stress being affected more than reactions during rest.

There are a number of pathophysiological events affecting the nervous system of older people that cause particular alterations in their motor functioning. Two such events are Parkinson's disease and the sequelae associated with a major cerebrovascular accident. The assessment parameters for such phenomena are those employed in the usual neurological examination, such as a history of tremors, weakness, and paralyses; an observed slowness in movement; inability to perform voluntary movements; and altered coordination.

The chronic brain syndromes are intrinsic events affecting the brain of the older person that alter his capacity for effective psychosocial functioning. The distinctive features of chronic brain syndrome are: impairment of intellectual functioning and comprehension, disturbance of memory, impairment of orientation and judgment, and labile or shallow affect. All of these signs may not be present to the same degree, however.[7]

The two major chronic brain syndromes affecting elderly people are the psychoses accompanying cerebral arteriosclerosis, which result from impaired blood flow to the brain arising from arteriosclerotic changes in the cerebral blood vessels, and the senile psychoses, also known as senile dementia, which result from atrophy and degeneration of the brain cells independent of vascular changes.[15]

In obtaining the nursing history from family or friends, the nurse should elicit information relative to any change in the client's mental functioning. It is also germane to evaluate those events in the client's life that may relate to an assessment of mental functioning. An individual who appears depressed may have a chronic illness or have recently experienced a death in the family. The clinical assessment parameters would include observing the client's experience, behavior, speech, and motor activity; assessing his intellectual functioning, insight, and judgment; and evaluating his emotional state.[18] Wandering attention also is an important clinical sign.[35]

In addition to implementing whatever rehabilitative nursing approaches may be appropriate, the nurse needs to educate the client's family as to the nature and probable course of his altered health status, and strategies they can employ in relation to the older person's changed behavior. Sometimes it is more difficult for family members to cope with the psychological alterations in an elderly family member than with the physiological changes of aging.

MUSCULOSKELETAL CHANGES

With aging, a general decrease in muscular strength and a wasting of the skeletal muscles is common. As a part of the general atrophy of the organs and tissues with aging, the number and bulk of muscle fibers decreases. Such changes particularly are conspicuous in the small muscles of the hands, which appear bony and thin, with marked interosseous spaces. The arm and leg muscles appear thin and flabby.[15]

An example of the loss of muscular strength with aging is exemplified by tests of hand grip strength. In one series, tests of the strength of the dominant hand revealed a decline from 44 kg of pressure at age 35 to 23 kg at age 90. Endurance, measured by the average grip pressure exerted for 1 minute, declined from 28 kg at age 30 to 20 kg at age 75.[4]

In disorders of the neuromuscular system, weakness is the usual initial complaint. Some of the more common forms of muscular disorders that affect elderly persons are upper motor neuron disorders, resulting from impairment to the motor cortex or pyramidal tracts from diseases such as vascular disorders, infections, or brain or spinal cord tumors; lower motor neuron disorders, including injury to the motor nuclei of the brain stem, the anterior horn cells of the spinal cord, or the anterior roots or motor nerves; disorders of the neuromuscular junction, such as myasthenia gravis; and muscle disturbances caused by electrolyte imbalance, such as hypokalemia or hyperkalemia. Other types of muscular disorders may be the result of inflammatory diseases and endocrine disorders.[15]

Skeletal changes

One of the most striking skeletal changes that one sees in the elderly person is the change in bodily configuration. The position that the older person assumes when attempting to stand erect may often be one of flexion, with some kyphosis of the dorsal spine, the head and neck held forward, the upper limbs bent at the elbows and wrists, and the hips and knees slightly flexed. The older person commonly exhibits a loss of stature. In part, these alterations of bodily configuration may be from age-associated changes in the vertebral column and intervertebral discs, sclerosis and shrinking of the tendons and muscles, and ankyloses of the ligaments and joints.[15]

Osteoporosis, a common skeletal disorder seen in the elderly, is characterized by a loss of skeletal mass. This disorder occurs more frequently in women past the age of 50 than in men. The ratio for the occurrence of osteoporosis is 2:1 with it gradually equalizing, however, to a 1:1 ratio by the eighth decade of life. The probable cause of osteoporosis is a hormone deficiency, particularly the decrease in estrogens and androgens seen in the elderly. Other factors leading to the development of osteoporosis include inadequate protein intake and a decrease in physical activity, since muscular stress on bone is an important stimulus for bone formation. A deficient calcium intake over a period of years also contributes to the development of osteoporosis in the elderly.[19]

The bones of older people appear to be more fragile than those of people in younger age groups. This fragility is selective, however, and appears primarily in those areas where the main bone structure is cancellous—the proximal femur, proximal humerus, distal radius, and vertebral bodies. Particularly common in elderly persons are fractures of the femoral neck and the proximal end of the humerus.[3] The occurrence of such fractures in the elderly may indicate generalized osteoporosis. Associated changes of aging, including diminished reaction time, visual changes, muscular weakness, and poor balance also contribute to the older person's probability of falling.[21]

A major assessment role of the nurse involves evaluating the hazards in the older person's environment and the older person's ability to manipulate himself in his environment with a reasonable assurance of safety. One should remove potential hazards in both home and institutional settings.

Part of the nurse's assessment should include eliciting information from the patient relative to articular symptoms, such as stiffness and joint pain occurring on motion and weight bearing. In a more objective assessment of the patient, the nurse should evaluate the presence of crepitation and limitation of joint motion. In osteoarthritis, weight-bearing joints are more commonly affected, particularly the hip joints, with a unilateral involvement in more than half of the cases; involvement of the hip joint occurs more frequently in men. The client may experience pain caused by motion, which may be located in the inner aspect of the knee, the thigh, the sciatic region, the buttock, or the groin. The client may exhibit limitation of motion, more often in internal rotation, extension, and abduction. The gait may be shuffling. Arising from a sitting position may be difficult.[22]

Assessment of ability to walk is particularly important in elderly persons since this is a critical variable influencing the degree of one's independence in the activities of daily living. Generally, elderly persons in good health stand erect, rise nimbly from chair or bed, walk at a brisk pace, and alter the rate or direction of gait in a natural manner. With the onset of the accumulated physiological changes associated with neurological, cardio-respiratory, and musculoskeletal disorders eventually affecting motor functioning, progressive changes in gait become more common. Gait disorders associated with spasticity are common, reflecting disease processes of many locations and causes. A spastic gait is short and narrow based. Defective hip flexion and abduction are caused by the weakness of these movements and exaggerated extensor reflex spasms. Commonly associated with extensor postures, abductor spasms reduce the breadth of the base on which the person walks. Amyotrophic lateral sclerosis is an example of a disorder that can cause a spastic gait.[53]

Other disorders seen in elderly persons that can affect gait are the basal ganglia diseases, including parkinsonism. In addition to gait disturbances, major features of basal ganglia disease include fixed postures and attitudes, heightened muscle tone, impairment of the initiation of movement, tremor, and dystonia.[23]

In assessing the musculoskeletal system, a clinically important concept is the distinction between upper and lower motor neuron involvement. Upper motor neurons are located in the cortex, with corticobulbar fibers terminating in the cranial nerve nuclei in the brain stem. The corticospinal fibers cross over in the anterior gray horn of the medulla, finally ending in the spinal cord. The term "pyramidal tracts" is given to the corticospinal axons passing through the medullary pyramids. With lesions of the upper motor neuron, one encounters spasticity or hypertonicity of the affected muscle, diminished muscle strength, brisk tendon reflexes, and the presence of a Babinski sign. Atrophy develops only in the presence of muscle disease. A cerebrovascular accident, for example, would result in an upper motor neuron lesion.[24]

The cranial nerve nuclei, their axons, the anterior horn cells of the spinal cord, and their axons comprise the lower motor neuron. Lower motor neuron lesions produce a loss of muscle tone, or flaccidity. This hypotonus leads to atrophy. Fasciculations are present. The tendon reflexes are absent or depressed.[24]

The nurse, in a subjective evaluation of the musculoskeletal system of the elderly person, should determine whether the older person complains of muscular weakness, drops objects, or falls easily, particularly if there is a suspicion the client may be experiencing some form of neuromuscular disorder. Objectively, the nurse would look for the presence of bruises and lacerations, indicating that the person has been falling, as well as evaluating his general muscular strength and coordination.

The gamut of alterations that occurs with aging in the neuromusculoskeletal system has the effect of diminishing the older person's reaction time, lessening his level of coordination, and augmenting the probability of accidents. Psychologically, the neuromusculoskeletal changes associated with aging tend to enhance the constriction of the older person's sphere of interaction with his environment, making social and sensory deprivation areas of concern to the nurse working with elderly people.

RESPIRATORY SYSTEM

The assessment of the effects of aging itself on the lungs is difficult because there are many other variables that affect the lungs. Such variables include exposure to environmental air pollution and respiratory diseases such as emphysema, bronchitis, lung cancer, and tuberculosis, all of which occur with increasing frequency with aging.

Most normal elderly people are free from chronic respiratory problems. Unless he is a smoker, the normal person should have no persistent cough or sputum production. However, the older person may seek medical attention because his ability to work, walk, or climb stairs has diminished.[25]

Anatomical alterations

The elderly person usually has a characteristic stoop of the shoulders and an increase in the anterior posterior diameter of the chest. Age-related changes contributing to this picture include osteoporosis, kyphosis, calcification of the costal cartilages, and reduced mobility of the ribs. The change in the shape of the thorax toward an enlargement of the anterior-posterior thoracic diameter is predominantly the result of degenerative changes of the intervertebral discs and increased spinal curvature.[25,26]

Structural and functional changes

With the process of aging, the amount of oxygen that the blood takes up from the lungs and transports to the tissues decreases. This decline in oxygen uptake partially reflects the decline in cardiac output occurring with aging, since less blood flows through the lungs of the older person at any given time. However, it also indicates marked changes in the lung tissue as well.[7]

The elasticity of the lung is partly dependent on the properties and arrangement of its connective tissue, consisting mainly of collagen and elastin. With aging, collagen becomes increasingly rigid, presumably because of the cross linking of its fibers. There also is an increased linking of collagen with elastin fibers, which are present in the large and small bronchi, the bronchioli, the aveolar ducts and walls, and the subpleural connective tissue.[1] With increasing age, the chest wall demonstrates a reduced compliance or distensibility and a decreased force of the expiratory muscles; the vital capacity also is decreased.[25]

Although considerable attention has been focused on the composition of pulmonary connective tissue, other factors may be significant in the decline of lung elasticity that accompanies aging. Most of the retractive force developed by the lung is the result of surface-active forces developed at the air tissue interface rather than tissue elasticity. Pulmonary surfactant maintains the stability of this interface and influences the elastic forces generated at the interface. Nothing is known about the influence of age on these factors. At the present time, the precise mechanisms responsible for the decreased lung elasticity that accompanies aging are unclear.[26]

The decreased capacity to cough is an important clinical consideration in elderly people. The reduced strength of the expiratory muscles, coupled with the increased rigidity of the thoracic wall, decreases the propulsive effectiveness of coughing. In addition to the reduction in the efficiency of the cough mechanism, an increased dead space and a decreased ciliary activity in the bronchial lining enhance the potential respiratory complications of enforced or prolonged bed rest for the older person.

For the subjective portion of the assessment, the nurse will want to elicit data relevant to those environmental factors affecting the lung in the aging process, such as exposure to sources of environmental pollution, smoking, and a prior history of respiratory disease. The nurse also will want to know about the older person's exercise tolerance, the amount of sputum production, and the presence of shortness of breath.

In the objective portion of the nursing assessment, the nurse should be aware that dyspnea may occur in conjunction with obesity. Dyspnea also may be symptomatic of lung disease and various types of heart disease. In left ventricular failure, dyspnea is a common symptom at night. Many elderly persons have learned that they breathe more easily at night if they are propped up with pillows without realizing why this maneuver is of clinical value.

An increase or change in the respiratory rate may be of major clinical significance in an assessment of the elderly person. In contrast to younger persons, elderly people may experience no rise in temperature with a respiratory infection. Therefore a slight rise in the respiratory rate of the older person is of clinical importance. In addition, when the older person is on bed rest, the nurse should check regularly to ensure that the position that the older person assumes permits adequate chest expansion and ventilation. When dyspnea is a problem, the nurse should evaluate the client's exercise and weight control pattern, and then establish an ongoing monitoring of these variables since obesity aggravates dyspnea.

Evaluating the mobility status of the elderly person is imperative, not only for the purpose of establishing regular exercise patterns, but also in protecting the elderly person from the hazards of immobility associated with enforced bed rest. In older persons, underventilation of the alveoli of the lower lung fields, or bases, occurs even during normal breathing. In older people, lung elasticity decreases to a point where the smaller bronchi are not held open by the diminished force of the lung recoil. Therefore bed rest and immobility particularly are hazardous to the elderly person.

One should encourage older people to breathe deeply at periodic intervals, even when ambulatory. When bed rest is required, regular coughing, deep breathing, and frequent changes of position are of utmost importance. A periodic evaluation of the patient's position in bed and the implementation of a regular coughing and deep breathing regimen are indicated.

A nursing assessment also would include an evaluation of those environmental stimuli that would be hazardous for an older person. Since a respiratory infection constitutes a major threat to the life of elderly persons, they should be shielded from exposure to persons with respiratory infection. Institutional staff and family members should be instructed about this potential health hazard. Older people should receive prompt medical treatment at the first sign of a respiratory infection. Influenza vaccine is a frequently used prophylactic measure.

Other objective factors that the nurse should include in an assessment of the respiratory status of the elderly person include color, use of accessory muscles of respiration, shape of thorax, symmetry of respiratory excursion, rate and rhythm of respirations, and auscultation of the lung fields for abnormal breath sounds.

GASTROINTESTINAL SYSTEM

The older person may experience a loss of teeth caused by changes in the aged gingival structures. This edentulous state makes it difficult for the older person to eat the same types of food he once enjoyed. The older person experiences a decline in taste sensation because of age-related atrophy of the taste buds. He also experiences a decline in his sense of smell. This change is significant, since a large part of taste is based on one's sense of smell. These factors contribute to a diminished enjoyment of food.

Gastrointestinal motility

With aging, defects in deglutition appear, along with relaxation of the lower esophageal sphincter, delay of esophageal emptying, dilatation of the esophagus, and an increase in its nonpropulsive contractions.[1,7]

Diminished peristalsis also affects the intestines, with both the small and large intestines exhibiting muscular atrophy and a diminution in secretions. Such events probably contribute to the frequent complaint of constipation by elderly people, in conjunction with other variables including weakness of abdominal muscles, inadequate fluid intake, and decreased activity.[28]

While the output of digestive secretions declines with aging, ample quantities remain available for digestive functioning. There is a reduction in gastric acidity with aging.

The liver decreases in size with aging. Unfortunately, data about the effects of aging on liver function are contradictory and meager, but apparently the functional capabilities of the liver remain within normal range. As is true for the liver, there is no significant alteration in the functioning of the pancreas that can be attributed exclusively to aging.[27,29,30]

Gallbladder functioning usually is normal in the elderly, although there is a higher incidence of gallstones with advancing age.[4,30]

Symptoms of disorder in the digestive tract are commonly encountered in the elderly and should be thoroughly evaluated. One may see functional disorders of the digestive tract in the older person that may be attributable to emotional antecedents such as loneliness, depression, and adjustment to a lower standard of living. The most important organic diseases affecting the gastrointestinal functioning in the elderly are neoplasms, particularly of the stomach, colon, and rectum. Since both gastric ulcers and carcinoma of the stomach increase with aging, their differential diagnosis is particularly important.

Because of the possibility of cancer of the stomach, colon, or rectum, it is important that complaints related to difficulty in swallowing, weight loss, pain, indigestion, anorexia, or a change in bowel habits or abnormal stools receive a thorough medical evaluation. Weight loss is the most common complaint in persons with cancer of the stomach. A change in bowel habits and rectal bleeding are the most common complaints of patients with carcinoma of the rectum.[31] Most physicians believe that a rectal examination should be a routine part of the physical examination of elderly patients. A rectal examination, however, will adequately cover only the lower 6 to 8 cm of the rectum. Since an x-ray examination is satisfactory only above the level of 15 to 20 cm, this leaves a segment of 8 to 10 cm in the upper portion of the rectum remaining, which can be adequately examined only with the sigmoidoscope.[31]

The nurse will want to determine the status of the elderly person's appetite, remembering that there are numerous psychosocial, as well as physiological variables that may affect the older person's appetite. Anorexia may result from decreased sensations of smell and taste and may be accentuated by physical illness and eating in a strange, institutional environment. An evaluation of the surroundings in which meals are served is important. Sometimes the anorectic elderly person who is confined to bed will eat better if he is gotten up in a chair and moved to another setting for the meal, such as the sun porch in a hospital or another room in the home.

The nurse working with older people will undoubtedly, at some time, be involved in assessing the problems of constipation and incontinence. Since constipation is a common complaint, the nursing history should include the regularity of the client's bowel movements and any psychological, physical, or environmental factors that may be contributing to an alteration in his usual pattern. For example, depression, inactivity, poor fluid intake, and lack of privacy may contribute to constipation. Determining the amount of bulk and fiber in the diet also is important in the assessment of constipation. It is also well to remember that during the childhoods of many older people today, considerable attention was focused on the relationship between regularity of bowel movements and a state of good health. Use of a laxative weekly or even more frequently may be a long-standing habit with many older people.

Fecal incontinence may be a symptom of carcinoma of the colon and rectum. It is sometimes associated with fecal impaction, and also may accompany other health problems affecting older people, such as diverticulitis. Fecal incontinence additionally may be related to loss of cortical control or spinal cord damage.[32,33]

Other diseases affecting the gastrointestinal tract that one may encounter in elderly clients include peptic ulcer disease, gallbladder disease, rectal polyps, diverticulosis of the colon, and hiatus hernia, all of which indicate that the gastrointestinal problems of the older patient do not differ greatly from those of younger patients. There is no disease directly attributable to a "wearing out" of the digestive tract. As noted earlier, the most common gastrointestinal disorder seen in an elderly population, as in any group of patients, is a functional disorder, although this diagnosis is made only after organic disease has been ruled out.

The most common nursing problems that are related to the gastrointestinal tract are those due to excesses or deficiencies of nutritional intake, with the latter problem probably being more common.

ASSESSMENT OF NUTRITIONAL STATUS IN ELDERLY PEOPLE

Assessment of nutritional intake is important, particularly for the nurse working with older people who live in a home setting. A good nutritional state can be defined as a physical and mental state of health that cannot be improved by providing or withholding food. At any given time, the nutritional state of an individual is the net of his intake, absorption, and utilization of nutrients.[34]

One should recognize that there is a 20% decrease in the basal metabolic rate from 25 to 65 years of age. After the middle years therefore caloric requirements are substantially reduced. As a result of these metabolic and physiological changes, body composition in older persons is altered. Both fat-free body mass and body weight are decreased. Total body potassium is reduced. Also reduced are total body water and oxygen consumption per unit of body water. In considering these changes in body composition with aging, one may infer that the number of cells in the body is reduced, with cell death being a significant concomitant of the aging process.[35]

An accurate diet history may be difficult to elicit from the elderly person, particularly when he lives alone. When the older person lives with a family member, reconstruction of a fairly accurate dietary intake is more feasible. In any event, the dietary history should be directed toward the person who purchases food, prepares meals, and controls the consumption of food. The diet history should include questions about intake of vitamins or food supplements. Supplemental vitamin intake usually shows no relation to need as determined by the amount obtained through food. Any changes in the older person's behavior, mental status, physical activity, and interpersonal relationships should be elicited in his diet history since these are key variables influencing the nutritional status. If the older person is overweight, assessment of his exercise patterns is particularly important. Feelings of depression, loneliness, social isolation, an inadequate income, and a reduction in mobility preventing the older person from shopping easily probably are the major causes of nutritional deficiencies in elderly individuals.[34]

An evaluation of the older person's mouth, the state of his teeth, and the comfort and fit of any dentures is important, since lack of teeth and poorly fitting dentures may alter his food intake. Adequate mouth care before meals is particularly important in the elderly person with a poor appetite.

Other parameters that should be evaluated in the nutritional assessment of an older person include the following.

An individual's *body weight* at age 25 is considered to be the norm, with weights 10% above the reference point for age considered to be evidence of overnutrition, and weights 10% below the reference weight evidence of undernutrition.[34] Obesity can be a serious problem for the elderly person and can aggravate many of the physiological problems that the older person may be experiencing, particularly osteoarthritis, cardiorespiratory disorders, and hyperglycemia. Again, a dietary history is a mechanism useful in obtaining baseline data preparatory to dietary counseling of the older person.

Some of the more salient physical and mental *signs of malnutrition* include apathy, pallor, irritability, muscle wasting, edema, glossitis, an atrophic tongue, breaking of the skin at the corners of the mouth, and hepatomegaly.*

Assessment of the client's swallowing ability also is important, since difficulty in swallowing may lead to serious problems such as inadequate food and fluid intake or aspiration pneumonia.[36]

URINARY TRACT

The reduction in renal mass with aging has been well documented. In one study, the average combined weight of the kidneys for different age groups has been cited as: 60 years, 250 gm; 70 years, 230 gm; and 50 years, 190 gm. This reduction in the weight of the kidneys corresponds to a reduction in the size and weight of all of the body's organs.[37]

Between the ages of 20 and 90, the glomerular filtration rate decreases 46%. Con comitantly, the renal blood flow decreases 53%.[27] Both the excretory and reabsorptive capacities of the renal tubules decrease as age increases. The capacity to concentrate the urine depends on the maintenance of the osmotic gradient of the renal medulla and the integrity of tubular cell function. Data indicate that, between youth and old age, the maximum specific gravity decreases from 1.032 to 1.024. Between the ages of 20 and 80 years, the maximum urinary osmolality decreases from 1040 to 750. The kidney of the older person is able to maintain a normal acid-base balance within a narrowed range of adaptability.[27]

Tubular function apparently is compromised more by the aging process than is glomerular function, resulting in a reduced concentrating ability. Nocturia frequently occurs in elderly people because of the kidney's reduced ability to concentrate urine. The decrease in the tubular and glomerular functioning of the kidney with aging is associated with a reduction in the number of functioning nephrons.[37,38]

Because of the renal changes accompanying the aging process, there is a danger of both adverse and cumulative effects from drugs. In the presence of reduced kidney function, drugs must be monitored carefully since they may be inadequately eliminated and overdosage may become a problem. Associated factors include the multiple pathology of the older person, which increases the likelihood of multiple drug prescriptions, and forgetfulness or confusion, which causes him to take incorrect dosages. Elderly people

---

*A more comprehensive list of the physical signs indicative or suggestive of malnutrition may be found in the American Journal of Public Health, Supplement, 63, November 1964.

metabolize certain drugs less rapidly than younger people, leading to a relative overdose with the drug.[3]

Elderly persons demonstrate an increased probability of developing an obstruction in the lower urinary tract and an increased susceptibility to urinary tract infections. For women over 65, the incidence of urinary tract infections is approximately 20%. In contrast, men have a relatively low incidence of urinary tract infection in their 60s, with a rising incidence in their 70s and 80s. For men in the eighth decade, the incidence of urinary tract infection hovers around 20%. This rising incidence for men may be related to prostatic problems. Older people living in residential homes and hospitals have a greater incidence of urinary tract infections (25% and 32%, respectively) than do older people living in their own homes.[40]

Urinary incontinence may be a significant problem for certain groups of older people. The urinary incontinence of old age may be viewed as resulting from a predisposing factor, such as damage to the micturition center at the frontal cortex or the spinal pathways; a precipitating factor depriving the older person of control of his environment, such as confinement to bed or admission to a health care facility; or an event impairing bladder control itself, such as an acute urinary tract infection.[40]

The forms of renal disease present in older people differ only quantitatively from those present in younger people. For elderly persons, chronic renal failure is a common terminal phenomenon. A large number of cases of renal failure in elderly persons are due to arteriosclerotic changes in the kidney caused by advancing age.[37,40]

Subjective data of interest to the nurse include a history of relevant health problems, such as a urinary tract infection, chronic renal disease, or a cerebrovascular accident, and symptoms such as dysuria, nocturia, hematuria, and frequency of urination. Objective data would include observation of the urine for color, sediment, and odor and relevant laboratory reports.

In taking a nursing history, the nurse will want to elicit information relative to the elderly person's usual fluid balance patterns prior to the onset of illness. Establishment of hospital fluid patterns similar to those prior to hospitalization reduces or eliminates many problems. Also such a history will reveal the older person's fluid preferences at home.

In the inpatient setting, an ongoing appraisal of the older person's clinical course would reveal whether particular therapies interfered with the patient's fluid intake as well as with the ongoing relation of intake to output; the presence of any atypical fluid gain or loss patterns, such as vomiting, diarrhea, blood loss, and intravenous fluid therapy should be noted. In this ongoing appraisal, the nurse also should assess the client's response to medications, particularly diuretic therapy, since excessive diuresis may result in electrolyte imbalance, particularly potassium loss. Dehydration and a rise in blood urea nitrogen may lead to mental confusion. Fatigue and weakness also may be symptomatic of excessive diuresis.

Assessment of the adequacy of the client's fluid-balance patterns is essential, particularly if fluid intake seems inadequate or incontinence is a problem. A fluid schedule may be established to ensure adequate intake. Assessment of the client's excretory patterns also is instructive since one may observe, for example, that even though a person often is continent during the day, he may be incontinent at night. In that case, restricting fluid intake in the evening or awakening the patient during the night to take him to the bathroom may be helpful. Incontinence during the day may be alleviated by offering the patient the opportunity to use the bedpan or go to the bathroom at specified intervals. The older person should be assessed for presence of an inadequate fluid intake that would lead to confusion, or a urinary tract infection, or for any other physiological problems that may contribute to an incontinence pattern.

SENSORY PROCESSES
Vision

With increasing age, the individual experiences a decrease in visual acuity. A decline in the ability to visualize distant objects becomes apparent between 40 and 50 years of age. At about the same time, the individual also experiences a decline in accommodation, evidenced by a diminished ability to focus on nearby objects, a condition known as presbyopia. In the mid-40s, the use of bifocal glasses becomes common. The pupil, with aging, becomes smaller and less responsive to changes in light. Consequently, older people need more illumination to see well. The older person also exhibits a decrease in peripheral vision. Because of the filtering effect caused by the yellowing of the lens with aging, color discrimination with respect to lights of shorter wave lengths becomes more difficult. Because of this alteration, older people may have difficulty in discriminating among the blues, blue-greens, and violets.[12,27,41]

Changes in the eye with aging. A number of changes occur in the eye with aging and only a few selected ones will be mentioned here. There is a loss of orbital fat, with the elderly person's eyes sinking into their orbits, producing a mild enophthalmos. As the tone of the levator palpebrae muscle diminishes, the upper lids develop a slight ptosis. Lacrimation decreases, the conjunctiva becomes thin or friable, and the aging cornea exhibits the arcus senilis or gerontoxon. A loss of corneal sensitivity with aging has been noted. The aging sclera becomes more rigid and may develop a yellowish tinge because of the deposition of lipids. Age changes interfere with the two functions of the lens, the transmission and the refraction of light. As noted earlier, an associated age change is the gradual loss of the capacity to undertake close range work. Also related to this change is atrophy of the muscles of the ciliary body. In almost all persons over the age of 80 years, lens opacities have been noted. Thus senile cataracts are associated with the normal aging process. With aging, the zonular fibers of the lens become more friable, thereby facilitating intracapsular lens extraction. The iris atrophies and demonstrates depigmentation, which is seen at the pupillary margin and is associated with a degeneration of the ectodermal epithelium. The aging eye exhibits an increased incidence of morbidity. The three most common eye problems of elderly people are glaucoma, cataracts, and macular degeneration.[41]

In evaluating the visual status of the elderly person, the nurse should be aware that spilling food, squinting, making missteps, and tearing are indications of the need for an eye examination. The nurse's subjective assessment of the eye would include eliciting a history of eye problems, diplopia, inflammation, decrease in visual acuity, rainbows around lights, pain, and headache. The nurse should inspect the structures of the eye, including the lids, conjunctiva, and sclera. The nurse may make a gross evaluation of intraocular tension by palpating the sclera. The nurse should also note whether the eyelids close properly, since serious damage may be incurred if they do not. The nurse may check visual acuity with the Snellen chart and visual fields by using the method of gross confrontation. Carefully observing the older person's behavior by watching, for example, how closely he holds a newspaper to read, often gives valuable data indicating the need for an eye examination. Making more sophisticated assessments of the eye is particularly valuable in situations in which the older person does not have ready access to a physician, for instance, in the home and certain long-term facilities.

The older person's environment should be modified to compensate for the visual changes of aging. Not only should it have brighter lighting but older people should be taught about the rationale for using brighter lighting. The decorating scheme should utilize bright colors. Signs should have large letters. Night lights are desirable. The nurse should evaluate the older person's environment for the adequacy of lighting and environmental features that, in conjunction with diminished visual acuity and diminished coordination and reaction time, may pose safety hazards.

Recently, low vision clinics have been established to aid older persons, with eye problems such as senile macular degeneration, cataracts, aphakia, and chronic glaucoma, who have not been helped by the usual eye examinations and conventional glasses.[43]

Hearing

Presbycusis, the hearing impairment associated with aging, becomes noticeable at about 50 years of age and is progressive. Hearing loss is more common than visual impairment and occurs in about 30% of the population over 50 years old. The hearing loss initially affects high-pitched sounds, with involvement of the lower frequencies as the impairment progresses. The hearing loss of older persons involves not only a decreased receptive capacity attributable to changes in the organ of Corti, but also a decreased capacity for the discrimination of sounds involving farther pathways in the brain. For this reason, the hearing loss associated with aging has been described as a sensorineural loss.[44]

Particularly for persons over 75 years old, a decline in hearing results from a deterioration of the neural pathways and a reduced receptor nerve cell population in the cerebral cortex, rather than from cochlear degeneration. Associated symptoms may include slowed physical and mental responses, such as speech interpretation. With more complex subject matter, the older person becomes more confused, experiencing increased difficulty in conducting a conversation. Although a hearing aid may be of value, the most effective approach is to speak distinctly and directly, so that the elderly person can see the speaker's face and his voice can be readily heard. Also, the conversation should be simplified and carried on in a quiet environment, free from interruptions.[45]

People younger than 75 years old who have a hearing impairment involving the basilar turn of the cochlea, where high tones are represented, have difficulty in distinguishing between certain consonants, such as ''s,'' ''z,'' ''t,'' ''f,'' and ''g.'' In contrast to the vowels, which are lower notes in the speech register and give power to speech, the consonants help to convey the distinctive meaning of words. Thus a person affected with this particular hearing impairment may be unable to differentiate between two similar words, thereby losing the drift of the conversation. Because consonants are weak sounds, incidental noise drowns them out, increasing the difficulty of discriminating among them. Conversation in the presence of company frequently is embarrassing to the older person. Under such circumstances, the older person may respond with inappropriate answers. Because of the reaction of his family to his inappropriate replies, he may realize that his family believes he is becoming ''old and incoherent,'' which adds to his diminished self-esteem. To compensate for his hearing loss, the older person should be instructed to look at the speaker, anticipate what he is about to say, and to try to acquire a facility for supplying missing conversational links. Such an approach may ameliorate the effects of presbycusis on the older person's personality.[45]

Even though the capacity for hearing high frequency sounds diminishes with age in civilized societies, apparently such decreases do not occur in primitive societies. This discrepancy evidently occurs because civilized populations are exposed to higher ambient noise levels. Other data have indicated that men have a greater incidence of high-tone deafness than women, presumably because they experience greater noise pollution. One can only speculate as to whether the current adolescent generation, because of their habit of listening to loud music, will experience a greater incidence of high-tone hearing loss with aging.[10,12]

Other factors and diseases contribute to a hearing loss with aging, including otosclerosis, a hereditary disease affecting the middle ear that first makes its appearance in middle age, and an accumulation of cerumen in the auditory canals.

When a hearing loss progresses to the point where it affects the older person's ability to hear accurately, he may become suspicious, almost to the point of seeming paranoid, or may act inappropriately since he cannot accurately hear what is being said.

Pertinent subjective data in the nurse's assessment include obtaining a history of ear infections, a family history of hearing loss, and the elderly person's subjective impression of a hearing loss or ringing in the ears. Rough objective techniques include the use of the whispered voice and a ticking watch, since both screen for the existence of a high-tone hearing loss. Several different screening tests for hearing loss involve use of the tuning fork. A hearing loss in elderly people may be associated with certain ototoxic drugs. Aspirin is a common offender in producing hearing loss and tinnitus in older persons since many elderly people take large daily doses of aspirin for arthritic problems. The effects of aspirin on hearing, however, generally are reversible once this medication has been discontinued.[44]

Everyone has the right to communicate with other people throughout his lifetime, and aging does not modify this right. There are a number of rehabilitative approaches that can be used to alleviate the effects of hearing loss in elderly persons, including surgical intervention, hearing aids, and lip reading.

Olfactory and taste alterations

As discussed previously, olfactory acuity and the sense of taste decline with aging. The latter alteration is accompanied by a decrease in the number of taste buds on the tongue.[27] This change undoubtedly contributes to the complaint of many elderly people in institutional settings that their food is "tasteless."

Touch and pain alteration

Touch and pain sensations also decline with age, with alteration in the pain threshold becoming obvious after age 60 years.[27] The loss of pain sensitivity has serious implications since the older person may suffer from accidents, such as spilling hot water on himself or touching a hot radiator, and not be aware of it. The older person also may be unaware of an illness in which pain is a major symptom. Because of a reduction in pain sensitivity, the older person may be unaware of the symptoms of an inflamed appendix and consequently experience a ruptured appendix. With aging, the symptoms seen in myocardial infarction may be altered, and prolonged ischemia may be associated with a painless infarction.

The nurse should ask the elderly person if he ever burned or injured himself and was unaware of it because of a decreased appreciation of pain. The nurse should observe the client's skin for evidence of burns or other injuries. One may evaluate the client's sensitivity to pain by touching the upper and lower extremities bilaterally with a sharp pin.

Temperature regulation

Temperature regulating mechanisms are less reliable in elderly persons. One may not encounter an elevation in temperature with an acute infection in elderly persons. In a pulmonary infection, for example, tachypnea and tachycardia are often more reliable signs than a temperature elevation. Pyrexia may be late in appearing or may never appear at all. When an elevated temperature is manifested, the level seldom rises to above 103° F. The oral temperature may be normal in some elderly persons, whereas the rectal temperature may indicate a febrile response. Therefore, whenever in doubt, one should take a rectal temperature. Fever in the elderly may give rise to symptoms such as headache, dizziness, restlessness, and confusion.[45,46] Thus the nurse caring for the elderly person needs to be an astute observer, attending promptly to subtle changes in the older person's appearance, behavior, pulse, and respiration.

SKIN AND RELATED APPENDAGES

The skin, man's interface with his environment, reveals a series of noticeable changes with aging. One sees a marked thinning of the epidermis, with the veins appearing more prominent. The function and number of adnexal structures decreases with aging. Apocrine glands atrophy. The function of the sebaceous glands decreases slightly. These glands contribute to the surface lipid layer that helps to prevent water loss. The dermis becomes dehydrated with aging, and this, along with the loss of subcutaneous fat and elasticity, contributes to the wrinkled, lined appearance of the older person's skin. The aging skin loses elasticity, does not exhibit the turgor of younger skin, and does not return to its original position quickly when picked up.[50]

Many of the skin changes associated with aging are related to chronic exposure to sunlight. Older persons who have worked outdoors much of their lives, such as farmers, exhibit more dryness and wrinkling of the skin than elderly persons who have pursued indoor occupations, such as housewives and businessmen. Repeated exposure to sunlight also predisposes one to development of skin cancers, which commonly develop on exposed areas of the body.[48]

Growths on the skin increase with aging. Seborrheic keratoses are common and appear as raised, flat, brown or warty areas, occurring primarily on the trunk, head, and neck.[48] Since early diagnosis is important to the outcome, skin lesions in the elderly population should be evaluated by a physician to rule out the possibility of precancerous or cancerous lesions. Any change in a preexisting lesion or a new cutaneous growth is suspicious in the older person. Because skin cancer is asymptomatic, it may be overlooked. Sometimes skin lesions are located in obscure areas and the older person may hide them out of fear.[47,49]

The most common dermatologic problem of persons past middle age is xerosis, or dry skin, which is more prevalent during the winter when the humidity is low. Increased wind velocity, which increases evaporative water loss from the skin, and rapid changes in humidity can also cause xerosis. Older persons tend to spend more time indoors than younger people. Both heat and air conditioning remove moisture from the air, making the environment artificially dry. The nurse therefore may wish to suggest a humidifier for the home. A vaporizer is a less expensive alternative if it is placed in the room where the elderly person spends most of his time.[45,50]

Since the production of natural protective body oils decreases with age, the older person should be taught that he does not need to bathe daily. Because most Americans customarily bathe daily, this may be a difficult habit for the older person to change. One also may prevent xerosis by using emollient creams and oils, which should be applied directly to the skin. The use of bath oil in tub water is contraindicated since it tends to make the bathtub slippery, thereby increasing the likelihood of an accident. Other factors that may aggravate dry skin include the use of cleansing agents that may be abrasive, defatting, or dehydrating.[47]

Nursing assessment of the elderly person should include eliciting a history of dryness and itchiness of the skin, frequency of bathing, and any changes in the size and appearances of growths on the skin. Like the other organs of the body, the skin requires the proper nutrition supplied by a balanced diet.[50] Since avitaminoses are more common in the elderly than in other age groups, the nurse should be alert to cutaneous signs indicating a deficiency of one or more vitamins.

Objectively, the nurse should examine the skin for color, turgor, dryness and any unusual growths. If lesions are present, one should describe them in detail. On admitting the older person to an institutional setting, the nurse should carefully inspect the skin for pressure areas and frank pressure sores, a particular problem with older persons who are experiencing decreased mobility. In institutional settings, the quality of nursing care and strategies of nursing intervention often determine the development or prevention of pressure sores.[48]

Hair

With aging, the hair pigment decreases, resulting in graying of the hair, a phenomenon that occurs most frequently between 45 and 55 years of age. The graying phenomenon, which is influenced by genetic background, customarily begins at the temples and moves toward the scalp's vertex.[50]

The quality, quantity, and distribution of hair also changes with aging. There is an increase in the number of vellus hairs on the scalp, a decrease in the facial hair of men, and an increase in the facial hair of women. The hair follicles in the scalp decrease by about one third. Pubic and axillary hair tends to decrease. Men often have coarse hair in the external ear canals, a secondary sexual characteristic.[49,50]

Nails

With advancing age, the rate of growth of nails also decreases.[50]

ENDOCRINE GLANDS

The endocrine glands do not cause senescence, but they participate in the same aging process affecting the rest of the body. I do not intend to embark on an inclusive presentation of aging changes in the endocrine system and their implications, but rather to point out some selected changes.

With advancing age, the size of the human pituitary gland decreases not more than

20%. The anterior portion of the pituitary secretes six well-recognized hormones: growth, or somatotropic, hormone (STH), thyroid-stimulating hormone (TSH), adrenocortico-tropic hormone (ACTH), follicle-stimulating hormone (FSH), lutenizing hormone (LH), and luteotropic hormone (LTH). The secretion of these hormones shows varying degrees of alteration with aging. The posterior portion of the pituitary secretes the antidiuretic hor-mone, with the secretion of this hormone changing little during aging. Physiologically and functionally, it apparently matters little whether the amount of a pituitary hormone changes with aging. The significant considerations pertain to the release of the hormone in response to appropriate stimuli that in turn relate to parameters such as age-determined changes in releasing-factor secretion, pituitary sensitivity to the releasing factor, and hy-pothalamic threshold to feedback inhibition.[5]

A decreased responsiveness of the pituitary to its physiological stimuli has been noted. For example, with aging, the pituitary fails to respond to stress with as rapid an increase in ACTH synthesis or release as it previously did. This may be a protective mechanism, however, since too rapid a change in the hormonal environment could be deleterious to the aging target organs.[52]

As measured by a variety of laboratory tests, generally there is little decrease in thy-roid functioning with aging. From a functional perspective, the thyroid function of even very elderly persons appears to be adequate.[51] When a thyroid disorder does occur in el-derly persons, however, it may go undiagnosed because the symptoms of thyroid disor-ders may differ in each aging person. In older persons, hyperthyroidism frequently results in cardiovascular symptoms, such as paroxysmal auricular tachycardia and congestive heart failure. The usual hypermetabolic symptoms, such as nervousness or sweating, may be inconspicuous. The signs of hypothyroidism in elderly individuals, such as a slowing mentation, elevated cholesterol, edema, and skin and reflex changes, may be attributed to "old age" or atherosclerosis and thus also pass undiagnosed.[52]

In women, the gonadotropic hormones remain at high but fluctuating levels through-out the reproductive years. After the menopause, however, they manifest changing rela-tionships. The follicle-stimulating hormone decreases in amount after the menopause, re-maining high for about 20 years and declining thereafter. The secretion of the lutenizing hormone declines slowly from middle or later middle life but is maintained in modest amounts into old age. The luteotropic hormone disappears shortly after menopause, ex-cept for small traces believed to be present for the rest of life.[50]

The menopause commonly begins in the late 40s and is one of the earlier signs of aging in women. Signs and symptoms associated with the menopause vary since ovarian hormone secretion ceases abruptly in some women and slowly in others. Sweating and hot flashes are among the more common signs and symptoms.[51]

While a decrease in the plasma testosterone level occurs in aging men, the degree of the decrease exhibits considerable variability. For men, the onset of the change of life (climacteric) takes place later than the menopause and occurs gradually. Common signs and symptoms of the male climacteric include mental depression, a lessening of self-esteem, easy fatigability, muscle weakness, and muscle aches and pains. Sexual behavior in elderly men and women generally corresponds to earlier life patterns.[51]

With aging, the secretion of aldosterone by the adrenals is apparently not well main-tained. Neither the urinary excretion of epinephrine nor excretion of norepinephrine, which reflects functioning of the adrenal medulla, changes with advancing age. Age ap-parently has a greater effect on adrenal androgen production than on the glucocorticoids.

The sensitivity of the adrenals to ACTH decreases with aging and the adrenal response to stress diminishes with aging.[52]

With aging, regressive changes in the islet cells of the pancreas and a decreased functional capacity for insulin synthesis and release may occur. When subjected to the usual glucose tolerance test, many older persons show varying degrees of carbohydrate intolerance. If not presented with unusual demands, however, the aging person is able to maintain carbohydrate metabolism at normal levels.[52]

Insulin has been the most extensively studied hormone in relationship to the aging process, undoubtedly because of the significance to health of an age-related insulin deficiency and possible diabetes mellitus. Diabetes has become the third leading cause of blindness and is present in about half of the patients with acute coronary disease.[52,53]

In elderly persons, the presence of diabetes may be overlooked because its onset generally is mild and gradual and the classic symptoms may be absent. Frequently elderly persons have hyperglycemia without glycosuria. Standard diagnostic criteria, however, may result in overdiagnoses because glucose tolerance decreases with advancing age. At present, authorities do not agree on the appropriate diagnostic criteria for diabetes in elderly persons.[50,52,53]

Obesity is common in elderly diabetics and it has been estimated that at least half of older diabetics are overweight. Pruritus vulvae is the most common symptom of diabetes in adult women and is usually associated with severe glycosuria. The glycosuria may develop only after a large carbohydrate load has been ingested and thereby may be overlooked if the urine is tested when fasting. Some older persons complain of blurred vision because of the acute myopia resulting from the refractive changes caused by the hyperglycemia. A few elderly persons demonstrate the sudden onset of ketotic diabetes with the accompanying classic symptoms of polyuria, polydpsia, weakness, and weight loss despite a good appetite. The most common signs of diabetic neuropathy are the loss of the Achilles reflex and of vibratory sensation in the feet. Long-standing mild diabetes may not become apparent until hyperglycemia is detected following a stressful event such as a stroke or a myocardial infarction. Atherosclerosis progresses twice as rapidly in individuals with diabetes as in persons without this disease.[53,54]

Regardless of their other physical complaints, screening tests for diabetes should be done on all elderly patients. The most sensitive test is a blood glucose determination 2 hours after a meal that includes at least 100 gm of carbohydrates. The patient should have been on a high carbohydrate diet of 300 gm for 3 days prior to testing. One should withhold all medications affecting blood glucose prior to the test.[54]

In obtaining the health history of an older person, the nurse should ascertain the existence of a family history of diabetes. One also should assess for the presence of the previously noted common signs and symptoms of diabetes in elderly persons.

In general, although aging affects many aspects of endocrine regulation, it does not affect all of the endocrine glands or all of the hormones secreted by the same gland to the same degree.[52]

SUMMARY

From reflection on the physiological alterations of the aging process, one can infer that the physiological balance of the older person is precarious because of an impairment of the homeostatic mechanisms and other changes associated with aging. As the functional performance of various systems declines with advancing age, along with the progressively more severe accumulation of pathological events affecting these systems, the ability of the elderly person to synchronize defensive and homeostatic mechanisms becomes impaired. The older individual's inability to adapt well to external and internal environmental alterations reflects more their inability to purposefully coordinate several functions involved in supporting homeostasis than the failure of any single function. The physiological changes of aging are universal and decremental, implying that they are inherent in the organism's structure and function. Thus the aging person exhibits the accumulation of multiple pathological processes, along with a progressively limited capacity to respond to stress—events leading to a logarithmically increasing probability of death.[7,27,56]

In using the data base obtained from any assessment of an older person, the nurse needs to view the older person holistically, taking into consideration behavioral, social, and cultural as well as physiological data, eliciting a history of the elderly person's prior patterns of behavior and evaluating his overall strengths and weaknesses and the probable influence his present environment of care has on his current level of functioning.

A recognition of the uniqueness of the older person, including his life history and responses to stressful events, should be incorporated into his health care plan. His care plan should not reflect discrimination on the basis of age. Health personnel interacting with the older person should convey feelings of hopefulness, concern, and caring to him, along with an appreciation of his past contributions to society.

REFERENCES

1. Zorzoli, A.: Biological aspects of the aging process, Public Health News, July, 1968, New Jersey State Department of Health. (Reprint.)
2. Goldstein, S.: The biology of aging, N. Engl. J. Med. **285:**1120-1129, Nov. 11, 1971.
3. Strehler, B. L.: Aging at the cellular level. In Rossman, I., Clinical geriatrics, Philadelphia, 1971, J. B. Lippincott Co., pp. 49-56.
4. Shock, N. W.: The physiology of aging, Sci. Am. **100:**100-110, Jan., 1962.
5. Stone, V.: Give the older person time, A. J. of N. **68:**2124-2127, Oct., 1969.
6. Harris, R.: Special features of heart disease in elderly people. In Chinn, A. B.: Working with older people, vol. 4, U.S. Department of Health, Education and Welfare Publication No. HRA 74-3119, 1971, pp. 81-102.
7. Timiras, P. S.: Developmental physiology and aging, New York, 1972, The Macmillan Co.
8. Caird, F. I., and Dall, J. L. C.: The cardiovascular system. In Brocklehurst, J. C.: Textbook of geriatric medicine and gerontology, Edinburgh, 1973, Churchill Livingstone, pp. 122-160.
9. Samorajski, T.: How the human brain responds to aging, J. Am. Geriatr. Soc. **24:**4-11, Jan., 1976.
10. Strehler, B. L.: Introduction: aging and the human brain. In Terry, R. D., and Gershon, S., editors: Aging, vol. 3, Neurobiology of aging, New York, 1976, Raven Press, pp. 1-22.
11. Tomlinson, B. E., and Henderson, G.: Some quantative cerebral findings in normal and demented old people. In Terry, R. D., and Gershon, S., editors: Aging, vol. 3, Neurobiology of aging, New York, 1976, Raven Press, pp. 183-204.
12. Botwinick, J.: Behavioral processes. In Gershon S., and Raskin, A., editors: Aging, vol. 2, Genesis and treatment of physiologic disorders in the elderly, New York, 1973, Raven Press, pp. 1-18.
13. Feinberg, I.: Functional implications of changes in sleep physiology with aging. In Terry, R. D., and Gershon, S.: Aging, vol. 8, Neurobiology of aging, New York, 1976, Raven Press, pp. 23-42.
14. Carter, A. B.: The neurologic aspects of aging. In Rossman, I.: Clinical geriatrics, Philadelphia, 1971, J. B. Lippincott Co., pp. 123-141.
15. Grob, D.: Common disorders of muscles in the aged. In Chinn, A. B.: Working with older people, vol. 4, U.S. Department of Health, Education and Welfare Publication No. HRA 74-3119, 1971, pp. 156-162.
16. Barbeau, A.: Aging and the extrapyramidal system, J. Am. Geriatr. Soc. **21:**145-149, April, 1973.
17. Butler, R. N., and Lewis, M. I.: Aging and mental health, St. Louis, 1973, The C. V. Mosby Co.
18. Prior, J. A., and Silverstein, J. S.: Physical diagnosis, ed. 4, St. Louis, 1977, The C. V. Mosby Co.
19. Spencer, H., Baladad, J., and Lewin, I.: The skeletal system. In Rossman, I.: Clinical geriatrics, Philadelphia, 1971, J. B. Lippincott Co., pp. 285-300.
20. Dequeker, J.: Bone and aging, Ann. of Rheum. Dis. **34:**100-115, Feb., 1975.

21. Birchenall, J., and Streight, M. E.: Care of the older adult, Philadelphia, 1973, J. B. Lippincott Co.

22. Grob, D.: Prevalent joint diseases in older persons. In Chinn, A. B.: Working with older people, vol. 4, U.S. Department of Health, Education and Welfare Publication No. HRA 74-3119, 1971, pp. 163-171.

23. Horenstein, S.: Managing gait disorders, Geriatrics, **29:**86-94, Dec., 1974.

24. Malasanos, L., et. al.: Health assessment, St. Louis, 1977, The C. V. Mosby Co.

25. Balchum, O. J.: The aging respiratory system. In Chinn, A. B.: Working with older people, vol. 4, U.S. Department of Health, Education and Welfare Publication No. HRA 74-3119, 1971, pp. 113-123.

26. Klocke, R. A.: Influence of aging on the lung. In Finch, C. E., and Hayflck, L.: Handbook of the biology of aging, New York, 1977, Van Nostrand Reinhold Co., pp. 432-444.

27. Goldman, R.: Decline in organ function with aging. In Rossman, I.: Clinical geriatrics, Philadelphia, 1971, J. B. Lippincott Co., pp. 19-48.

28. Straus, B.: Disorders of the digestive system. In Rossman, I.: Clinical geriatrics, Philadelphia, 1971, J. B. Lippincott Co., pp. 183-202.

29. Kampman, J. P., Sinding, J., and Moler-Jorgenson, I.: Effect of age on liver function, Geriatrics **30:**91-95, Aug., 1975.

30. Sklar, M.: Gastrointestinal diseases in the aged. In Chinn, A. B.: Working with older people, vol. 4, U.S. Department of Health, Education and Welfare, Publication No. HRA 74-3119, pp. 124-130.

31. Peterson, M. L.: Neoplastic diseases of the alimentary tract. In Beeson, P. B., and McDermott, W.: Cecil-Loeb Textbook of Medicine, ed. 13, Philadelphia, 1971, W. B. Saunders, pp. 1358-1376.

32. Agate, J.: Natural history of disease in later life. In Rossman, I.: Clinical geriatrics, Philadelphia, 1971, J. B. Lippincott Co., pp. 115-122.

33. Brocklehurst, J. C.: The bladder. In Brocklehurst, J. C.: Textbook of geriatric medicine and gerontology, Edinburgh, 1973, Churchill Livingstone, pp. 298-320.

34. Weir, D. R., Houser, H. B., and Davy, L.: Recognition and management of the nutrition problems of the elderly. In Chinn, A. B.: Working with older people, vol. 4, U.S. Department of Health, Education and Welfare Publication No. HRA 74-3119, 1971, pp. 267-278.

35. Shonk, R. E.: Nutrition and aging. In Ostfeld, A. M., and Gibson, D. C.: Epidemiology of aging, U.S. Department of Health Education and Welfare Publication No. (NIH), 75-711, 1975, pp. 199-214.

36. Caird, F. I., and Judge, T. G.: Assessment of the elderly patient, London, 1974, Pitman Medical.

37. Sourander, L. B.: The aging kidney. In Brocklehurst, J. C.: Textbook of geriatric medicine and gerontology, Edinburgh, 1973, Churchill Livingstone, pp. 280-297.

38. Kahn, A. I., and Snapper, I.: Medical renal diseases in the aged. In Chinn, A. B.: Working with older people, vol. 4, Department of Health, Education and Welfare Publication No. HRA 74-3119, 1971, pp. 131-140.

39. Davison, W.: The hazards of drug treatment in old age. In Brocklehurst, J. C.: Textbook of geriatric medicine and gerontology, Edinburgh, 1973, Churchill Livingstone, pp. 632-648.

40. Brocklehurst, J. C.: The urinary tract. In Rossman, I.: Clinical geriatrics, Philadelphia, 1971, J. B. Lippincott Co., pp. 219-228.

41. Kornzweig, A. L.: The eye in old age. In Rossman, I.: Clinical geriatrics, Philadelphia, 1971, J. B. Lippincott Co., pp. 229-246.

42. Leopold, I.: The eye. In Freeman, J. T.: Clinical features of the older patient, Springfield, Ill., 1965, Charles C Thomas, Publisher, pp. 420-427.

43. Kornzweig, A. L.: A low-vision clinic at a home for the aged, J. Am. Geriatr. Soc. **24:**538-541, 1976.

44. Ruben, R.: Aging and hearing. In Rossman, I.: Clinical geriatrics, Philadelphia, 1971, J. B. Lippincott, Co., pp. 247-252.

45. Sataloff, J.: Otolaryngologic problems. In Freeman, J. T.: Clinical features of the older patient, Springfield, Illinois, 1965, Charles C Thomas, Publisher, pp. 428-434.

46. Wollner, L., and Spalding, J. M.: The autonomic nervous system. In Brocklehurst, J. C.: Textbook of geriatric medicine and gerontology, Edinburgh, 1973, Churchill Livingstone, pp. 235-253.

47. Ogawa, C. M.: Degenerative skin disorders: toll of age and sun, Geriatrics, **30:**65-69, Feb., 1975.

48. Hanna, M., and Macmillan, A.: Aging and the skin. In Brocklehurst, J. C.: Textbook of geriatric medicine and gerontology, Edinburgh, 1973, Churchill Livingstone, pp. 593-617.

49. Tindall, J. P.: Geriatric dermatology. In Chinn, A. B.: Working with older people, vol. 4, U.S. Department of Health, Education and Welfare Publication No. HRA 74-3119, 1971, pp. 3-27.

50. Knox, J. M.: Common-sense care for aging skin, Geriatrics **30:**59-60, Feb., 1975.

51. McGavack, T. H.: Endocrine changes with aging significant to clinical practice. In Chinn, A. B.:

Working with older people, vol. 4, U.S. Department of Health, Education and Welfare Publication No. HRA 74-3119, 1971, pp. 194-216.

52. Gregerman, R. I., and Bierman, E. L.: Aging and hormones. In Williams, R. H.: Textbook of endocrinology, ed. 5, Philadelphia, 1974, W. B. Saunders Co., pp. 1059-1070.

53. Stahl, N. L., and Greenblatt, R. B.: Geriatric practice: age and the endocrine system. In Busse, E. W.: Theory and therapeutics of aging, New York, 1973, Medcom Press, pp. 62-71.

54. Gutman, L.: Diabetes mellitus and the aged. In Chinn, A. B.: Working with older people, vol. 4, U.S. Department of Health Education, and Welfare Publication No. HRA 74-3119, 1971, pp. 219-224.

55. Duncan, T. G.: Diabetes: diagnosis and management in the older patient, Geriatrics **31:**51-55, Oct., 1976.

56. Exton-Smith, A. N., and Windsor, A. C. G.: Principles of drug treatment in the aged. In Rossman, I.: Clinical geriatrics, Philadelphia, 1971, J. B. Lippincott Co., p. 389.

4 Drugs for the aging: use and abuse

ALAN CHEUNG

Victor R. Fuchs in his book *Who Shall Live? Health, Economics, and Social Choice* states, "Drugs are the key to modern medicine and the ability of health care providers to alter health outcomes depends primarily on drugs."[1] Since the beginning of man, drugs have fulfilled two of the most basic human needs — alleviation of suffering and protection against disease.

Even though drugs have been proved to be beneficial and sometimes life saving, they also may cause many drug-induced complications and may even cause death. In our drug-oriented society, consumers and some health care providers are led to believe that there is a pill for every complaint or symptom regardless of the diagnosis. Increased drug utilization results in increased drug-induced diseases and drug-related problems. Cluff states, "Consumption of drugs represents an important form of environmental chemical exposure and pollution. It is probably a more important cause of environmentally induced disease than other forms of environmental exposure which receive greater attention. . . ."[2]

The cost of drugs accounts for approximately 10% of the total health care expenditure. This figure does not include costs incurred as a result of treatment of adverse drug reactions and interactions, drug-induced diseases, and problems that arise from the misuse of drugs. In addition, the psychological traumas associated with drug-induced complications of disease states, income loss, and partial loss of work capability are impossible to measure.

Elderly individuals are especially prone to drug-induced complications. They often have a number of chronic diseases that may require long-term and continuous drug therapy prescribed by one or more physicians. Alterations in physiological states caused by aging affect drug absorption, distribution, metabolism, and excretion. In addition, changes in psychosocial and economic aspects of aging as well as a general lack of standards for prescribing and monitoring drug therapy in the geriatric population contribute to serious drug use problems. Therefore those health care providers involved in direct or indirect care of geriatric patients should have some fundamental training in geriatric pharmacology, especially in the areas of adverse drug reactions and interactions.

DRUG USE PROBLEMS

Use of illegal or street drugs and abuse of some addicting prescription drugs have attracted national attention, resulting in the development of the National Institute on Drug Abuse, the Drug Enforcement Administration, and other organizations to provide some solutions to these problems. Abuse and misuse of legal prescription and nonprescription drugs is a more important health hazard affecting far more people, yet it has received very little notice. In the last decade, a number of reports on the problems of drug utilization and drug-induced diseases have appeared in medical and scientific literature. Data from studies in countries such as the United States, Canada, and Australia show the problems and alarming statistics of adverse drug reactions in hospital settings[3-8]:

1. Fifteen to thirty percent of hospitalized patients experience one or more adverse drug reactions.
2. Three to five percent of hospital admissions to medical services are a result of adverse drug reactions.
3. The average hospital stay is nearly doubled for patients who suffer an adverse drug reaction.
4. The majority of adverse drug reactions are preventable.
5. The national cost of drug-induced hospitalization is close to $3 billion per year (1969).

Cluff quotes Alfred Stille, who states, "The virtues of a medicine depend less upon its intrinsic properties and powers than on the capacity of the physician who administers it—or the person who uses it—just as the efficiency of firearms depends less on the explosives and missiles they contain than on the judgment and accuracy of aim of the man who discharges them."[9]

Age is one of the predisposing factors in adverse drug reactions. The U.S. National Center for Health Statistics reported in 1966 that "Americans aged 65 and over acquired about 22 percent of all prescription drugs though constituting only 9 percent of the population." It further stated that there was a direct association among chronic illness, limitation of activity, and number of drugs acquired. Those individuals no longer able to carry on a "major activity" were getting 13 times the number of prescribed medicines that were acquired by those with no chronic illness.

In a study of long-term care institutions, such as nursing homes, Cheung and Kayne found that an average nursing home patient received seven medications, and that there were 122 adverse drug reactions detected in the 453 patients who were intensively monitored for early detection and prevention of adverse drug reactions.[10] Major tranquilizers, diuretics, digitalis and insulin preparations were responsible for 50% of all these adverse drug reactions. Fifty percent of those reactions were found to be of clinical significance. If left undetected, the reaction might result in serious harm to the patient or might necessitate readmission to the general hospital.

Learoyd reported that in a review of 236 consecutive patients admitted to an Australian psychogeriatric unit, 37 (16%) were found to suffer from the adverse effect of psychotherapeutic medications.[11] Seven patients were excessively sedated or confused, 16 had hypotensive episodes resulting in falls and fractures, and 14 had behavioral disturbances.

Cheung and Koga, in reviewing the drug utilization of 26 home care patients, found that 50% of these patients manifested adverse drug effects.[12] Cardiovascular, analgesic, and central nervous system and other neurological drugs accounted for nearly 90% of all drugs causing adverse effects.

These data demonstrate how important it is that the drug therapy of each elderly patient be continuously monitored, so that potential drug-induced complications can be prevented or detected early. The Federal Register for Skilled Nursing Facilities regulations on January 17, 1974 (paragraph 405.1127a), stated, "The pharmacist reviews the drug regimen of each patient at least monthly, and reports any irregularities to the medical director and administrator. . . ." This is the first indication of concern by a federal governmental agency on drug use in the elderly.

Noncompliance with proper drug utilization is as important as, if not more important than, the problems of adverse drug reactions and interactions. Hussar stated, "Considerable time, energy and expense have often gone into the diagnosis of a patient's illness and the development of his treatment program. Yet the goals of therapy will not be reached unless the patient understands and follows the instructions for the use of drugs prescribed.''[13] Blackwell, in reviewing more than 50 studies, found that ''complete failure to take medication often occurred in more than one-half of all outpatients. Other types of poor compliance, which may be more frequent, include taking medication for wrong reasons, errors in dosage and mistakes in timing or sequence.''[14]

There are two types of medication noncompliance. One is caused by the drug distribution system within an institution and generally occurs in a hospital situation. The patients usually do not assume any responsibility for their own care because the hospital staff are doing all they can *to* and *for* the patient. This type of noncompliance or medication error is staff initiated and can easily be corrected. The other type of noncompliance occurs in an outpatient setting, where the patients must assume the responsibility for coordinating their own care. Complexity of treatment plans, strange drug names, and complicated or inadequate instructions from health care providers are the major reasons for noncompliance in the outpatient setting. It can be confusing for an elderly patient to take a number of medications unless he has been clearly informed, which includes written instructions. Schwartz, in her study of medication errors, found:

> Three-fifths of all the elderly respondents were found to err in taking their medications properly. Their error-making patients averaged 2.6 errors each. . . . The type of error that occurred most frequently was ommission of a medication. Next most frequent was inaccurate knowledge, followed by errors in self-medication, inaccurate dosage, and lastly, improper timing or sequence of drugs that were to be taken in a definite order.[15]

Major consequences of noncompliance are summarized below:

1. Worsening of the condition being treated
2. Necessity for prescribing larger doses of the same agents or prescribing more potent drugs
3. Increased risk of adverse drug reactions and interactions
4. Escalated cost of care

Complete drug use records, patient education on the proper use of drugs, and patient involvement in the decision making of his or her care will greatly alleviate the problems of noncompliance in taking prescribed medications.

Most elderly patients receive medications over a long period of time, sometimes months and years. Narcotic and nonnarcotic analgesics, sedative-hypnotics, antidepressants, and major tranquilizers are among the drugs most commonly prescribed. Most of these drugs can cause psychological and physical dependence or addiction, and their cessation may induce withdrawal symptoms. Some prescribers may rationalize that prescribing these medications is appropriate because the patients are old and should be allowed to enjoy the effects of the medications.

The instinct to self-medicate is basic to human nature. An abundance of medicinal preparations such as folk medicines, herbs, and homeopathic remedies are available for self-treatment. The therapeutic value and active ingredients of many of these preparations remain unknown. In addition, a large number of over-the-counter drugs are available in drug stores and supermarkets. Elderly patients, even though they may be under regular care by their physicians, are especially prone to try these medications, because they do not like to impose on busy physicians and may feel that they can manage their symptoms through self-medication. Use of these medications may interfere with the therapeutic management of the patients and may result in a higher incidence of adverse drug interactions.

ALTERED PHYSIOLOGICAL RESPONSES TO DRUGS IN AGING

The aging process causes changes in major organ functions that may alter the physiological responses to drug effects. The activities of the gastrointestinal tract, liver, and kidneys may be modified, thereby changing drug absorption, drug metabolism, and drug excretion. Total body water, lean body mass, and body fat may decrease with advancing age, affecting the amount of free drugs in the circulation and the distribution of drugs in body tissues. Tissue sensitivity to drugs seems to differ in older individuals, especially in tissues of the central nervous system. This can be attributed to altered response by the receptors and to changes in homeostatis mechanisms.

Drug absorption

Absorption and transport of some drugs are likely to occur at a slower rate in older patients. Factors that influence and control absorption are as follows:

1. Decrease in acid output with a corresponding decrease in drug solubility
2. Reduced level of mesenteric blood flow
3. Reduction in size of the absorbing surface
4. Impairment in enzyme systems responsible for transport across the intestinal epithelial membrane[16]

It should be emphasized that a decrease in absorption with age is not a definitive finding. Evidence has been found that suggests that absorption of some sugars, minerals, and vitamins is diminished in the elderly.

Drug metabolism and excretion

Once a drug is introduced into the circulation, its concentration in the blood reflects the rate at which it is eliminated. In general, drugs are either excreted unchanged by the kidney or are metabolized in the liver into less active or inert compounds. With advancing age, renal excretion and liver metabolism become less efficient. The plasma half-life of drugs such as antipyrine, phenylbutazone, phenobarbitol, paracetamol, and diazepam have been found to be significantly increased in older patients when compared to younger patients.[17] The degreased ability of elderly patients to metabolize these drugs and the resultant increase in blood levels may contribute to the known high incidence of adverse reactions in the elderly.

The aging process reduces glomerular filtration and tubular secretory capacity of drugs. Those drugs that are highly polar or low in lipid solubility, such as aminoglycosides (gentamicin, kanamycin, etc.), are generally excreted by the kidney. Drugs such as penicillin and tetracycline that are excreted through the tubular secretory mechanism are found to have higher blood levels and longer plasma half-lives.[18,19] With the occurrence of diminishing renal function, overdosage may be a serious problem for the elderly, especially if they take drugs with high potential for adverse effects such as digoxin, chlorpropamide, and lidocaine. It is a good practice to individualize the dosage of drugs that are excreted mostly through the kidneys in elderly patients.

Drug distribution

Elderly patients usually have a smaller lean body mass as well as decreased total body water. As a result, drugs such as digoxin may be expected to have a higher level in the blood of older patients than in younger patients if both are given the same dosage. In addition, plasma albumin levels are lower in older individuals. Drugs such as warfarin and phenytoin that are highly bound to protein may have a higher free drug concentration in the circulation of older patients. Other factors that may influence drug distribution are caused by changes in the systemic blood flow and in the ability of the drug to pass through various membranes such as the blood-brain barrier. All these factors may lead to altered or exaggerated pharmacologic effects.

Changes in receptors and homeostatic mechanisms

Changes in the pharmacologic effects of drugs on the elderly cannot always be explained by pharmacokinetic principles because there may not be resultant changes in plasma or blood levels. These pharmacologic changes can be attributed to the alteration of a number of receptors as well as to the homeostatic capacity. This may partially explain why many elderly patients are very sensitive to the central nervous system effects and the orthostatic hypotensive actions of many drugs. These are important considerations in the prescribing and monitoring of drug therapy in geriatric patients.

CLINICAL USES OF DRUGS IN THE ELDERLY

Most elderly persons have multiple pathological conditions or chronic illnesses that necessitate drugs as part of the treatment. Often elderly patients may have a different response to drugs than do younger patients. Therefore it is important to know the clinical indications and the potential hazards of drugs used in the treatment of common chronic conditions in the elderly.

Cardiovascular drug therapy

Digitalis preparations. Digitalis preparations are usually recommended for the treatment of congestive heart failure and certain types of supraventricular arrhythmia. This group of drugs probably causes the highest incidence of adverse drug reactions in the elderly. The difference between the therapeutic and the toxic dose of digitalis is small. The elderly patient often has decreased lean body mass, impaired renal function, multiple cardiovascular problems, and a possible electrolyte abnormality while taking potentially interacting drugs. Therefore the dosage of digitalis preparations, for example, digoxin or digitoxin, should be individualized and carefully monitored for each geriatric patient.

Diuretics. Diuretics such as thiazides, furosemide, and ethacrynic acid are important therapeutic agents in the management of congestive heart failure and hypertension. Because the glomerular filtration rate decreases with age, diuretic therapy in the elderly patient may cause a decrease in blood volume and may further compromise renal function. In aged men with prostatic hypertrophy, diuretics can cause urinary retention, especially when combined with drugs having anticholinergic properties. Diuretics can also precipitate urinary incontinence in elderly patients of both sexes.

It is important to monitor the effects of diuretic therapy. Regular weighing usually is a good monitoring device. Both furosemide and ethacrynic acid are potent, short-acting diuretics and they are more likely to cause dehydration and hypotension. Longer acting diuretics such as chlorthalidone, if given in the late afternoon and evening, may induce nocturia and insomnia. Therefore the elderly patient should be advised to take these medications in the daytime to avoid the predictable undesirable effects and to assure proper compliance.

Other major complications of the thiazide group of drugs, including furosemide and ethacrynic acid, are electrolyte disturbance, acid-base imbalance, impaired glucose tolerance, and hyperuricemia. Because they are often given with digitalis, a potassium supplement, preferably in liquid form, should be added to the treatment and serum potassium should be checked periodically.

Potassium-sparing diuretics, including spironolactone and triamterene, are given in combination with thiazides to reduce hypokalemia. These diuretics should be used with great caution in elderly patients with impaired renal function.

Antihypertensives. Even though hypertension is a common condition in the elderly, inappropriate and irrational use of antihypertensive agents can cause more harm than good in the geriatric patient. The incorrect lowering of blood pressure may precipitate cerebrovascular and coronary insufficiency.

Thiazides are usually the first choice for management of hypertension. Other drugs such as methyldopa, hydralazine, reserpine, clonidine, and guanethidine may be added to the diuretic therapy. Because of different sites of pharmacologic actions, antihypertensive treatment is one of the few situations where multiple drug therapy is justified.

Hydralazine and methyldopa are usually preferred for patients with renal insufficiency. Methyldopa and reserpine are more prone to cause drowsiness, depression, and other psychiatric disturbances in the elderly. Hydralazine may aggravate coronary ischemia and it is often given with a beta receptor blocker (propranolol). Guanethidine has a potent postural hypotensive effect that may be sufficiently severe to cause unconsciousness. This effect is potentiated by other drugs and accentuated by hot temperature and exercise.

Lethargy and drowsiness in the initial treatment and impotence or decreased libido in the long-term use of guanethidine and methyldopa may account for some noncompliance by the elderly patient. Geriatric patients on antihypertensive therapy should be monitored closely and regularly. Patient education and counseling should be provided continuously.

Psychotherapeutics

Sedative-hypnotics and major tranquilizers are among the most abused prescription drugs. They are often used for the treatment of acute confusion states, insomnia, and mental disturbances associated with cerebral arteriosclerosis and senile psychosis in the aged patient. They are often overprescribed to patients in long-term care facilities as a substitute for attention by health care providers. As a result, elderly patients with behavioral or mental disturbances are usually treated with one or more psychotropic drugs.

Long-term and regular use of sedative-hypnotics may lead to psychological and physical dependence, and the abrupt cessation of these agents may induce withdrawal symptoms. Sedative-hypnotics can cause syncope, drowsiness, and hypotension, which are common and may have serious complications in the elderly. Geriatric patients are very sensitive to the effects of these drugs. Excessive dosages may lead to immobility and may result in stasis pneumonia and urinary retention.

Parkinsonian rigidity as well as dyskinesia are common in phenothiazine therapy; dyskinesia is more common in the aged. The dosage regimen should be selected cautiously and should be individualized for each geriatric patient. Regular monitoring is required to prevent potential serious adverse effects.

Insulin and oral hypoglycemic agents

The elderly diabetic patient is prone to develop a hypoglycemic reaction, which may result in an acute brain syndrome and other mental changes. If this reaction is not recognized, the patient may receive a psychotropic agent for the management of mental disorder. Hypoglycemia usually results from a long-acting preparation of insulin or an oral hypoglycemic agent, for example, chlorpropamide. The dosage of insulin or an oral hypoglycemic agent is usually regulated in conjunction with dietary control. Because of poor dietary habits, inadequate resources, or loss of appetite, the elderly diabetic patient may fail to eat properly and subsequently may develop a hypoglycemic reaction. Many elderly patients do not manifest a classic hypoglycemic syndrome; by the time the hypoglycemic symptoms do appear, the reaction may be very severe. Therefore the geriatric diabetic patient should be closely monitored.

Analgesic and antiarthritic therapy

Pain, arthralgia, and myalgia are common symptoms in the elderly and have a variety of etiologies. The most popular preparations for their treatment are the salicylates, acetaminophen (paracetamol), indomethacin, phenylbutazone (Butazolidin), and narcotic analgesics for severe pain. Salicylates, indomethacin, and phenylbutazone have analgesic, antipyretic, and antiinflammatory properties. They all cause gastrointestinal distress and hemorrhage. In addition, phenylbutazone has serious hematologic adverse effects; regular complete blood counts are necessary to detect and prevent these adverse reactions. Phenylbutazone should be reserved for use in acute and short-term therapy in conditions in which other agents are not effective.

Acetaminophen, propoxyphene, and pentazocine do not have anti-inflammatory activities. They are not irritating to the gastrointestinal tract. Long-term use of high dosages of acetaminophen by patients with renal impairment may further aggravate the renal abnormality. Many experts consider propoxyphene and pentazocine to be weak narcotic analgesics, equal to salicylates in effectiveness. Narcotic analgesics are usually reserved for severe pain. Patients with terminal illnesses such as cancer often become addicted to narcotic analgesics through regular long-term use of these preparations.

Drugs with anticholinergic effects

Geriatric patients often receive a variety of medications that may have anticholinergic properties. In addition to the parasympatholytic preparations, drugs such as major tranquilizers, tricyclic antidepressants, antiparkinsonian agents, and antihistamines all have anticholinergic characteristics. Alone, most of these drugs have weak anticholinergic effects. But if the drugs are used in combination, these effects will be prominent, especially in the elderly. The more serious effects are acute brain syndrome, hypotension, tachycardia, urinary retention, and constipation. Without proper monitoring and recognition of the adverse effects, elderly patients may receive other medications to treat this drug-induced complication.

It is not possible to cover all drugs that may affect the geriatric patient. A standard textbook of pharmacology will serve as a good reference source.

DESIRABLE GUIDELINES FOR DRUG PRESCRIBING AND MONITORING IN THE ELDERLY

To assure the proper drug utilization and to prevent drug misuse in the elderly, the following guidelines are suggested.

Establish and maintain a complete up-to-date drug profile. Many geriatric patients take medication prescribed by more than one physician. In addition, they may self-medicate with over-the-counter drugs, folk remedies, or leftover prescription drugs. A medical history is not complete without an adequate drug history. A good drug profile will enable the provider to recognize potential drug prescribing problems such as duplication of prescriptions, inappropriate drug combinations, and noncompliance with instructions for drug administration. The drug profile needs to be continuously updated.

Develop a pathophysiological profile. It is important to understand the pathophysiological process occuring in the elderly patient, especially those physiological functions that may affect or modify the effects of drugs. This is where the therapeutic plan and objectives can be realistically established and drugs can then be rationally prescribed and monitored.

Acquire knowledge of geriatric pharmacology and clinical pharmacokinetics. The elderly patient reacts to drugs differently from the younger patient, especially in relation to drug absorption, distribution, metabolism, and excretion. Background and training in geriatric pharmacology and clinical pharmacokinetics can prepare the providers to predict the effects of drugs more rationally and scientifically in the elderly patients. It is important to individualize the drug dosage in the elderly. Some advances in this area are the development of computerized dosage programs and certain drug assays to measure the concentration of drugs that are toxic or require a constant therapeutic concentration to produce the desired response.

Develop drug monitoring plans and criteria. Criteria for monitoring the patient's response to drug therapy should be developed. (See the section on drug therapy monitoring, p. 72.) Plan when, how often, and what aspects of the patient's drug therapy to monitor. The monitoring of drug therapy has to be continuous and organized.

Outline social, psychological, and economic profile. Health is more than physical well-being. The social, psychological, and economic profile of the elderly patient is important for developing a complete treatment plan and therapeutic approaches. Only by considering the psychosocial and economic factors of the patient can the optimal therapeutic benefit be realized.

Provide patient education and counseling. The main reasons for patient noncompliance are inadequate patient communication, education, and counseling on the proper uses of drugs. Written educational material should be made available to reinforce the oral instruction; an example is given on p. 73. The information should include how the drug works, instruction as to how and when to take the drugs, possible drug interactions to avoid, and cautions concerning major adverse effects.

Documentation and communication. Significant findings relating to drug responses and drug use problems should be recorded and documented in the drug profile as well as in the patient's chart and should be communicated directly to those responsible for the care of the patient.

Drug utilization review. Procedures and standards should be established to evaluate the pattern of drug utilization. If the drug utilization review is properly organized and implemented on a continuous basis, it will assure a high level of drug therapy and patient care to the elderly. The problems of drug use in the elderly cannot be solved overnight. It takes the combined efforts of the health care providers and the patient to improve the effectiveness of drug therapy through communication, patient counseling, and education.

DRUG THERAPY MONITORING
Signs and symptoms of digitalis toxicity

A. Central nervous system
  1. Headache, fatigue, malaise, drowsiness (common and early)
  2. Neuralgic pain (similar to trigeminal neuralgia)
  3. Mental symptoms — disorientation, confusion, aphasia, delirium, hallucination, and rarely convulsion (in elderly atherosclerotic patients)
B. Eye
  1. Blurred vision — white borders or halo on dark objects
  2. Disturbed color vision — chromatopsia, most common for yellow and green
  3. Transitory amblyopia, diplopia, and scotomata
C. Throat: Salivation associated with nausea
D. Cardiovascular
  1. Arrhythmia of all types
     Extrasystoles — most frequent (ventricular is greater than atrial, coupling or bigeminy)
  2. A-V block
  3. Others — sinus arrhythmia, paroxysmal atrial or ventricular tachycardia, atrial tachycardia, ventricular tachycardia, atrial fibrillation, and ventricular fibrillation
E. Gastrointestinal
  1. Anorexia, nausea, and vomiting (earliest signs of digitalis toxicity)
  2. Abdominal discomfort or pain
  3. Diarrhea
F. Renal: Diuretic effect
G. Hematological: Eosinophilia (rare)
H. Metabolic-endocrine: Gynecomastia (rare)
I. Skin: Skin rash — urticarial (rare)

Comparison of digitoxin and digoxin

	Digitoxin	*Digoxin*
Absorption (oral)	90% to 100%	60% to 85%
onset (IV)	½ to 2 hours	15 to 30 minutes
peak (IV)	4 to 12 hours	1 to 5 hours
Distribution		
protein-binding	97%	25%
V_d	40.9 liters/kg	5.27 liters/kg
Metabolism	Extensively by liver	
Renal excretion	Inactive metabolites	60% to 90% unchanged form
Plasma T½	5 to 7 days	36 hours
Plasma concentration		
therapeutic	14 to 26 ng/ml	0.8 to 1.6 ng/ml
toxic	>34 ng/ml	>2.4 ng/ml
Optimal tissue store		
congestive heart failure	8 to 10 μg/kg	8 to 10 μg/kg
atrial arrhythmia	13 to 15 μg/kg	13 to 15 μg/kg
Daily oral maintenance dose (adult)	0.05 to 0.2 mg	0.125 to 0.5 mg
Daily loss (percentage of tissue store)	10%	37%

Drug interactions of digitoxin and digoxin

A. Pharmacodynamic effect
   1. Diuretics (electrolyte disturbances)
   2. Calcium
   3. Sympathomimetic
B. Decreased absorption
   1. Antacids (nonabsorbable)
   2. Antidiarrheal (adsorbent-type)
   3. Cholestyramine
C. Increased absorption: anticholinergic drugs
   Accelerated hepatic metabolism: phenobarbital, phenylbutazone, phenytoin

DIGITALIS PREPARATIONS

- This drug is used in heart conditions to eliminate shortness of breath, tiredness, and general swelling. It works by increasing the strength of the heartbeat so that more blood is pumped to the body tissues.
- This is an important medication; therefore, follow the directions on the label carefully. DO NOT exceed the dosage specified on the label.
- If your physician has prescribed diuretics (water pills) or potassium supplements (KCl, Kaon) it is very important that you take these medications while on digitalis or digoxin.
- Contact your physician or clinical pharmacist if you develop severe nausea and/or vomiting while taking this drug.
- If you DO NOT understand the instructions or want further information on the drug, contact your physician or pharmacist.

REFERENCES

1. Fuchs, V. R.: Who shall live? Health, economics, and social choice, New York, 1974, Basic Books, Inc., Publishers, p. 105.
2. Cluff, L. E., Caranasos, G. J., and Stewart, R. B.: Clinical problems with drugs, Philadelphia, 1975, W. B. Saunders Co., p. 2.
3. Ogilvie, R. I., and Ruedy, J.: Adverse drug reactions during hospitalization, Can. Med. Assoc. J. **97**:1450-1456, 1967.
4. Hoddinott, B. C., et. al.: Drugs reactions and errors in administration on a medical ward, Can. Med. Assoc. J. **97**:1001-1006, 1967.
5. Smith, J. W., Seidl, L. G., and Cluff, L. E.: Studies on epidemiology of adverse drug reactions, Ann. Intern. Med. **65**:629-640, 1966.
6. Hurwitz, N.: Admissions to hospital due to drugs, Br. Med. J. **1**:539-540, 1969.
7. Melmon, K. L.: Preventable drug reactions—causes and cures, N. Engl. J. Med. **284**:1361-1368, 1971.
8. Task Force on Prescription Drugs: Final report, U.S. Department of Health, Education, and Welfare, Washington, D.C., 1969.
9. Cluff, et. al., p. 3.
10. Cheung, A., and Kayne, R. C.: An application of clinical pharmacy services in extended care facilities, Calif. Pharm. **23**(3):22-43, 1975.
11. Learoyd, B. M.: Psychotropic drugs and the elderly patient, Med. J. Aust., **1**:1131-1133, 1972.
12. Cheung, A., Koga, P. Y., and Mitchell, A.: A survey of drug utilization of patients, referred by a home health agency, Unpublished report, 1976.
13. Hussar, D. A.: Patient noncompliance, J. Am. Pharm. Assoc. **NS15**(4):133-139, April, 1975.
14. Blackwell, B.: Patient compliance, N. Engl. J. Med. **289**:249-252, 1973.
15. Schwartz, D.: The elderly patient and his medications—chance and mischance, Geriatrics **20**(1): 517-520, June, 1965.
16. Bender, A. D.: Effect of age on intestinal absorption and implications for drug absorption in the elderly, J. Am. Geriatr. Soc. **16**:1331, 1968.
17. Avery, G. S., editor: Drug treatment, principles and practice of clinical pharmacology and therapeutics, Sydney, 1976, Publishing Sciences Group, Inc., p. 126.
18. Leikola, E., and Varitia, K. O.: On penicillin levels in young and geriatric subjects, J. Gerontol. **12**:48, 1957.
19. Varitia, K. O., and Leikola, E.: Serum levels of antibiotics in young and old subjects following administration of dihydrostreptomycin and tetracycline, J. Gerontol. **15**:392, 1960.

5 Nutritional needs and effects of poor nutrition in elderly persons

SHERMAN R. DICKMAN

Although good nutrition for the aged does not differ in principle from good nutrition for the young, it *does* differ in detail. These differences are listed as follows:

1. Calorie requirements for the elderly are usually less. This is because most of them engage in much less physical activity than younger people do.
2. Elderly people are likely to require more vitamins and essential elements in their diets than do younger people since they are much more likely to suffer from digestive disturbances that will affect absorption, storage, and utilization of nutrients.
3. Elderly people use more medication (drugs) than any other group. As will be discussed later, this practice can result in serious nutritional problems.

Although nutritional needs of human beings may be grossly similar, the foods that satisfy those needs probably vary more widely among the elderly than in younger age groups. Swanson states, "A person at 70 is an historical record of all that has happened to him — injuries, infection, nutritional imbalances, fatigues, and emotional upsets. Old people, therefore, differ from each other much more than do younger folks."[1] In practical terms, this means that generalizations as to what dietary regime is satisfactory is less apt to be applicable for a group of elderly persons than for other groups.

This chapter covers two broad topics, components of a balanced diet and causes and effects of imbalance.

COMPONENTS OF A BALANCED DIET

A balanced diet contains (1) sufficient calories to meet the energy requirements of an individual but not enough to lead to obesity, (2) essential amino acids, (3) essential fatty acids, (4) vitamins, (5) essential elements, (6) dietary fiber — indigestible material, and (7) water.

Calories. Calories are provided by proteins (12%), fats (30%), and carbohydrates (58%). These percentages are considered an optimum daily diet. This diet suggests more carbohydrates and less fats than are ordinarily found in the typical American diet. This proportion decreases tendencies towards atherosclerosis and makes the diet less fattening since carbohydrates furnish 5 kcal per gm versus 9 kcal per gm for fat.

In addition to providing calories, proteins also furnish the ten dietary essential amino acids: arginine, histidine, isoleucine, leucine, lysine, methionine, phenylalanine, tryptophan, tyrosine, and valine.

Proteins. In this country, most people habitually fulfill their protein requirements by eating meat. Meat is a complete protein in that it contains all ten essential amino acids. Six to eight ounces per day of lean meat (beef, pork, lamb, fowl, or fish) will satisfy the recommended daily allowance (RDA). The RDA can also be supplied through a variety of vegetable, grain, and milk combinations.[2] However, no one of these sources contains all ten essential amino acids, and combinations are necessary. When using combined sources, it is important that all ten essential amino acids be consumed in less than 3 hours. For example, cereal with milk for breakfast provides adequate protein, but toast with coffee at 8 AM and bean soup or bean salad at 1 PM does not.

Fats. Fats should contain an essential fatty acid, such as a linoleic or arachidonic acid. These occur in many plant oils and are included in the chemical class called poly-unsaturated fatty acids (PUFA).

Carbohydrates. There is no essential dietary carbohydrate comparable to dietary essentials of amino acids or fatty acids. However, a diet lacking in starchy foods would necessarily be high in fat and low in fiber, water-soluble vitamins, and mineral elements. These imbalances would have serious consequences on health. In addition, carbohydrates add variety, flavor, and interest to our diets.

Vitamins. There are 13 known vitamins. These are organic substances that the body cannot manufacture and therefore are required in the diet in small amounts. Vitamins are divided into two classes: (1) water-soluble; this group includes ascorbic acid, vitamin C; thiamin; riboflavin, pyridoxine, or pyridoxal; vitamin B_{12}; niacin, pantothenic acid; folic acid; and biotin, and (2) fat-soluble; vitamin A, retinol; vitamin D, cholecalciferol; vitamin E, alphatocopherol; and vitamin K, a napthoquinone derivative.

Elements. The essential elements are also divided into two groups. The seven macroelements — calcium, magnesium, potassium, sodium, iron, sulfur, and phosphorus — are present in the body in relatively large amounts. The 14 known essential microelements — chromium, cobalt, copper, manganese, molybdenum, nickel, selenium, tin, vanadium, zinc, chloride, fluoride, iodine, and silicon — are found in the body in small amounts. It should be emphasized that in most cases the ionic form — cation or anion — of the element is meant, not the pure element. For example, phosphate anion and not elemental phosphorus is the biologically active form.

Fiber. Dietary fiber has long been recognized as important in contributing to regular bowel movements. Recent studies have suggested that fiber may also be important in prevention of a number of diseases of the intestine, such as diverticulitis, hiatus hernia, and polyps.[3]

Liquid. Water or aqueous liquid is often omitted from such lists. This is unfortunate since a regular intake of about 8 glasses (2 quarts or 2 liters) per day is necessary for good health.

For the past 30 years the food and nutrition board of the National Academy of Sciences–National Research Council has published a table that contains the RDAs of a variety of nutrients for men and women of different ages.[4] The allowance levels are intended to cover individual variations in 95% of the U.S. population. An abbreviated form of the 1974 allowances is presented in Table 1. These RDAs apply to persons over age 51 years.

Nutrient density — nutritional quality. The concept of nutrient density is important in regard to weight control. The term nutrient density refers to the content of different nutrients in a foodstuff or combination of foods in relation to the caloric content of the same foodstuff or combination. Foods that are relatively low in nutrients compared to their caloric content are said to possess "empty calories"; that is, these foods have a low nutrient density. Refined sugar is a prime example of this group. Table sugar contributes 13 kcal per teaspoon (4 gm) but contains no nutrients whatsoever! Enriched white flour is similar, except that three vitamins and iron have been added during its processing. It

Table 1. Recommended daily allowances (RDAs) for Americans over 51 years old*

Nutrient	Man†	Woman‡
Energy	2,400 kcal	1,800 kcal
	10,080 k joules	7,560 k joules
Protein	56 gm	46 gm
Vitamin A	5,000 IU	4,000 IU
Vitamin D	—	—
Vitamin E	15 IU	12 IU
Ascorbic acid (vitamin C)	45 mg	45 mg
Folacin	400 μg	400 μg
Niacin	16 mg	12 mg
Riboflavin (vitamin B_2)	1.5 mg	1.1 mg
Thiamin (vitamin B_1)	1.2 mg	1.0 mg
Pyridoxine (vitamin B_6)	2.0 mg	2.0 mg
Vitamin B_{12}	3.0 μg	3.0 μg
Calcium	800 mg	900 mg
Phosphate	800 mg	800 mg
Iodine	110 μg	80 μg
Iron	10 mg	10 mg
Magnesium	350 mg	300 mg
Zinc	15 mg	15 mg

*Modified from Recommended dietary allowances, ed. 8, Washington, D.C., 1974, National Academy of Sciences. Reproduced with permission of the National Academy of Sciences.
†Needs based on a man 70 kg (154 pounds) weight and 172 cm (69 inches) height.
‡Needs based on a woman of 58 kg (128 pounds) weight and 162 cm (62 inches) height.

is difficult to obtain the RDA of the essential nutrients without ingesting excess calories if the diet contains a high proportion of low-density nutrient foods. This is the justification for advising people who are concerned about being or becoming overweight to eat foods that possess high essential nutrient–calorie ratios.

Recently an interesting and valuable application of nutrient density was suggested by the Utah State University's nutrition group.[5] They suggested a new term, the Index of Nutritional Quality (INQ). This is defined as the percentage of a particular nutrient requirement supplied by a certain quantity of food divided by the percent of the energy requirement supplied by the same quantity of food. An INQ of 1.0 for a particular essential nutrient, for example, vitamin A, indicates that a food that contributes 10% of the daily energy requirement would also contribute 10% of the RDA for that nutrient. INQ values higher than 1.0 indicate that a certain food would supply more than the required amount of a nutrient relative to that food's energy contribution. Conversely, any INQ less than 1.0 indicates that the food in question supplies a greater proportion of energy than it does of a certain nutrient. Thus the protein in 1 cup of skim milk calculates to an INQ of 3.5, but the vitamin A in the skim milk has an INQ of less than 0.1. This tells us at a glance that skim milk is an excellent source of protein and a poor source of vitamin A.

This concept can be used to represent the nutritional quality for any number of nutrients of any food or food combination for which there are data. These values are being coded for computers, and thus information will be directly available to nutritionists and dieticians who have access to a computer terminal that is connected to a nutrient data bank. This combination of nutritional information and sophisticated technology will make meal planning and evaluation much easier than in the past.

The essential nutrients are all required for the maintenance of good health. The RDAs of many nutrients are known (Table 1). However, values for most of the 14 essential microelements are unknown. One can define a satisfactory diet for an individual as one that contains adequate amounts of the essential nutrients and of calories in well-prepared, appetizing foods. It is generally agreed amongst nutritionists that this objective is most readily obtained by eating a wide variety of foods including fresh fruit, vegetables, and other unprocessed foods.

COMMON IMBALANCES IN DIETS OF ELDERLY PEOPLE

Few people in America eat a balanced diet every day. Many essential nutrients are not stored, although some are stored for brief periods. There is a calcium reserve in bone and a vitamin A reserve in liver. Thus most people can endure fairly long periods of low intake without exhibiting deficiency symptoms. The elderly, however, possibly because of the time factor, may be closer to the "edge" than younger people and the effects of dietary imbalances may be evident sooner in them. Symptoms may vary from abnormal EKGs to abnormal or strange behaviors.

Calories

Overingestion. It is often said that the most common example of malnutrition in the U.S. is overnutrition. It is estimated that 37% of persons over 60 years old are obese.[6] If the inconvenience of lugging 25 to 150 pounds of extra weight were the only consequence of obesity, the subject would merit little medical interest; but obesity shows a high correlation with a number of serious diseases, including later-onset diabetes, hypertension, and cardiovascular disorders.[7] These three diseases are cripplers, and any one of them can turn a pleasant and benign old age into a ghastly horror.

Overeating can result from habit or from psychological reasons. In either case, it requires extensive therapy and training for the elderly to learn to control their appetites. In mild diabetes, alteration of the diet by increasing carbohydrate and fiber content has been shown to reduce or remove the daily insulin requirement.[8] Hypertension is commonly controlled with drugs, although meditation or other forms of relaxation techniques are occasionally effective. If diuretics are being used, foods high in potassium and low in sodium, such as halibut, potatoes, asparagus, bananas, and citrus fruits, should be recommended and eaten.[9] If this is not sufficient to maintain serum K^+ in the normal range, 3.5 to 4.5 mEq per liter, a K^+ supplement should be given.

A high blood cholesterol (greater than 250 mg per 100 ml) is generally considered a risk factor for cardiovascular diseases. In persons over 65 years old, however, a high value is not taken as seriously as it is among younger people.

Underingestion. Occasionally older people lose interest in food and eat much less than their requirements. This condition can result from loneliness, depression, bereavement, loss of a job, or, not uncommonly, ill-fitting or absent dentures. If underingestion is not corrected promptly, loss of weight, lack of energy, or multiple nutrient deficiencies may develop.

Alcohol

Alcoholism plagues a large number of Americans and the elderly are not immune. Alcohol in excess of 1.5 ounces of 190 proof per day can damage a number of organs, including the liver, pancreas, and brain. In addition, since ethanol furnishes calories but is deficient in nutrients, its chronic overingestion often leads to multiple vitamin deficiencies and/or obesity.

Amino acids

Meat is the most common source of essential amino acids among Americans. There is little difference in nutritive values of the proteins of different cuts or species of meats. The recommended amount for a man, 56 gm, is equivalent to about 2 ounces of dry protein. Since meat contains about 60% water and 40% fat, a person would need to eat about 7 ounces (200 gm) of meat to obtain his entire protein RDA. An average woman can satisfy her protein RDA with approximately 80% of these amounts. Most middle-class Americans eat far more protein than is necessary.

Vegetarians who eat dairy products and/or eggs have few problems in obtaining the essential amino acids. Those, however, who eat only plant proteins need to plan their menus more carefully. The ten dietary essential amino acids can be obtained by combining foods. A number of satisfactory combinations are rice plus legumes, corn plus legumes, and soybeans plus sesame seeds plus peanuts or wheat. Many recipes that include these and other tasty vegetable combinations are presented in *Diet for a Small Planet*[2] and *Recipes for a Small Planet*.[10]

Fatty acids

Most Americans not only eat too much fat, but this fat is largely animal fat that contains mostly saturated fatty acids and few polyunsaturated fatty acids. This long-standing situation is of course perpetuated by the American's overconsumption of meat as a source of protein. A high proportion of saturated fatty acids in the diet has been strongly implicated as a contributing factor to high serum cholesterol levels and consequently to the high incidence of cardiovascular diseases in this country.[11]

Polyunsaturated fatty acids (PUFA) serve as essential components in cell membrane structures and as precursors of prostaglandins, which act as hormone modulators. The relative proportions of PUFA are high in many plant oils such as corn, safflower, soybean, and cottonseed. It is now possible to purchase margarine that contains large amounts of corn or safflower oil that has not been completely hydrogenated and therefore contains a much higher proportion of PUFA than ordinary margarines or butter.

An average ratio of polyunsaturated to saturated fatty acids (P/S ratio) in meats and dairy products is approximately 1/30, in corn oil 1/0.2, and in corn oil margarine 1/0.45. It is considered desirable to eat foods with an overall P/S ratio of about 1. In addition to increasing the amount of PUFA in the diet, one can decrease the saturated fatty acids by removing excess fat from meats and by substituting low-fat dairy products, such as low-fat milks, cottage cheese, and frozen desserts. The P/S ratio can also be increased by eating more poultry, fish, and vegetable proteins as substitutes for beef, pork, and lamb. It is recommended that vitamin E intake be increased concomitantly with that of PUFA. This is readily accomplished since most plant oils that are high in PUFA are also high in vitamin E. The extra vitamin E helps in protecting the PUFA from peroxidation, which destroys their activity. Although agreement has not been reached on the vitamin E requirement under these conditions, Witting and Lee[12] recommend 0.6 IU vitamin E per gm linoleate in 100 gm adipose tissue fatty acids.

Vitamins

There are many contributing causes for vitamin deficiencies. They may be listed as (1) an inadequate diet, (2) incomplete digestion or absorption, (3) loss of vitamins by processing or storage of foods, and (4) destruction by cooking and short-term warming before serving. Additional problems are vitamin deficiencies in the elderly and the advisability of vitamin supplements. Each of these will be briefly discussed.

Inadequate diet. Elderly people who live alone or who are subject to chronic depression may lose interest in food preparation and may consume inadequate diets because they have no motivation to purchase and prepare nutritious meals. Others may be unable to cook satisfactorily because of physical disabilities. Ill-fitting dentures, or none at all, may severely limit food selection. This group obviously needs support in meal preparation on a temporary or permanent basis and is the object of Meals on Wheels and similar programs. Alcoholism is probably the most common reason for severe, multiple vitamin deficiencies in Americans.

Incomplete digestion and absorption. This medical complication can lead to serious deficiencies if not diagnosed and corrected. Food allergies that may have resulted in a chronic inconvenience at a younger age, for example, gluten intolerance, may assume more serious proportions in later years and may necessitate major shifts in food selection. Digestion of fats seems to lose efficiency with age more than does digestion of carbohydrates and proteins. This can affect absorption of fat-soluble vitamins.

Food preservation. The term "food preservation" includes canning, freezing, drying, milling, pickling, smoking, and so forth. Most of the food consumed by Americans has been processed to some extent. The most common procedure used in the preservation of foods is the application of heat. Heat inactivates enzymes and, in canned goods, sterilizes them as well. Frozen vegetables are blanched, that is, heated before freezing. Dehydration is often accomplished by blowing warm dry air over the foodstuff. In general, it has been found that the shorter the heating time to accomplish the objective desired, the lower the loss of vitamins. Ascorbic acid, thiamin, and pantothenic acid are the most heat-labile vitamins.[13] Significant losses of water-soluble vitamins occur during the washing and blanching steps prior to canning.[14]

Despite the known losses of vitamins, commercially canned or frozen foods that were picked at their peak of maturity, cooled immediately, and processed probably contain more vitamin C than "fresh" products do that have a long period between harvesting and consumption and that may not have been stored under optimal conditions. Leaching of elements into the packing medium from canned products occurs in storage at a slow but significant rate. To reduce this loss as much as possible, the packing medium should not be discarded, but used as part of the food.[15]

Food storage. In recent years, the word "fresh" as applied to vegetables, fruits, and so forth, has come to signify that the product is unprocessed rather than that it has been recently harvested. Most of the fresh fruits and vegetables that are consumed in this country are grown in districts far removed from population centers and must be transported long distances. Consequently, there may be a delay of weeks or even months between harvesting and eating of many fruits and vegetables. Conditions of temperature, moisture, and atmospheric composition during storage have been demonstrated to play key roles in the vitamin content of a wide variety of plant foods.[16]

Research by the U.S. Department of Agriculture and the U.S. food industry has found optimum conditions for storage, transportation, and handling of a wide variety of foodstuffs. Fortunately those characteristics that make a fruit or vegetable attractive to the consumer are maintained longer under the same set of conditions that preserves nutrient content. Conditions of home storage are, of course, just as important as those in the store. Fresh vegetables should be stored in the refrigerator at a high humidity and with minimum air movement. For example, lettuce lost half of its vitamin C in 24 hours at room temperature, but less than half in 72 hours in the refrigerator.[16]

Cooking and short-term warming. Since water-soluble vitamins readily leach out of vegetables and may be destroyed in the "pot liquor," it is imperative to cook for as short a time as possible in a minimum volume of water. Excess liquid should be saved and utilized in sauces or soups.

Large-scale preparation and serving of meals may necessitate keeping foods warm or hot for hours after cooking. This practice may result in large losses of vitamins, especially ascorbic acid. For example, baked potatoes with jackets lose 20% of their ascorbic acid. After holding for 60 minutes, the loss is increased to 40%. Mashing or pan frying potatoes results in an immediate loss of 80% of their vitamin C, which increases to 100% in 30 minutes. French fried potatoes have lost 60% of their ascorbic acid and this increases to 80% after 1 hour. Similar data for other vegetables and other vitamins are available.[17] These losses may be counter-balanced by the inclusion of fresh fruits and vegetables in salads and by serving orange juice frequently. Many canned vegetables are quite appetizing when served cold in a salad.

Occurrence of vitamin deficiencies in the elderly. Since World War II, white flour has been enriched in vitamins B_1, B_2, niacin, and iron. As a result of this public health measure, pellagra has become a rare disease in the South, where it was once endemic. Extreme thiamin deficiency is now almost entirely restricted to some alcoholics. Despite these advances, however, subclinical deficiencies are often discovered in surveys, particularly among the elderly. The Health and Nutrition Examination Survey (HANES) of 1971-1972[22] found that in people over 65 years old, 50% of diets included less than two-thirds the RDA of vitamin A and 31% had similar deficiencies of vitamin C. In 1973, investigators from the Gerontology Research Center of the National Institute of Child Health and Human Development showed that with advancing age in middle income men there was a reduction in blood levels of thiamin, riboflavin, and pyridoxine. Solomon[27] states that deficiencies of calcium, iron, and vitamins A, B_1, B_2, and C are common in the aged. Thus it would be invalid for public health or gerontological nurses to assume that their patients or clients had received adequate amounts of all the essential nutrients. If vitamin shortages are suspected in the absence of overt symptoms, vitamin analyses may be run on blood samples and appropriate dietary changes may be suggested.

Should one recommend vitamin supplements to the elderly? Multi-vitamin preparations seem an easy solution to a complicated problem, and they are used widely. In my opinion, they are not a satisfactory substitute for a varied diet high in unprocessed foods unless special conditions or limitations prevail. The reasons are as follows: (1) The practice may lead to a false sense of security. No single supplement contains all the essential nutrients, but the elderly person, dietician, nurse, or physician may forget this and consider the diet solely as a source of calories. In time, the missing nutrients will become deficient. (2) The person may forget to take the pill. (3) Many drugs adversely affect vitamin and nutrient absorption (see Table 4, p. 86). (4) Many elderly persons or nursing homes simply cannot afford routine supplements.

Elements

Macroelements. Calcium is the macroelement most likely to be deficient in numerous diets because many people do not drink milk. It is difficult to obtain the RDA for calcium (800 mg) solely from vegetables, grains, and meat products. Dried milk can be incorporated into many recipes. This serves as a good source of both calcium and protein. When a supplement is necessary, I recommend bone meal tablets. Many nutritionists, however, consider this RDA too high. Apparently some humans can adapt to much lower calcium intakes than 800 mg per day with no effects on bone cortical thickness.[18]

The nutrients most likely to be taken in excess are sodium and chloride, in the form of sodium chloride (common table salt). It has been estimated that the average American uses 10 to 15 gm per day of this substance, which is far more than necessary. Excess salt intake is a major contributing factor to hypertension, one of the most common conditions of old age. Since low-salt or salt-free diets are not considered palatable by many people, a variety of diuretics and other drugs are available as controllers of essential hypertension. Many diuretics have the disadvantage of depleting body stores of potassium and magnesium ions. This question has been discussed previously. Other types of antihypertensive drugs may produce different, nonnutritional side effects.[19]

Ingestion of sulfate and phosphate depends on protein intake and deficiencies are seldom encountered in this country. On the other hand, phosphate is present in many soft drinks in fairly high concentrations. Thus it is frequently over-consumed in relation to calcium. A balanced diet contains approximately equal amounts of both elements.

Although magnesium deficiency is probably not widespread in the elderly population, there are certain specific situations in which magnesium deficiency should be suspected. These are:

1. Chronic loss from the gastrointestinal tract caused by vomiting or diarrhea.
2. Surgical trauma followed by prolonged intravenous feeding with magnesium-free solutions.
3. Alcoholism: This is probably the most general cause of magnesium deficiency in adults and is caused both by improper diet as well as by increased excretion rate. Cessation of drinking also often triggers an abrupt and significant drop in serum magnesium concentration. This coincides with the neuromuscular hyperexcitability that characterizes the withdrawal state.
4. Malabsorption due to a variety of causes; chronic steatorrhea may result in hypocalcemia as well as hypomagnesemia.
5. Diuretics: Magnesium deficiency can occur as readily as that of K^+ in diuretic usage; therefore analyses for both elements should be run routinely.[20]

Although severe hypomagnesemia may be totally asymptomatic, many patients exhibit one or more of a wide variety of symptoms. Some of these are (1) muscular twitching and tremors, (2) convulsions, (3) sweating and tachycardia, (4) apathy, depression, and memory loss,[21] and (5) confusion, disorientation, hallucinations, and paranoia. For a person who has one of the five causes listed above and one or more of the symptoms, it is advisable to think of magnesium deficiency as a possibility.[20]

For any case of hypocalcemia that does not respond to calcium therapy, magnesium deficiency should be considered. Magnesium repletion is usually accomplished by intramuscular or intravenous routes for at least 4 days.[20] Good food sources of magnesium are nuts, seeds, wheat germ, oatmeal, corn, and peanut butter.[21]

Microelements. White flour has been enriched in this country since the early 1940s. The essential nutrients, thiamin, riboflavin, niacin, and iron, have been restored to their original levels in whole wheat flour. However, these are the only four nutrients that are replaced. The percentage of losses of microelements in milling are chromium, 40%, manganese, 85%; cobalt, 88%; copper, 68%; zinc, 78%; selenium, 16%; and molybdenum, 38%.[13] None of these are restored in enriched white flour. Vitamin losses in milling are vitamin B_6, 70%; pantothenic acid, 50%; folacin, 66%; and tocopherol, 86%.[13]

The recent HANES survey has revealed that many people are anemic, as determined by hematocrit or blood hemoglobin levels. However, this anemia is probably not caused by insufficient dietary iron. The cause of the anemia is not known at present.[22]

For cases of iron deficiency, iron absorption from foods can be increased two- to three-fold by dietary or supplemental ascorbic acid.[23] This alternative may be preferred to that of iron pills.

In recent years chromium has been suggested as a micronutrient that may be quite widely deficient because much of it is removed in the manufacture of white flour. The main condition linked to chromium deficiency to date is a diabetic-type glucose tolerance curve. This condition is so common among the nation's elderly that it has been considered a normal counterpart of aging. The recent elucidation of the role of a chromium–nicotinic acid–amino acid complex (GTF, glucose tolerance factor) acting in conjunction with insulin to increase glucose transport into cells in some people suggests a nutritional deficiency as a possible factor in the development of a diabetic-type glucose tolerance curve in the elderly. Results with chromium supplementation, however, have been equivocal. Unfortunately, GTF, which is much more efficiently absorbed than Cr^{3+}, is not yet available for clinical trials. Good sources of GTF are beef, pork, liver, whole wheat bread, beer, and mushrooms.[24] In conclusion, preliminary surveys have revealed a chromium deficiency among the American elderly in relation to comparable groups in the Middle and Far East and in Africa. The data raise the possibility that a prolonged marginal chromium deficiency may contribute to the widespread occurrence of chronic diseases frequently associated with impaired glucose utilization in the American elderly population.

The other microelements are seldom deficient except in special situations. Since a number are iatrogenic, it may be relevant to mention them here. Dunlap et al.[25] have reported on two patients who developed copper deficiency as a result of long-term hyperparenteral alimentation after bowel surgery. The neutropenia, anemia, and other symptoms disappeared after oral copper was taken. Sandstead[26] has mentioned the occurrence of zinc deficiency in some institutionalized people and among some low-income populations. Animal products in general are good sources of zinc as are whole grains. Asymptomatic zinc-deficient people are less able to handle trauma or disease than are normal people.

The safety factor, that is, the spread between adequate and toxic amounts of a substance, is quite small for selenium and fluoride. Therefore I do not recommend the purchase of "trace element" supplement combinations. It is far more desirable to obtain the microelements from whole grains, meat products, and vegetables.

Fluids

Although water does not furnish calories or vitamins, it is as essential as any nutrient. It comprises about 70% of the weight of a person and, since it is excreted daily in urine and sweat, these losses must be replenished by daily intake. Six to eight glasses (1½ to 2 quarts or 1.5 to 2 liters) should be consumed daily. This can, of course, be in the form of milk, soups, drinks, and so forth as well as plain water.

In some institutions or situations the evening meal may be served as early as 5 pm. A long period may intervene before breakfast is served, especially if the person eats a late breakfast or brunch. This may produce an unhealthy overnight dehydration. Every person who is unable to obtain his own liquid should routinely be offered a pre-bedtime drink.

Dietary fiber (roughage)

Dietary fiber, roughage, or indigestible material is now considered an essential component of the diet, primarily due to the publicizing endeavors of Burkitt and Trowell.[3] The "fiber hypothesis" is based on their observations of native African diets and the health of those natives compared to the health of those who eat a "Western" diet. From a chemical standpoint, fiber can vary widely. Some types are primarily composed of cellulose, others of hemicellulose (which, despite the name, is quite different from cellulose) and still others of materials called pectins and lignins. What these substances have in common is their indigestibility. In the digestive tract, however, they act quite differently. Thus, since analyses are not yet performed on the amounts of these four types of fibers in foodstuffs, it is advisable to eat a diet that contains them all. This calls for a widely varied diet that contains unprocessed grains, vegetables, and fruits. There is no fiber in animal products.

Besides its role in preventing constipation, hemorrhoids, and probably other digestive disorders and diseases, dietary fiber, because it is filling, also helps in reducing caloric intake. Thus it is of value in controlling obesity. Burkitt estimates that an adequate diet should contain a minimum of 10 to 15 gm of dietary fiber daily. To ingest this quantity, it is necessary to eliminate non-fiber-containing carbohydrates such as white flour and white sugar. Fortunately, many food products are now labeled with respect to their fiber content. If it is not feasible for an elderly person to obtain sufficient fiber in his daily food, a supplement of bran may be added to cereals, yogurt, soups, milk, or vegetables. Above all, a fiber supplement should be palatable.

In conclusion, although the hypothesis of the contributions of dietary fiber in helping to prevent a number of the "diseases of civilization" is far from being proved, it is evolutionarily sound and reasonable. According to current knowledge, including more fiber in our diets is not likely to hurt anyone and probably will improve the functioning of our digestive apparatus.

EFFECTS OF NUTRITION ON BEHAVIOR

There is no question that a significant number of elderly persons in the United States routinely eat nutritionally deficient diets. This may be caused by ignorance, low income, habit, or a variety of other factors. It is widely recognized that nutrient deprivation can lead to a variety of clinical or subclinical behavioral symptoms. Some of these have been identified as anxiety, apathy, distractability, fatigue, loss of appetite, loss of recent memory, irritability, insomnia, and even mild delusions.[28] This is not to say that these symptoms are necessarily caused by nutritional inadequacy. I wish to emphasize, however, that when an older person presents a number of these symptoms, his diet and dietary habits should be carefully examined and, if necessary, improved before the final judgment of "semi-senile," depressed, or moody is pronounced. It is encouraging to state that a number of reports show that many of these symptoms are reversible or ameliorated by dietary improvements.

Alcoholics with psychiatric symptoms and elderly patients with mental deterioration often have lower than normal blood levels of vitamin C. Kinsman and Hood[29] have re-

Table 2. Drugs known to cause vitamin deficiencies*

Deficiency	Drug or drug class	Deficiency	Drug or drug class
Folic acid	Anticonvulsants	Niacin	INH
	Methotrexate		
	Pyrimethamine	C	Aspirin
	Aspirin		Indomethacin
B_{12}	Metformin	D	Anticonvulsants
B_6	INH (isonicotinic hydrazide)		Diphosphonates
	Thiosemicarbazide	K	Coumarin anticoagulants
	Hydralazine		Cholestyramine
	Penicillamine		
	L-Dopa		

*Modified from Roe, D.: Drug induced nutritional deficiencies, Westport, Conn., 1976, Avi Publishing Co.[19]

ported on the "neurotic triad"—hypochondriasis, depression, and hysteria—that often accompanies moderate ascorbic acid deficiency. The same triad was found by Brozek[30] to occur in experimental thiamin deficiency (0.6 mg per day) in young men. The symptoms were readily reversed when adequate thiamin was restored to the diet.

Altman et al.[31] carried out an interesting double-blind study with psychogeriatric inpatients. They were treated for 6 weeks with a multivitamin supplement that contained B vitamins plus ascorbic acid. Each capsule contained thiamin, 15 mg; riboflavin, 10 mg; pyridoxine, 5 mg; niacinamide, 50 mg; calcium pantothenate, 10 mg; and ascorbic acid, 300 mg. One clinically and statistically significant finding emerged: there was a striking decrease in pathological manifestations, as measured on the Missouri Inpatient Behavior Excitement Scale, for a nonschizophrenic subgroup receiving the vitamin supplement when compared to a control group.

DRUG-INDUCED NUTRITIONAL DEFICIENCIES

It is widely recognized that, as a group, the elderly are the largest consumers of drugs in this country. Many of these drugs are used to help control chronic conditions such as hypertension, angina, and arthritis. It is not as widely recognized that many drugs exert marked effects on absorption, digestion, excretion, or function of both vitamins and mineral elements. Drug-induced nutrient deficiencies can occur even in the presence of an adequate diet.[32] Once the relationship between the drug and the particular deficiency is worked out, a satisfactory solution can generally be found by changing the drug or the diet. If changing the drug is not feasible, increasing intake of the vitamin in the diet often alleviates the problem.

Table 2 lists some vitamin deficiencies and the drugs that induce them. Long-term therapy with anticonvulsant drugs often results in megaloblastic anemia due to folate deficiency. If the anemia is treated with supplementary folate, the number of seizures increases. Extra vitamin B_{12}, in addition to folate, improved mental condition without increasing the number of seizures.[32] The cytotoxic drug methotrexate is used both in the chemotherapy of cancer as well as for psoriasis. Methotrexate acts as a folic acid antagonist that decreases thymidylate synthesis and thus inhibits cell division. The anemia that frequently results responds to supplementary folate. Even aspirin may lead to folate deficiency. In one study, a majority of patients with rheumatoid arthritis who were taking

Table 3. Drugs affecting vitamin D, calcium, and phosphate transport*

Drug	Usage	Malabsorption	Mechanism
Prednisone (other glucocorticoids)	Allergic and collagen diseases	Calcium	Calcium transport[1]
Phenobarbital	Anticonvulsant	Calcium	Accelerated catabolism of vitamin D and active metabolites
Phenytoin	Anticonvulsant	Calcium	
Primidone	Anticonvulsant	Calcium	
Glutethimide	Sedative	Calcium	
Diphosphonates	Paget's disease	Calcium	1,25-DHCC formation[1]
Aluminum hydroxide	Antacid	Phosphate	Precipitation

*Modified from Roe, D.: Drug induced nutritional deficiencies, Westport, Conn., 1976, Avi Publishing Co.[19]

aspirin were found to have subnormal serum folate levels. Table 3 lists drugs that affect vitamin D, calcium, and phosphate transport. A wide variety of commonly used drugs reduces calcium absorption either directly or by accelerating the catabolism of active vitamin D metabolites. Included in Table 4 are many other drugs that decrease absorption of other vitamins or elements. In summary, drug usage leads to drug side effects that can complicate or render inadequate otherwise satisfactory diets. It is to be hoped that in the near future the drug regimen of each person can be placed in a computer so that nutritional and other side effects can be predicted and avoided.

OBESITY

Too many Americans are overfed and underexercised. Dealing with the obese on an individual basis is often more of a psychological problem than a nutritional one. The first step is to find out why the person overeats. Does he have a poor self-image, does he feel sorry for himself, does he feel unloved or lonely, or has he had a recent loss of a loved one? If the motivation can be brought out and discussed, then other means of satisfying the psychological problem, besides overindulgence in food, may be found.

On the other hand, obesity may result gradually, from a small but increasing reduction in physical activity over the years with no decrease in food consumption. Most people do not realize that eating an extra piece of toast with margarine and jam daily, about 100 kcal, can add 10 pounds to their weight in a year. This slight amount of overingestion can easily be counteracted by exercise. But if exercise has decreased, the person may hardly be aware of any significant changes in his weight until he is 20 to 40 pounds overweight. Such a person may respond positively to dietary counseling. A reduction of 500 kcal per day will result in a weight loss of about 1 pound per week. This reduction can best be achieved by cutting out the ''empty calorie'' foods — pastries, candies, sweet desserts, carbonated drinks, etc. It is important that the diet not be changed too drastically or the person will not follow it. He should realize and cooperate with the objective of a gradual weight loss and stabilization at a desirable level. Moderate exercise, in accordance with the person's physical condition, is helpful in two ways: it burns off some calories directly and it also reduces the appetite.

Obesity slows therapy and complicates management of a number of common illnesses of the elderly, such as osteoporosis, arthritis, hypertension, diabetes, and coronary disease. Old age and joie de vivre are not incompatible. Old age cannot be avoided, but obesity often prevents the enjoyment of it.

Table 4. Drug-induced nutritional deficiencies: primary intestinal absorptive defects induced by drugs*

Drug	Usage	Malabsorption or fecal nutrient loss	Mechanism
Mineral oil	Laxative	Carotene, vitamins A, D, K	Physical barrier Nutrients dissolve in mineral oil and are lost Micelle formation
Phenol-phthalein	Laxative	Vitamin D, Ca	Intestinal hurry K depletion Loss of structural integrity
Neomycin	Antibiotic to "sterilize" gut	Fat, nitrogen, Na, K, Ca, Fe, lactose, sucrose, vitamin B_{12}	Structural defect Pancreatic lipase Binding of bile acids (salts)
Cholestyramine	Hypocholesterolemic agent Bile acid sequestrant	Fat, vitamins A, K, B_{12}, D, Fe	Binding of bile acids (salts) and nutrients, for example, Fe
Potassium chloride	Potassium repletion	Vitamin B_{12}	Ileal pH
Colchicine	Anti-inflammatory agent in gout	Fat, carotene, Na, K, vitamin B_{12}, lactose	Mitotic arrest Structural defect Enzyme damage

Biguanides
  Metformin
  Phenformin
	Hypoglycemic agents (in diabetes)	Vitamin B_{12}	Competitive inhibition of B_{12} absorption

Para-amino-salicylic acid	Antituberculosis agent	Fat, folate, vitamin B_{12}	Mucosal block in B_{12} uptake
Sulfasalazine (Azulfidine)	Anti-inflammatory agent in ulcerative colitis and regional enteritis	Folate	Mucosal block in folate uptake

*Permission granted for reprint by Biomedical Information Corporation, publisher of *Drug Therapy* Medical Journal, **3(4)**:130, April, 1973.[32]

INDIVIDUAL REQUIREMENTS

To say that we are all individuals is a cliché. To realize what this means at the nutritional level is not so obvious. Individual requirements for an essential nutrient such as calcium, tryptophan, or vitamin B_1 may vary by as much as a factor of 4. Consequently, one should be alert to the possibility that the RDA may not meet the requirements for an essential nutrient for a few people. This may explain the feeling of well-being of someone who likes to eat a lot of a particular food. Conversely, a person with an abnormal requirement may be suffering a deficiency on a supposedly adequate diet.[33,34] Older persons should experiment with their diets as long as fundamental nutritional principles are not violated. Even though it may be difficult or impossible to distinguish a placebo effect from a real physiological need, the peace of mind and other psychological benefits that result may justify a dietary quirk.

If only one physician, nurse, or attendant recognizes that the irrational, irascible behavior of one older person may be due to nutritional factors and acts accordingly, it will have been worthwhile writing this chapter.

REFERENCES

1. Schroeder, H. A.: Nutrition, In Steinberg, F. U., editor: Cowdry's care of the geriatric patient, ed. 5, St. Louis, 1976, The C. V. Mosby Co., p. 191.
2. Lappé, F. M.: Diet for a small planet, New York, 1974, Friends of the Earth/Ballantine Books, Inc.
3. Burkitt, D. P., and Trowell, H. C.: Refined carbohydrate foods and disease, New York, 1975, Academic Press, Inc.
4. Recommended dietary allowances, ed. 8, Washington, D.C., 1974, National Academy of Sciences.
5. Wyse, B. W., Sorenson, A. W., Wittwer, A. J., and Hansen, R. G.: Nutritional quality index identifies consumers' nutrient needs, Food Tech., **30:**22-40, 1976.
6. Mayer, J.: Obesity. In Goodhart, R. S., and Shils, M., editors: Modern nutrition in health and disease, Philadelphia, 1973, Lea & Febiger, p. 629.
7. Watkin, D. M.: Old Age, Fam. Health **2:**34, 1970.
8. Kiehm, T. G., Anderson, J. W., and Ward, K.: Beneficial effects of a high carbohydrate, high fiber diet on hyperglycemic diabetic men, Am. J. Clin. Nutr. **29:**895-899, 1976.
9. Wyse, B. W., Sorenson, A., Wittwer, A. J., and Hansen, R. G.: Foods instead of drugs to offset diuretic potassium losses, Utah Sci. **37:**86-90, 1976.
10. Ewald, E. B.: Recipes for a small planet, New York, 1971, Friends of the Earth/Ballantine Books, Inc.
11. Levy, R. I., and Ernst, N.: Diets, hyperlipidemia and atherosclerosis. In Goodhart, R. S., and Shils, M., editors: Modern nutrition in health and disease, Philadelphia, 1973, Lea & Febiger, p. 895.
12. Witting, L. A., and Lee, L.: Recommended dietary allowances for vitamin E: relation to dietary, erythrocyte and adipose tissue linoleate, Am. J. Clin. Nutr. **28:**577-583, 1975.
13. Nesheim, R. O.: Nutrient changes in food processing, Fed. Proc. **33:**2267-2269, 1974.
14. Lund, D. B.: Effects of blanching, pasteurization and sterilization on nutrients. In Harris, R. S., and Karmas, E., editors: Nutritional evaluation of food processing, Westport, Conn., 1975, Avi Publishing Co., p. 205.
15. Kramer, A.: Storage retention of nutrients, Food Tech. **28:**50, 1974.
16. Krochta, M., and Feinberg, B.: Effects of harvesting and handling on fruits and vegetables. In Harris, R. S., and Karmas, E., editors: Nutrition-al evaluation of food processing, Westport, Conn., 1975, Avi Publishing Co., pp. 98-117.
17. Lachance, P. A.: Effects of food preparation procedures on nutrient retention with emphasis upon food service practices. In Harris, R. S., and Karmas, E., editors: Nutrient evaluation of food processing, Westport, Conn., 1975, Avi Publishing Co., p. 463.
18. Garn, S. M.: The earlier gain and later loss of cortical bone, Springfield, Ill., 1970, Charles C Thomas, Publisher.
19. Roe, D.: Drug induced nutritional deficiencies, Westport, Conn., 1976, Avi Publishing Co.
20. Flink, E. B.: Magnesium deficiency and magnesium toxicity in man. In Prasad, H. S., and Oberloes, D., editors: Trace elements in human health and disease, vol. 2, New York, 1976, Academic Press, Inc.
21. Solomon, N. S.: Easy no-risk diet, New York, 1976, Warner Books, p. 165.
22. First health and nutrition examination survey (HANES), U.S. 1971-1972.
23. Cook, J. D., and Monsen, E. R.: Vitamin C, the common cold and iron absorption, Am. J. Clin. Nutr. **30:**235-241, 1977.
24. Hambridge, K. M.: Chromium nutrition in man, Am. J. Clin. Nutr. **27:**505, 1974.
25. Dunlap, W. M., Jones, G. W., and Hume, D. M.: Anemia and neutropenia caused by copper deficiency, Ann. Intern. Med. **80:**470-474, 1974.
26. Sandstead, H. H.: Zinc nutrition in the U.S., Am. J. Clin. Nutr. **26:**1252-1260, 1973.
27. Solomon, N. S., p. 176.
28. Howell, S. C., and Loeb, M. B.: Diet and the nervous system: effects on emotions and behavior in the older adult, Gerontologist Suppl. **9:**53-56, 1969.
29. Kinsman, R. A., and Hood, H.: Some behavioral effects of ascorbic acid deficiency, Am. J. Clin. Nutr. **24:**455-464, 1971.
30. Brozek, J.: Psychological effects of thiamin restriction and deprivation in normal young men, Am. J. Clin. Nutr. **5:**109-201, 1957.
31. Altman, H., Mehta, D., Evenson, R. C., and Sletten, I. W.: Behavioral effects of drug therapy on psychogeriatric patients. II. Multivitamin supplement, J. Am. Geriat. Soc. **21:**249-252, 1973.
32. Roe, D.: Drug induced vitamin deficiencies, Drug Ther. pp. 23-33, April, 1973.
33. Scriver, C. R.: Realized and potential neutralization of mutant genes in man by nutritional selection, Fed. Proc. **35:**2286-2290, 1976.
34. Williams, R. J.: Biochemical individuality, New York, 1956, John Wiley & Sons, Inc. (ch. 10).

part III
SOCIOCULTURAL IMPLICATIONS OF ADVANCED MATURITY

"One's chances of being on the outside are greatly enhanced if one is born into a minority group. . ."[1]

The need to understand and be understood by other cultures can no longer be treated lightly. The richness that can evolve from such understanding cannot be measured in dollars and cents but could result in a stronger, more cohesive society with an increasing level of stability. It is now recognized that the aged of all cultures need assistance in coping with the many problems of aging.

Part III deals with three ethnic groups of color* and with the subculture of the aging, analyzed as a subcultural group in Caucasian society.

In Chapter 6 Therese Sullivan points out that, according to observational studies and research, "individual variations exist among the elderly. The findings have pointed to a number of different kinds and degrees of variation that exist between the behavior patterns of the elderly and those of the younger general society." This chapter provides the reader with some understanding of the subculture of the aged. Much is yet to be learned about the beliefs, values, and practices of the elderly. Although more extensive research is proposed, the variables pointed out in this paper should assist the nurse in planning, with the elderly and others, to aid the elderly in maintaining the highest level of wellness possible within the limits that have already been imposed by the aging process.

In Chapter 7, Growing Old in the Black Community, Lillian Stokes emphasizes that "the process of aging is dynamic, thus indicating a process of growth and evolving, or a becoming, which begins very early in life, e.g., with birth and ends with death." Stokes deals with a number of problems faced by elderly blacks and she has described various support systems in addition to reviewing beliefs, customs, and practices that surround illness and death. Also included are descriptions of some rituals that surround death and burial in the black community.

Chapter 8, by Felipe Castro and Nathaniel Wagner, focuses on the Chicano community and its aged. The authors have pointed out ways of developing understanding for the similarities and differences among elderly Chicanos. Customs, practices, and beliefs surrounding growing old, illness, and death are described here in considerable detail. Castro and Wagner note that these customs and beliefs serve as a basis for the attitudes of many aged Chicanos toward living and dying.

---

*See WCHEN Position Paper: The phrase ethnic people of color, Western Interstate Commission for Higher Education, P.O. Drawer P., Boulder, Colo. 80302.

Martha C. Primeaux, author of Chapter 9, Health Care and the Aging American Indian, focuses on the historical background of the American Indian health care system, and their customs and rituals surrounding death and burial. Primeaux shares both generalities and specifics relating to American Indian medicine so the readers may understand better the social forces that shape the behavior and attitudes of the elderly native American population.

REFERENCE

1. Teaching the culturally disadvantaged, Palo Alto, Calif., 1970, Science Research Associates, p. iii.

6 The subculture of the aging and its implications for health and nursing care to the elderly

THERESE SULLIVAN

During the past 70 or more years, the total U.S. population has tripled, while the age group of 65 years old and older has grown to almost seven times its former size. Currently, about 10% of our population is at least 65 years of age and about one third of this aggregate is 75 years old or older. It is predicted that this age group will comprise an increasingly larger proportion of the population and will expand to 29 million by the year 2000.[1]

This pronounced change in the age distribution of our population is creating new and complex problems. While modern knowledge and technology have aided man's search for a longer life and thus resulted in more people reaching old age, they have also created many difficulties in aging, both personal and social. However, it is not the number of aged persons that has produced this contemporary problem. Rather, it is the lack of adequate preparation by our society for this increase in the elderly population.[2,3] In part, the problems of the aging are also a consequence of the fact that the aged in our society are defined socially rather than biologically or functionally. This definition bars full participation in community life for many persons once they reach the age of 65 years.

THE ELDERLY AS A SUBCULTURE

In response to their exclusion from effective participation in the major social systems and from interaction with other groups of the larger society, the aged are forming a distinctive subculture, a group that encompasses members of all other minorities as well as of the majority. References are made in literature to the "subculture of the aged," "aging group consciousness," and the aged as a "minority group."[48]

The issue of the aged as a minority group was first raised in the early 1950s by Barron.[7] He presented the following reasons for viewing this age category as a minority group: they are stereotyped by the majority group; they suffer subordination, discrimination, and prejudice; and they exhibit hypersensitivity about their status, self-hatred, and defensiveness. Barron noted, however, that at that time the elderly did not seem to be organized into functioning subgroups. Recently, Brotman supported Barron's observation regarding the minority status of the elderly.[8] He contended that the newest and most rapidly growing minority is the elderly. Unlike the militant struggle of the other minorities, Brotman asserted, the struggle among the aging is different, because for most it is a battle for economic survival, for many it is a battle for some social status, and for all it is a struggle against being forced out of the larger society into a subculture of poverty and social uselessness.

In the 1960s Rose proposed that age acts as a unifying principle leading to the development of a subculture of the aged.[3-5] He suggested that a subculture develops as a result of two conditions. First, the members have an attraction for each other on some basis, such as common backgrounds and interests or common problems and concerns. Second, the members of the subgroup are to some extent excluded from interaction with the rest of society. He believed that both conditions are increasingly being met by a growing number of older people. Rose referred to the growth of this new phenomenon as "aging group consciousness" or "aging group identification." He contended that some older people have begun to talk over their common problems and have begun to think of themselves as members of an aging group. The following social conditions have been suggested by Rose as causes of the emergence of a subculture of the aged: the large number of people over 65 years old; improved health of older people; shared grievances; segregation in retirement communities and apartments; retirement at younger ages and the consequent dissociation from major social institutions; opportunities to interact and identify with each other in increasingly numerous clubs for senior citizens; and decreased contact with the younger generation.

Rose speculated that the subculture is characterized by a distinctive set of values and behaviors, such as less emphasis on occupational prestige; more emphasis on physical and mental health and social activity as status factors; increased interaction with each other and less with younger persons; increased emphasis on leisure activities; and increased identification with members of their own age group. He stated that these characteristics did not present a comprehensive picture of the subculture of the aging and he suggested that the whole subculture needed objective investigation.

Clark and Anderson's major sociocultural study of the elderly concluded that the aged are functioning independently within the network of the American society as a deviant group.[9] They identified the aged as members of our society who, by force of circumstances, deviate from cultural norms. These investigators contended that if the aged are to assume a role in our public life today within terms acceptable to them, it will be necessary for them to function as deviant private citizens, since we have no well-developed institutional roles for them. They found that those in their sample who survived best were those who had been able to drop their pursuit of the primary values of American culture and had gone on to pick up alternative values. These alternative values include conservatism instead of acquisition and exploitation; self-acceptance instead of self-advancement; being, rather than doing; and congeniality, cooperation, love, and concern for others instead of control of others. In addition, according to Clark and Anderson, although the elderly function as a deviant group, they appear to lack a strong sense of being a cohesive social group. Their findings revealed that only where goals were directly concerned with immediate difficulties would the aged band together for their own protection and that the aged preferred to communicate with others face-to-face, not through group action.

Palmore examined the issue of whether or not it is useful to view the aged as an emerging minority group; he deduced that the aged already possess many minority group characteristics and that they are becoming increasingly like other disadvantaged groups.[10] Busse and Pfeiffer also believe that the status of the aged as a deprived minority group is substantiated and that retired persons in particular rarely share the advantages enjoyed by the majority of our society.

A report based on research materials from the Gerontological Society concluded that several conditions in our society have prompted the emergence of a subculture of the elderly. These conditions are as follows: the elderly appear to be more aware of themselves as a group and are starting to think of their problems less in individual terms and more in collective terms; interest is evident by the elderly's protesting against discrimination under which they have had to live and in their taking positive action to reduce their problems; and new values concerning social status, personal worth, interpersonal relations, and other important aspects of life are emerging among this group of citizens.[11]

Others, however, question the existence of an aging subculture in the United States. Neugarten and Moore stated that it may be too soon to speak of a subculture of the aged.[12] Streib asserted that the aged are to be seen as a statistical aggregate or social category and not as a genuine social or cultural group.[13] Rosow denied the existence of an aged role and suggested that the aged are essentially a social category rather than a viable group because they experience their common fates separately and alone, not with each other.[14]

Yet, despite these frequent references to a subculture and despite the rapid growth in the number and proportion of older people in our population, which creates new and complex personal and social problems, a paucity of research exists regarding the phenomenon of a subculture of the aging. Since one of the major problems facing the elderly is the inevitable change that occurs in their health status, as health problems become more frequent and acute when physical and mental processes change, this phenomenon is a matter of social and professional concern.

HEALTH AND ILLNESS STATUS OF THE ELDERLY

The issue of a subculture of the aging has significance for the provision of health and nursing services to this segment of the population. I believe that nurses and other health professionals must consider the social and cultural context in which health is maintained or in which illness occurs. The health and illness behaviors of people are not isolated physical or psychological phenomena. They encompass a broad and complex framework closely related to economic, political, religious, and other social and cultural practices. Therefore the better that health professionals understand the elderly's values, beliefs, and practices, the better they will be able to determine, plan, and provide services to assist elderly persons in achieving and maintaining the highest level of wellness possible.

Acute illness conditions account for more disability days among the elderly than among younger age groups.[15] Moreover, it is estimated that 25% of the total aged population, about 5 million people, require some type of care for chronic illnesses. Two million are presently receiving care in institutions and the needs of the remaining three million have been assessed as follows: nursing homes, 600,000; home health care, 1.3 million; congregate living facilities or help in preparing meals, another 1.1 million.[16]

Hospitalization and visits to the doctor provide other measures of health status. The elderly utilize facilities and services more frequently than persons under 65 years old. Older people have a one in four chance of being hospitalized during a year, twice as great as for people under 65 years. Once in the hospital, elderly people stay twice as long as do younger people, 17.5 days versus 8.7 days. The elderly have 50% more physician visits than younger people, with a higher proportion of the visits being within the 6 months since the last visit.[1]

Presently, a little more than 5% of the elderly are in institutions. This figure, however, is deceptive since it is not a definitive measure of the number of older people who have chronic illnesses and may need treatment. The 5% figure represents only the number of elderly in institutions on any given day, and recent studies indicate an 80% or higher turnover rate.[18,19]

According to the Subcommittee on Long-Term Care of the Special Committee on Aging, United States Senate, long-term care for Americans stands as the most troubled, and troublesome component of our entire health care system today.[19] The subcommittee further contended, "It appears evident that if the 2.4 million elderly in the community do not have their needs for home health care, supportive services and meal services met, they will deteriorate to the point where institutionalization will be necessary, or they will die."[19]

Philblad and McNamara's study of the social adjustment of older persons disclosed that health status influences almost every aspect of the older person's life: his income and expenses, the degree to which he can remain independent, his type of residence, his degree of mobility, the extent of his participation in the life of the community, and his association with other people.[17] In addition, Loether stated that from the social and psychological standpoints, the physical evidence of illness or disease may be largely irrelevant because the person's beliefs about his health may be more significant than his actual health status.[18]

Health care

Systematic planning for the health care of the aged has progressed slowly in the United States because of the low esteem in which the elderly have been held, the negative attitudes of health professionals, and the lack of communication between the various groups who care for the elderly.[20-22] The medical profession, to a large degree, appears to be disinterested in the problems of the aged and in their care.[19,20,22]

Nursing has cared for the elderly in general and psychiatric hospitals and has provided quality care where staffs have been adequately prepared and in sufficient numbers. On the other hand, few professional nurses have practiced in nursing homes. A number of factors have interfered and are continuing to interfere with the development of adequate nursing services to the elderly.[23] These factors include ambiguities in the role of the nurse relative to that of other health care professionals; a nursing literature on geriatric nursing that lacks a scientific base of knowledge gathered through systematic research with insights from the social sciences; and professional education that has not kept pace with the increasing demands placed on nursing personnel by the elaboration of their roles in nursing homes, retirement apartments and communities, outpatient departments, and community health centers.

Lately, however, advances have begun to relieve the bleakness of this picture. During the past decade nursing has become increasingly sensitive to the elderly's needs for comprehensive, coordinated, and continuing short- and long-term care in the community and in institutions. The American Nurses Association has established a division on geriatric nursing practice; standards of practice have been developed and are beginning to be applied, tested, and evaluated by those who care for the aged.[25,26]

Nursing has also been accepting greater responsibility for preparing individuals to care for the elderly. New concepts of gerontological nursing practice are presented to nurses through continuing education programs, in curricula of schools of nursing, and in a few universities now offering a speciality in gerontological nursing.[27]

It is becoming increasingly evident that if nurses are to provide more comprehensive, coordinated, and continued care for the elderly, the professional preparation required needs to have a gerontological frame of reference so that the nurses can assist the elderly in maintaining or attaining the highest possible level of functioning.[22,24,26,28] This conclusion is in keeping with the intense movement in nursing to expand the range and function of nurses and to broaden the scope of practice to meet the needs of the public for quality health care. The attempts to meet these needs have resulted in the emergence of new categories of nurses with expanded education and responsibilities.[29-32]

If the challenge of providing health care that fully considers the elderly person's world is to be accepted, it appears imperative that nurses and other professional health workers obtain a more complete understanding of the subculture of the aging. This includes an understanding of the values, beliefs, and practices of the elderly, particularly regarding health and illness and the seeking of health care services.

THE PACIFIC NORTHWEST STUDY: COMPARISON OF OLDER AND YOUNGER ADULTS

The theory of older people as a subculture has fostered little research and little empirical knowledge exists regarding the values, beliefs, and practices of the elderly pertaining to health, illness, and the seeking of health care. Therefore I conducted an exploratory study to provide initial insights into the differences among expressed values, beliefs, and practices that might exist between the older adults (over 64 years old) and the younger general population.[33] I thought that these insights might have important implications for the provision of health care and might provide a basis for future explanatory studies.

Interviews were conducted with residents of a large metropolitan city in the Pacific Northwest. The subjects' responses to open-ended questions were studied and critically examined for major themes that recurred with some frequency. The investigator was interested in the kinds of emphasis the older adults and the younger adults gave to a particular category. This was to differentiate patterns characteristic of the older adult subjects from those more characteristic of the younger adult subjects. Because the idea of a subculture of the aging had not been put into operation, the investigator identified from the literature a number of variables as criteria for delineating the subculture.[3,10,34-42] The variables identified were daily life style, leisure, social interaction and group identity, work and employment, health and illness, politics, religion and world view, status system, socialization processes, and language patterns. The respondents' expressed values, beliefs, and practices were measured by their answers to items on an interview guide that had been selected as an indicator of the variables.

Since the sick and institutionalized aged have been the major subjects in reported research and form the basis of many of our conceptions of the elderly, this study attempted to help provide a more realistic picture of the elderly and their values, beliefs, and practices.

In selecting the target population, therefore the investigator wanted to focus on persons living in the community since, even though most aged persons have one or more chronic conditions, a relatively small percentage of the elderly are institutionalized.[1]

The first variable on which the members of the age group of 65 years and older and the members of the younger age group were compared on was daily life-style, the characteristic way an individual spends a typical day, or his generalized pattern of daily living. As the literature suggests, the daily life-style of the aged is that of a leisure participant.[39] Almost all of the older adults described a leisurely style of daily living with only

3% describing a combined leisurely and occupational style. The majority of the younger adults described an occupational daily life-style. The remainder described either a student daily life-style or a combination student and occupational daily life-style. Differences were also found regarding the preference of a routine or of regularity in their daily life. Most of the older adults preferred a lack of regular routine or a somewhat flexible routine whereas the majority of the younger adults favored a routine combined with some flexibility.

Leisure, defined as either the time not needed for practical pursuits or the pleasurable activities engaged in during such time, is becoming increasingly available in the lives of most Americans. It has been suggested that the elderly may have their own distinctive beliefs, values, and practices concerning leisure. The older as well as the younger adults did exhibit some leisurely behaviors that were distinct in style. The majority of the elderly indicated they had much leisure time, or at least all that they wanted, and that they spent it alone equally as often as with others; the younger adults had only a few hours of leisure time daily and spent most of it with others. Older adults seemed to enjoy and to engage actively in a wide variety of leisure pursuits. Playing cards appeared to be an important activity and there seemed to be little interest in sports, whereas younger adults appeared to enjoy actively and passively participating in sports and did not indicate an interest in card playing. More of the elderly than the younger adults also reported participating in church activities and working around the house during their leisure time.

Rose suggested that the elderly interact more often with members of their own age group than with members of other age groups and many have begun to think of themselves as members of an aging group.[5] The findings on the variable of social interaction and group identity provide evidence in support of Rose's proposal. The older adults reported associating more frequently with friends, usually at age-graded groups and organizations. They also interacted frequently with relatives, customarily on holidays, at lunches or dinners, and on visits. The aged had a high rate of membership in and also attendance at groups and organizations in general, and age-graded ones in particular. Their principal reasons for participating in groups and organizations and for attending their meetings and activities were to be with people and to work with people. The elderly believe that some of the conditions that make living hard, as well as easy, for them in this society are related to their age.

On the other hand, the younger adults appeared to be divided more in their frequency of interaction with members of their own age group and with members of other age groups. They came in contact as often with members of other age groups as they did with their own age group and a number of them believed that being with their own age group was too limiting. Younger people also interacted frequently with their friends, but it was usually at school and in their homes or at the homes of friends. They interacted less frequently with relatives and when they did so it was principally during visits. The younger adults less frequently belonged to and attended groups and organizations and did not report membership in any age-graded groups or organizations. Whereas about half of the younger adults said that what they enjoyed about participating in groups and organizations and about attending their meeting and activities was working with people, the other half indicated it was because they were interested in the causes and in the activities. The younger adults mentioned only one age-related condition that made life hard for them in this society and that was the difference in values among different age groups.

Employment status was found to be another attribute that differentiated the two groups. A major part of most members of a group's time and attention is usually spent on economic pursuits,[35] but in our society most people over 65 years old are now classified as retired and retirement is becoming recognized as an emerging status. Yet, it has been observed that many people in this age group actively work either full time or part time because they prefer the activity involved in gainful employment to other possible ways of spending their time.[34] Only 3% of the older adults said they were working. When they were employed, the principal reason given for liking their jobs was that they provided an opportunity to work with people and to help people. Working or holding down a job meant a livelihood and a sense of security to them. In contrast, most of the younger adults were participating in the labor force or were in the process of preparing for occupations or professions. The main reasons they gave for liking their job was that it was interesting or challenging and that it provided an opportunity to work with people and to help people; their jobs supplied a sense of satisfaction and accomplishment and also a livelihood and security.

One of the most important aspects of any group is their health and illness behaviors. Individuals and groups must be concerned with health and illness since both individual functioning and social processes are disrupted by the onset of illness. In later life declining health frequently cuts across all social, political, and economic lines in later life and health becomes a major influence on the older person's situation. Health becomes a primary influence on participation in the family, the job, the community, and leisure pursuits, and health needs absorb a larger amount and proportion of most individuals' incomes as they grow older.[17,43,44]

Members of the two groups were asked to evaluate their present health status. About half of the aged rated their health status as fair or poor; the others rated theirs as "good for my age," or as good or very good. Most of the older adults reported experiencing health problems, the majority of which were chronic conditions. With regard to preventive health care measures, some emphasized using good judgment and common sense to guide behavior. Although the greater part of the older adult group went to a doctor when ill, a few stated that they utilized such persons and places as a naturopath, a chiropractor, an osteopath, a hospital emergency room, and a health maintenance organization. Their reasons for using such persons and places were the good care and coverage provided, the convenience, the time taken to listen to them, and the use of natural ways rather than drugs. Suggestions concerning ways in which our health care system could be improved to meet more adequately their health care needs were by providing more free services for senior citizens and the handicapped and by expanding Medicare to include office visits, drugs, and better nursing home coverage.

The older adults also expressed specific opinions concerning doctors and nurses in the health care system. The response given by the largest number of the aged with regard to beliefs concerning doctors was that many doctors do not take time to listen to the patient and consequently the patient frequently ends up going through unnecessary suffering and expense. Some classified two kinds of doctors: "good" ones who take an interest in the person and his problems and "poor" ones who are only interested in money. Others stated that generally doctors are helpful and give good care. Some of the comments concerning doctors that were characteristic of the aged were (1) they changed from doctors with high and mighty attitudes; (2) they thought that those at the county clinics told them something different each time they went, and (3) they believed some doctors did not want to be bothered with older people.

Regarding nurses and the care they provide, the majority of the elderly stated that nurses treat you nicely and do a good job of helping you. Some of the older adults emphasized that better care was given by educated or trained nurses than by those functioning in nursing homes.

Most of the younger adults rated their present health status as good or very good and they did not report experiencing health problems. The younger adults placed more emphasis than did the older adults on preventive health practices such as adequate exercise, keeping busy and active, cleanliness, and regular check-ups by a doctor. Some also reported taking vitamins. Although the majority of the younger adults said they went to a doctor when ill, a few mentioned utilizing such places as free student health services and clinics.

With regard to their beliefs concerning doctors and nurses and the care they provide, the majority of the younger adults agreed with the older adults that many doctors do not take time to listen to the patient and consequently the patient frequently ends up going through unnecessary suffering and expense. A large number also agreed with the older adults that there are two kinds of doctors: "good" ones who take an interest in the person and his problems and "poor" ones who are only interested in money. The other beliefs about doctors given by the younger adults involved the following convictions: they were leery of small-town doctors because they frequently missed important symptoms; too many have negative attitudes; they tend to be pill pushers and to treat symptoms instead of looking for causes; many are "quacks" who give out all kinds of medicine and charge outrageous prices; and many do not promote preventive medicine because they want the money involved in future treatment.

With regard to nurses and the care they provide, the younger adults reported the following beliefs: some nurses are too busy to spend time with or to listen to patients; nurses are necessary, and doctors could not do their job without them; nurses are the ones who make you well; they provide the bulk of the care; they are a great help in relieving anxiety when going to the doctor's office; many are not as empathetic and compassionate as they should be; some are more concerned with patients as persons than doctors are; they provide an important service and within the scope of their ability they come closer to doing what they "should be doing than doctors; and some of them go out of their way to be kind." The younger adults did not provide any age-related suggestions on how our health care system could be improved to meet more adequately their health care needs.

Another significant facet of any group is their political behavior. The older adults demonstrated some political behaviors that were different from those of the younger adults. The differences noted on this aspect of behavior, however, were of degree only. A few more of the older adults than the younger adults believed that individual political action does have, or can have, an influence on government. In addition, a few more of the older adults reported voting in both the last national and the last city elections than did the younger adults. Slightly more of the younger adults than the older adults believed that group action on government is effective.

Many groups also have their own special way of viewing life and the total environment. This world view serves as a framework for fitting their experiences into a general, ordered set of ideas that makes their experiences credible and relevant in their efforts to survive. A good deal of any group's world view is inseparable from its religious view.

Some research findings indicate an increased interest in and concern about religion as people age in our society.[45] Some differences were displayed between the older and younger adult groups concerning their behaviors in dealing with religion and world view. With regard to what they believed helped people discover meaning, peace of mind, or other values in life, a few more of the aged emphasized religion and prayer and more of them stressed treating others as one would like to be treated. The older adults reported additional beliefs that seemed to center on unselfishness, giving of oneself to help others, and living according to the dictates of one's conscience or what one was raised to believe. The younger adults, in addition to religion and prayer, seemed to stress self-understanding, and knowing one's own strengths and weaknesses and accepting them when explaining what they believed helps people discover meaning in life. Their other beliefs appeared to concentrate on meaningful relationships with others and education.

Values between the two groups also differed concerning organized religion. The majority of the elderly stated that they were involved in religious organizations and activities. Church services were attended by most of the older adults and about one fourth of them reported participation in age-graded groups that were church affiliated. In contrast, only half of the younger adults reported involvement in religious organizations and activities. They did not report belonging to any age-graded church-affiliated groups.

The life perspective or outlook of many of the elderly seemed more oriented to the present and some of them expressed cognizance of the fact that their future is limited. A few seemed to have come to terms with approaching death. The life perspective of the younger adults, however, was more optimistic and future oriented. Only a few expressed pessimistic outlooks on life.

Rose suggested that the aged have their own separate status system. Even though education carries over from middle age as a significant component of the system, social activity and good health are not as widely distributed among the aged and thus take on special significance as determinants of status among them.[5] Rose proposed that distinctive factors, such as physical and mental health and social activity, help to create the separate status system for older Americans. With respect to the characteristics that they believed gave members of their own age group social status, the older adults appeared to place more emphasis on personal qualities, such as integrity, knowledge, contentment, friendliness, warmth, leadership ability, agility, independence, and personal appearance. Education was also mentioned by a few. In general, the older adults appeared to have discarded criteria such as money and jobs or positions when assessing social success within their own age group.

Conversely, a number of the younger adults listed social status criteria that were not mentioned by the older adults, such as money, ability and drive, job or position, and community involvement. More of the younger adults also cited ability to get along with people, unselfishness, and willingness to help others than did the older adults.

Socialization processes are another characteristic of a group. It is through such processes that the individual is inducted into membership in the group and learns its preferred values, beliefs, and behavior patterns. The activity of socialization is also the means whereby a group preserves it norms and perpetuates itself.[36] Rose suggested that an age-graded subculture must necessarily be limited in its socialization processes as compared to a subculture that has members who live most or all of their lives in it. The time it takes to be socialized into an age-graded subculture and the limited period an individual is expected to remain in it are factors that prevent the subculture from completely enveloping most of its members.[5]

Some differences were found between the two groups on the variable of socialization processes. Most of the older adults stated they learned to function as a member of their present age group principally through trial and error and from friends and associates in their own age group. A number of them also specified observation of younger people and reading. A few mentioned that they had not yet learned to function as a member of their own age group since they were not quite used to it. The majority of older adults received publications written specifically for members of their own age group from a variety of age-graded groups and organizations.

Parents and family were the socializing agents reported by the largest number of younger adults. Trial and error and friends and associates in their own age group were mentioned by fewer of the younger adults. The younger adults also cited distinctive socializing agents such as education and psychotherapy. Only a few of the younger adults reported receiving publications written specifically for members of their own age group and these publications were identified as fashion magazines.

Within each society, subgroups also develop their own special systems of communication in the form of a unique vocabulary, slang, or technical terminology. One of the important social effects of such language systems is the strengthening of group solidarity; use of the terms reminds users of their affiliation with the special group, especially in the presence of nonmembers.[38,46] However, the older adults did not display any language behaviors different from those of the younger adults. The majority of subjects in both groups stated that they did not use certain words or expressions exclusively with their own age group. Members of both groups also denied that the style of speaking of their own age group differed from that of members of other age groups.

In summary, while the exploratory nature of this study necessitates careful interpretation, the data reveal that it is possible to identify some areas of life in which the behavior of the elderly is different from that of the younger general population. Subcultural differences that characterize the aged included some of the following variables: daily life-style, leisure, social interaction and group identity, work and employment, health and illness, religion; social status; and socialization processes. In politics the elderly displayed some slight behavioral differences that were differences of degree only and not of kinds of behavior. The Older Adults and the Younger Adults were quite similar with regard to the variable of language patterns.

POSSIBLE IMPLICATIONS FOR HEALTH AND NURSING CARE

These findings concerning the existence and characteristics of the subculture of the aging substantiate some of the observations and opinions stated in the literature and appear to have some possible implications for nurses and other health personnel in their planning and administering of health and nursing services to the elderly.

Health professionals should take special efforts to discover and understand the daily life-style of the older person since this affects the acceptance and efficiency of the care plan. Because many of the elderly prefer freedom from set routines or prefer routines with some flexibility, health care professionals should reconsider the ritualization of certain practices such as strict adherence to time scheduling in care planning. Health care workers should attempt to individualize care and adapt to the patient whenever possible. An example of such personalization of care would be consideration of the patient's preferences in the timing of his activities of daily living.

The findings indicate that the elderly spend their leisure time alone equally as often as with others and that they engage actively in a wide variety of leisure pursuits. Therefore, when planning diversional activities, health care workers should determine what the patient wants and needs and which activities help make his life meaningful. Opportunities for both group and solitary activities should be provided.

These older people living in the community displayed patterns of frequent interaction with members of their own age group, usually at age-graded groups and organizations. These occasions provide an excellent opportunity for health care personnel to encourage each individual to continue his health care education. Such health education should be of value in increasing the elderly community's awareness of physical symptoms indicative of diseases. These signs and symptoms should not be just tolerated and accepted but should be investigated since they might be caused by incipient disease. Health education or preventive measures should also include knowledge of home safety and of sources of illness and injury. Within the home, increasing illumination levels, using large readable labels on containers of dangerous products, and keeping electrical and gas equipment in good repair all serve to protect the aged against serious accidents. Information about community agencies and resources should also be provided.

The data show that the elderly have relinquished their work role and thus their productive status. In addition, the majority of them stated that they did not agree with the practice of forced retirement. For some older persons this change in status may lead to a decrease in self-esteem and to an altered self-image. Health care professionals should keep in mind the relationship between a person's feelings of dignity and self-respect and the state of his health as they attempt to assess and meet his needs.

Religion appeared to play an important part in the lives of the elderly. Their life perspective was present oriented, with some of them expressing cognizance of the fact that, for them, time is limited. It is apparent that the health and nursing care planned and administered should be provided in a form consistent with the elderly's world views and orientations toward life.

Since all of the elderly stated that good health was important to them yet many of them perceived their present health status to be fair or poor, I think that one of the first steps in planning a health program for community-based older people should be further study of the needs, fears, and desires of these consumers of health services. If this is not done, it is doubtful that the health services planned will be helpful. Availability and accessibility of services do not always guarantee utilization of services. Acceptibility of services is also important.

The majority, 81%, of this group of elderly persons, reported having one or more health problems. Most of the problems listed were chronic. At this particular time, this group of elderly subjects appeared to be coping fairly well with these conditions; however, this observation raises the question of how long they will be able to cope with these health problems. If health care personnel are to provide health maintenance and comprehensive health care services from both a wellness and an illness frame of reference, a continuum of services for older persons is needed. Such a continuum of services should include services for community residents that could help to prevent deterioration and breakdown before crises arise. Such services might include health education and counseling, referral services, preventive health services, and health screening. As their health needs change, the elderly could then utilize health and nursing services in their homes, in day centers and hopsitals, in outpatient clinics, and in hospitals and long-term care facilities. Health education and counseling services could be of particular value in motivating people to seek health and to understand the functions and services of health care personnel and facilities. A good deal of fear, ignorance, and misunderstanding concerning their health problems and health services might then be eliminated.

The majority of the aged reported going to a doctor when they were ill. Some also indicated that they used a health maintenance organization, and a few mentioned going to a naturopath, a chiropractor, an osteopath, and a hospital emergency room. The elderly's reasons for their particular choices were numerous and varied. These findings suggest that the elderly use a number of different criteria in selecting the people and places they utilize when seeking health care. In health care practitioners they seem to look principally for knowledge, honesty, understanding, and listening skills. Good care, coverage, and convenience also seemed to be important. The implications of this data for those attempting to meet the needs of the elderly are that, in addition to possessing the necessary knowledge for meeting their needs, the elderly also consider the interpersonal skills of the practitioner important. The location and the cost of services should also be given serious consideration in the planning of health and nursing care for the elderly.

The response given by the largest number of the aged with regard to their specific beliefs about doctors and the help they do or do not provide was that many doctors do not take the time to listen to the patient and consequently the patient frequently ends up going through unnecessary suffering and expense. These findings seem to further substantiate that the services provided for the elderly should be more personalized since impersonality breeds resentment.

When asked their beliefs about nurses and the care they provide or do not provide, the majority of the elderly stated that nurses treat patients nicely and do a good job of helping them especially, some believed, if they are educated, trained, or public health nurses rather than those functioning in nursing homes. Therefore, to continue to improve nursing practice, it seems that all nursing personnel need to become informed about the elderly's perceived needs and desires and about the aging process itself and the needs created by it.

It is becoming increasingly clear that good health care requires a satisfactory partnership between the patient and the professional health care worker. An open and interested attitude on the part of the health care professional is necessary to avoid problems in interpersonal relationships. In addition, the provision of more complete explanations along with the elderly's participation in the design of their care plans might lead to more successful health care. Moreover, additional knowledge and understanding of the physical, mental, and sociocultural changes that accompany aging, as well as the expectations of the elderly themselves, should assist health care practitioners in meeting more effectively the needs of people in this stage of the life span.

In conclusion, the data substantiate some of the observations of Rose and others that are stated in the literature. Although individual variations exist among the elderly, the findings have pointed to a number of different kinds and degrees of variation that exist between the behavioral patterns of the elderly and those of the younger general society. This study provides a beginning understanding of the subculture of the aged and suggests that there is much to be learned about the values, beliefs, and practices of this age group. In light of the current and the predicted population distribution, I believe that continued research with larger probability samples and more direct indicators of these variables will assist nurses, through cooperative planning with both the elderly and with other health professionals, in helping people at this stage of life achieve and maintain the highest level of wellness possible.

REFERENCES

1. U.S. Department of Health, Education, and Welfare, Office of Human Development, Administration on Aging. New facts about older Americans, Washington, D.C., June, 1973, U.S. Government Printing Office.
2. Neugarten, B.: The aged in American society. In Becker, H. S., editor: Social problems: a modern approach, Chicago, 1968, The University of Chicago Press, pp. 20-21.
3. Rose, A. M.: Future developments in aging-perspectives. In Hoffman, A. M., editor: The daily needs and interests of older people, Springfield, Ill., 1970, Charles C Thomas, Publisher, p. 449.
4. Rose, A. M.: The subculture of the aging: a topic for sociological research, The Gerontologist **2:** 123, 1962.
5. Rose, A. M.: The subculture of the aging: a framework for research in social gerontology. In Rose, A. M., and Peterson, W. A., editors: Older People and Their Social World, Philadelphia, 1965, F. A. Davis Co., pp. 3-16.
6. Palmore, E.: Sociological aspects of aging. In Busse, E. W., and Pfeiffer, E., editors: Behavior and adaptation in late life, Boston, 1969, Little, Brown & Co., pp. 33-57.
7. Barron, M. L.: Minority group characteristics of the aged in American society, J. of Gerontol. **8:** 477-482, 1953.
8. Brotman, H. B.: The fastest growing minority: the American aging, Am. J. Public Health **64:** 249, 1974.
9. Clark, M., and Anderson, B. G.: Culture and aging, Springfield, Ill., 1967, Charles C Thomas, Publisher, p. 431.
10. Palmore, E., p. 56.
11. U.S. Department of Health, Education, and Welfare, Public Health Service: Working with older people: a guide to practice, vol. 2, Washington, D.C., 1969, U.S. Government Printing Office.
12. Neugarten, B., and Moore, J.: The changing age status system. In Neugarten, B., editor: Middle age and aging, Chicago, 1968, The University of Chicago Press, pp. 20-21.
13. Streib, G. F.: Are the aged a minority group? In Goulder, A. W., and Miller, S. M., editors: Applied sociology, New York, 1965, The Free Press of Glencoe.
14. Rosow, I.: The social context of the aging self, The Gerontologist, Spring, 1973, p. 84.
15. U.S. Department of Health, Education and Welfare, National Center for Health Statistics: Vital and health statistics, Washington, D.C., 1973, U.S. Government Printing Office.
16. Dunlop, B. D.: Long-term care: need versus utilization, The Urban Institute, June 1974, pp. 2, 11, 19.

17. Philblad, T., and McNamara, R.: Social adjustment of elderly people in three small towns. In Rose, A. M., and Peterson, W. A., editors: Older people and their social world, Philadelphia, 1965, F. A. Davis Co., p. 57.
18. Loether, H. J.: Problems of aging: sociological and social psychological perspectives, Belmont, Calif., Dickenson Publishing Co., Inc., 1967, p. 22.
19. Introductory report prepared by the Sub-committee on Long-Term Care of the Special Committee on Aging: Nursing home care in the United States: failure in public policy, United States Senate, Washington, D.C., 1974, U.S. Government Printing Office, p. 15.
20. Wright, I. S.: A look into the future of geriatric medicine, J. Am. Geriatr. Soc. **21**(2):55, Feb., 1973.
21. Field, M.: Aging with honor and dignity, Springfield, Ill., Charles C Thomas, Publisher, 1968.
22. Brown, E. L.: Nursing reconsidered: a study of change, Philadelphia, 1970, J. B. Lippincott Co., pp. 201-202.
23. Schwartz, D. R.: Aging and the field of nursing. In Riley, M. W., editor: Aging and society, vol. 2, New York, 1969, Russell Sage Foundation.
24. Brown, M. I.: Nursing of the aging and aged, In Chinn, A. B., editor: Working with older people: clinical aspects of aging, vol. 4, Washington, D.C., U.S. Government Printing Office, July 1971, p. 355.
25. Standards for geriatric nursing practice, Am. J. Nurs. **70**(9):1894-1897, Sept., 1970.
26. Knowles, L. N.: Symposium on putting geriatric nursing standards into practice, Nurs. Clin. North Am. **7**(2):201-202, June, 1972.
27. Department of Baccalaureate and Higher Degree Programs: Masters education in nursing: route to opportunities in contemporary nursing, 1974-1975, New York, 1974, National League for Nursing.
28. Stone, V.: Nursing services to meet the needs of the aged. In Field, M., editor: Depth and extent of the geriatric problem, Springfield, Ill., 1970, Charles C Thomas, Publisher, p. 108.
29. Lambertson, E. C.: The changing role of nursing and its regulation, Nurs. Clin. North Am. **9**(3): 395-402, Sept., 1974.
30. Huether, S. E.: "The clinical specialist in action," Nurs. Clin. North Am. **8**(4):683-764, Dec., 1973.
31. Lewis, E. P.: The clinical nurse specialist, New York, 1970, American Journal of Nursing Co.
32. Lysaught, J. P.: From abstract into action, The National Commission for the Study of Nursing

and Nursing Education, New York, 1973, McGraw-Hill Book Co., p. 171.

33. Sullivan, R. T.: The subculture of the aging and its implications for health and nursing care to the elderly, Unpublished doctoral dissertation, University of Washington, Seattle, 1974.

34. Back, K.: The ambiguity of retirement. In Busse, E. W., and Pfeiffer, E., editors: Behavior and adaptation in late life, Boston, 1969, Little, Brown & Co., p. 95.

35. Clifton, J. A.: Introduction to cultural anthropology, Boston, 1968, Houghton Mifflin Co., p. 184.

36. Chinoy, E.: Sociological perspective, New York, 1968, Random House, p. 129.

37. Hoebel, E. A.: Anthropology: the study of man, New York, 1966, McGraw-Hill Book Co., p. 491.

38. Lindesmith, A. R., and Strauss, A. L.: Social psychology, New York, 1956, Holt, Rinehart, & Winston, pp. 56-57.

39. Mercer, B. E., and Wanderer, J. J.: The study of society, Belmont, Calif., Wadsworth Publishing Co., Inc., 1970, p. 152.

40. Miller, W. B.: Subculture, social reform and the 'culture of poverty,' Hum. Organization **30(2):** 111-125, Summer, 1971.

41. Valentine, C. A.: Culture and poverty, Chicago, The University of Chicago Press, pp. 104-189.

42. Yinger, J. M.: Contraculture and subculture. In Yinger, J. M., editor: The sociology of subcultures, Berkeley, 1970, The Glendessary Press, p. 123.

43. Smelzer, N. J., and Davis, J. A., editors: Sociology, Englewood Cliffs, N.J., 1969, Prentice-Hall, Inc., p. 95.

44. Hammerman, J.: Health services: their success and failure in reaching older adults, Am. J. Public Health **64(3):**253, 1974.

45. Moberg, D. O.: Religiosity in old age, The Gerontologist **5(2):**78-87, June, 1965.

46. Rose, A., and Rose, C. B.: Sociology: the study of human relations, New York, 1969, Alfred A. Knopf, p. 595.

7 Growing old in the black community

LILLIAN G. STOKES

Growing old is a natural, inevitable, and gradual occurrence. It may be considered a stage or part of the continuum of human development. The process of aging is dynamic, thus indicating a process of growth, of evolution, or of becoming, which begins with birth and ends with death.

The process of growth may reach different levels of development in the same person. To specify at which point one "grows old" is difficult, if not impossible. The concept of "being old" differs from the concept of "growing old" in that being old indicates that one has become or has evolved to a defined point.

Several approaches have been used to define old. One approach is chronological, for example, the sixty-fifth birthday. There are rules that support this approach, such as retirement at age 65 years, income tax regulations, and Social Security requirements. Although not accurate in its use, chronological age does give a definition to the concept of old. Knowledge of chronological age can provide a means of understanding aging, as it can provide clues to the phases of the individual's life cycle.[3]

Present knowledge indicates middle age, later maturity, and old age to be stages of advanced adulthood. These stages are thought to encompass specific and easily identifiable aspects of the growing old process. Middle age has been identified as the period when the individual first becomes aware that he is growing old. The 40s and 50s have been equated with this phase. Chronologically, later maturity correlates with the 60s and 70s and is characterized by a greater awareness of aging. Old age, as defined by Atchley, is the beginning of the end.

Knowledge of these stages helps to relate the effect the earlier years may have had on the individual once he has grown old. This is to say that one should not consider the chronological age of 65 years in isolation. Consideration must be given to what happened earlier in life. Munnichs summarizes this concept aptly:

> Life develops through time, in which the past acts as the basis of experience, which influences future plans, and which in turn become manifest in the present. There always is a lively interaction between past (experience) and future (plans, expectations), the resultant of which will be apparent in the present.[25]

When consideration is given to the black aged, for example, those over 65 years old, it is necessary to consider factors that may have influenced their lives during the early stages of adulthood. According to the National Urban League, blacks bring to their older years "a lifetime of economic and social indignities, a lifetime of struggle to get and keep a job, a lifetime of overcrowded substandard housing, of inadequate medical care, of unequal opportunities for cultural and social activities, and a lifetime of second class citizenship."[26] Therefore to understand aspects of growing old in the black community, one must be aware of these factors. However, one must also be cognizant that *the black aged, as any group, are not a homogenous group*. Among the variables that account for the heterogeneity are sex, and socioeconomic factors such as income, education, social class, and residence. Because of the diversity, life-styles and attitudes and beliefs about health and illness may differ. For example, the life of an elderly black who lives in a rural area is likely to be different from that of one who lives in a large city. Much of the material that has been written documents some of these differences. A great deal of the material is impressionistic, but nonetheless, it clearly describes some of the attitudes and beliefs held among the black elderly.

PRESENT AND HISTORICAL ASPECTS OF AGING
Common themes

Several themes are evident when one views aging among blacks: *acceptance, respect, tolerance, independence,* and *supports* (for example, family and religion). These themes will be evinced throughout in relation to how the black aged view themselves, as well as to the types of relationships they have with others. The tendency of aged blacks to accept old age better than their white counterparts has been documented. They tend to look forward to the advanced years. As reported by Messer, old age is perceived by blacks "as a reward in itself."[21] Such feelings might be related to their having had to struggle hard to survive until old age. Thus they are less likely to deny their advanced years. A statement such as "I'm glad I have lived long enough to be considered old" is commonly expressed. Their morale has also been documented to be higher.[21]

Traditionally, there has been evidence of the elderly being highly regarded, respected, and treated with dignity. African culture has historically included a high regard for the Council of Elders, a group of elderly men who serve in an advisory capacity on business and concerns of the villages. The "griot," or oral historian, is old and highly respected in the village, and the elderly, especially men, are reported to be the most revered individuals in the Ibo culture.[2] Shelton reports the high level of involvement of elderly Igbo men in community affairs.[29]

After the period of slavery, elderly women along with their daughters formed one household, often with the elder women at the head.[34] This rule was associated with added dignity and tended to enhance the grandmother's position. At the present time, although the supports are often reciprocal, (that is, there is a tendency of the elders to help their children and vice versa) older family members tend to have less power over matters related to family decisions.[8] However, respect is evident in the day-to-day dealings with them.

Demographic patterns and economics

The black elderly comprise approximately 7% of the total black population. The number of blacks 65 years old and over totaled 1.2 million in 1960 and 1.6 million in 1970; the majority were women.[6] To grow old in the black community means that one is faced with problems in many ways similar to those of the rest of the aging population, one of which is income. Since there are problems, a number of support systems are also evident.

Reports have indicated that the majority of elderly members of the black community have incomes below the poverty level of approximately $2,000 per year. As reported by the Committee on Aging, seven out of every ten elderly black couples have income of less than $3,000 a year; one in two couples have less than $2,000, and one couple in ten must live on less than $1,000 a year. When income is viewed on the basis of sex, the situation seems just as grave. For example, in 1968 the median annual income for black elderly males was $1,470. The majority of females had an annual income of less than $2,000.[17]

Relationship of educational patterns to economics

The basis for such low income can perhaps be related to educational attainment. Many blacks who are now elderly received no education beyond elementary school. Because of this, many of their jobs (domestic service, food service, housekeeping, agricultural work, and janitorial services) were low paying jobs and Social Security benefits for them are low. It was not until the 1950s that these jobs were among those covered by Social Security. Even those who made plans for their retirement three to four decades ago discover that, once they reach retirement age, their pensions are no longer adequate income. The Department of Health, Education, and Welfare confirms the fact that a large percentage of elderly blacks do not receive benefits sufficient for maintenance and that most receive additional aid through old age assistance programs. Even incomes from more than one source are not enough to make ends meet.

Again, one must not forget the diversity among the black elderly. Some, perhaps a minority, are economically independent.

Despite the majority's low incomes, the black aged tend to take pride in their "independence." They try to manage on their limited incomes. There is a distinct preference to be able to support themselves with their own money and not be dependent on someone else or even on the menial benefits from Social Security. Gifts (for example, in the form of money) from children and relatives are accepted, but not often solicited. Many do not ask for help. Incidentally, Jackson[12] reports that many black elderly refuse benefits for fear of degrading themselves by receiving welfare. She also reports that middle income parents tend to receive assistance from their children more so than do lower income parents.

Many elderly blacks enjoy maintaining, or find it necessary to maintain, "small jobs," thus trying to remain employed as long as they can. It is not uncommon to see elderly black women maintaining babysitting jobs, either full- or part-time, to supplement their income. Programs such as foster grandparents are utilized. Although most black elderly are not gainfully employed, it has been reported that elderly black women work outside their homes more often and longer than their white counterparts. Employment is usually confined to domestic work.[30] Men may also maintain part-time jobs. Many participate in senior citizen groups. Often the crafts made in senior citizen classes are sold to supplement income.

Despite the problems associated with limited income, a contention of happiness and a desire to survive is often expressed. Comments such as "I'm happy to be alive" or "Thanks to God for allowing me to live long enough to be considered old" are not uncommon. These feelings might be evident because of the conditions in which many have had to work and live, or the feeling of having lived "through the worst conditions," and within well-defined limits all their lives.

Supports for the black elderly

Family support. Many elderly blacks live alone, especially women. Kent reports that more black women live alone than white women.[17] Among the black elderly Mosser states that the National Urban League reported that 44% of the men and 75% of the women are alone.[24] This possibly reflects the greater life expectancy of women. Those who live alone, men or women, are frequently assisted by family members, friends, and neighbors with their housework and transportation. Grandchildren also play a big part in assisting their elderly grandparents, especially when the school session is over. This is a common practice if the elderly person lives in the home with the family. Many children are required to help out while the parents work.

Another worthwhile point is that in many black homes an aged relative, usually a woman, lives with a younger couple and takes care of the children or performs household chores. This practice is in keeping with the extended family pattern, which was, and to a certain extent still is, so prevalent in early black households. Such an arrangement not only builds strengths but provides social, economic, and emotional support for both age groups.[31]

Support by youth. A large portion of elderly blacks live in areas that are considered high crime areas: urban ghettos and rural areas of the South. In 1969 Brotman reported that 60.7% of the black population 65 years old and over lived in metropolitan areas. For those who have economic security, residence in the inner city area is usually by choice. However, many live in these areas because of circumstances that are beyond their control, such as low income and lack of transportation. Although many elderly people have been mugged, militant young blacks have been reported to exhibit a certain degree of support and protection for the elderly by escorting them to shopping areas and in the community to prevent their being robbed.

Professional support. The National Caucus on the Black Aged was established in 1971. This group serves as an advocate of the black elderly. The group concerns itself with bringing attention and giving visibility to the plight of the black elderly in areas such as income, housing, and health and with stimulating other organizations to join in the efforts to effect changes.[12]

Religious support. Religion frequently remains a part of elderly persons' lives. Many elderly actively participate in church activities, enjoy going to church, and attend when health allows. Although church attendance may decrease, feelings and beliefs about religion do not change with increasing age. As reported by Heyman, "The church has long exerted a dominant influence in both personal and group life, thus serving as a social, educational and recreational center, as well as the source of great personal support and comfort."[11]

Many elderly spend time, usually daily, reading the Bible or taking advantage of religious programs through radio or television or participating in religious activities in the community. To many the scriptures offer a source of consolation. Prayer traditionally has been a way of dealing with problems. It is not uncommon for churches and community groups to hold weekly prayer meetings. This is a tradition that has survived. In addition to daily individual prayer, a group of friends may get together periodically to engage in prayer. There is a belief that prayer and faith have a positive influence on illness. Prayer is often expressed by some as an attempt to solve problems and raise their spirits. It is not uncommon to hear comments such as "I pray and ask God to help," or "I talk with the Master about problems of concern. . . . He gives me the strength that I need." There is usually heavy reliance on "the Master" and prayer in dealing with problems. Many elderly believe that their trust in God has helped and continues to help them survive the hard times. This was true in the days of slavery and persists today. The clergyman is highly regarded among the elderly. Close contacts are often made with clergy, as they serve as excellent resource persons with whom to discuss various problems.

Support from outside activities. When health allows, much enjoyment is obtained from engaging in outside activities. Frequent visits with families and friends are highly regarded. Close contact is usually maintained by telephone with relatives and friends.

Many communities have organized senior citizen groups that meet regularly. Members of these groups often participate in craft classes, games, religious activities, and recreational outings. In addition to the socialization that these groups afford, they also enable the elderly to participate in organized activities, create new interests, or revive old ones.

Health status

Elderly blacks are affected more by chronic illness than their white counterparts. Many did not receive adequate medical care early in life. When acute illness occurred, their choice was often to continue work so that day-to-day needs could be met. Often medical care was not sought until it interfered with their ability to maintain their jobs. Such differences might also be related to the accessibility of health care, which is largely affected by socioeconomic conditions.

The life expectancy of blacks is shorter than that of whites, and black women tend to live longer than black men. The life expectancy for black women is 67.5 years, 7.4 years less than for white women. For black men the life expectancy is 60.1 years, and therefore many black women are widowed much earlier than white women. Black men who are over 75 years old are in better health than black women.

Arthritis, heart disease (hypertensive heart disease), and diabetes are the most common chronic illnesses that individuals over 45 years old experience. Arthritis is more common among black women.

Beliefs about illness

Feelings expressed about health and illness are varied. Many of the problems are associated with increasing age, of which physical deterioration is considered a natural part. Some relate conditions such as arthritis and loss of teeth as necessary components of aging. Others relate personal habits such as improper diet, drinking, smoking, and keeping late hours as a basis for problems. Hypertension, for example, is often equated with ingesting too much meat, especially pork. Blacks who are in fairly good physical condition generally feel that they took good care of themselves during the younger years, or that they lived a lifetime of moderation. By the same token, those whose health is bad often attribute ''not taking care of themselves during their youth'' as being responsible. For example, one may hear the black elderly relating the aches and pains of arthritis specifically to events of their youth, such as being out in cold, damp weather without proper clothing. Statements such as ''Exposing yourself (improper clothing) will catch up with you when you get old'' are common. Such statements are often given as advice to younger people to encourage them to take care of themselves while they are young. ''The will of God'' may also be related to illness. These examples demonstrate what Snow classifies as natural causes of illness.[29]

Reports have also indicated that some elderly blacks attribute illness to unnatural causes or external forces that are beyond the control of an individual. Terms commonly used are voodoo, the evil eye, and roots.[14] There are also reports that do not support this contention.[18]

Just as there are beliefs about the cause of illness, there are also beliefs about prevention and management of it. Many blacks, despite hardships, place a high value on preventive care. Preventive measures as expressed by the elderly include good self-care, appropriate medical attention, and assistance of God.

Patterns and practices of illness management

Once an illness occurs, there is a tendency to regard it as a problem to be solved; the specific approach utilized often depends on what the person believes is the cause. For example, those who see illness as a part of the aging process have a tendency to take the illness in stride and accept the disability as a part of growing old. Another attitude of acceptance, often expressed as "God's will" or "if you have an illness you should live with it" is frequently evident.

The use of home remedies and patent medicines are practices that perhaps date back to the time of slavery or immediately after slavery. The older person, for example, a grandmother, was the storehouse of knowledge about medicine and gave advice and instructions about specific remedies for certain ailments, many of which were passed on by word of mouth. Even today grandmothers may make suggestions concerning remedies for minor problems.

Those who believe in self-treatment may or may not seek medical assistance until the condition becomes serious or the home remedy seems to fail. Home remedies may be utilized for prevention of illness, maintenance of health, and cures. For example, a certain type of bracelet worn around the wrist is said to prevent arthritis. Substances that have been reported to be used for hypertension include vinegar, lemon juice, pickles, and epsom salts;[29] honey and water have also been reported. Each of these is believed to have the potential for bringing the blood pressure down. Bicarbonate of soda is used for problems associated with the stomach and a number of rubbing compounds, including rubbing alcohol, are used for problems associated with the joints. The basis for self-treatment is perhaps economic; to have to pay professionals for their service means an added bill, which only serves to compound already existing financial problems.

Those who believe in folk medicine may seek help from a number of practitioners such as faith healers, spiritualists, or root doctors.[14]

There are many black elderly, perhaps a majority, who believe in medical science to the fullest. These people will not take medicines or follow any treatment regime unless they are prescribed by a doctor. They keep doctor and clinic appointments and closely follow prescribed therapies. Some, because of religious or cultural influences, trust God over medicines, therapies, and so forth; they may take medications until they feel better, then stop and not follow through fully.

Practices related to care

Themes that have been identified in regard to illness are acceptance and tolerance. This is evident in the fact that there is a tendency for many to remain at home until the discomfort is so great that there is no choice other than to seek medical assistance. It is not uncommon to see a relative or another significant person travel long distances for the sole purpose of trying to convince the older person either to go to the hospital or to seek medical assistance. The tendency of many elderly blacks to not seek medical care until the disease is advanced may be related to their view of a hospital as a place to die. There is also a belief held by some that "troublesome patients in hospitals are killed by being given a 'black pill' or a liquid poison from a 'black bottle.'"[20]

There is also a tendency for blacks to provide care at home for the aged family member. Such practice could be related either to tradition or to limited resources. As reported by the National Urban League around 1968, only 2.8% of all women and men in homes for the aged were black. Factors such as inadequate income to cover the expense or unavailability of adequate homes could account for this. Some institutions have been established for the care and protection of the black elderly. Church groups, womens' clubs, and fraternal organizations have provided most of the leadership for this support.

Because of the tradition of the extended family, the necessity of sending the elderly person to a nursing home often creates guilt feelings. The desire to have them in a supportive environment around individuals who are significant and close is great. The practice of the elderly person being taken in by a son, daughter, or close relative is not uncommon. A close relative, such as a widowed or divorced daughter or niece, may leave home for brief (or sometimes extended) periods of time to care for an elderly family member. Another option that is frequently evident is the employment of someone, for example, a sitter, to take care of them. During an acute state of an illness, family members and neighbors may take turns at night in assisting with care. Often when the necessity for a nursing home arises, all other physical resources have been used. The family physician often convinces the elderly and family of the need for a nursing home. If a nursing home becomes necessary, the proximity of the facility to family members and the concern of the personnel for comfort and care are priority factors in the selection.

As attitudes about other facets of life are changing, so are attitudes about chronic care. For some the theme of independence is quite evident, as many do not want to be a bother or burden on family members. Therefore the thought of going to such facilities is more readily accepted.

CUSTOMS SURROUNDING DEATH AND BURIAL

One might assume that the elderly would likely have well-defined attitudes about death. Themes that have been evident in literature discussing death among elderly blacks include "not being fearful of death" and the view of death as "God's will." Perhaps these themes are evident because of their religious orientation. Jeffers found that few religious people admit fear of death.[15] A recent conversation with a hospitalized black elderly man revealed this orientation. His comments were based on this strong religious belief: If he gets well and returns home, it will be God's will, or if he dies, that, too, is His will.

These observances following the death of an individual usually involve relatives, friends, and acquaintances of the deceased or the family. From the time of death, and even during the period of illness prior to the death, relatives, neighbors, and friends join in to assist the family or to offer services. Assisting with housework and assisting with younger children if they are in the home are two examples. The practice of preparing food either in the home of the family or in their own homes is common. Several individuals may drop by at regular intervals to leave various foods.

Arrangements are usually made for the funeral the first or second day after the death. These arrangements are made by close family members; usually the next person in line takes the leadership. For example, on the death of the father, the wife usually is automatically viewed as the head of the family. However, consultation with other family members is generally the rule. As arrangements are being made, close contact is maintained with the funeral director and often with the minister.

One of the first observances in which rituals are evident is the *wake*. The wake, often referred to as the lying in state, is the period during which the embalmed body lies in the casket to be viewed by those in attendance.[5] Those who come (friends, employers, representatives of fraternal organizations, and church members) do so to pay last respects and to express sympathy to the family. This visit may be either brief or extended. Those who remain may engage in quiet conversation with others in attendance or may sit quietly and wait. A minister may be in attendance. If so, he may offer a prayer and condolences to the family and friends. If the deceased were a member of a specific organization (fraternity, sorority, or lodge), it is during the wake that special ritualistic services are conducted by members of the group.

The wake is held the day prior to the funeral, usually in the evening or night. It has been customary for some family members and visitors to sit up all night with the body. This was particularly true when the body was taken back to the home to "lie in state." However the period of time presently set aside for the wake is generally limited to 2 to 4 hours, since the majority are held at a mortuary. Some are held in churches. When this is the case, family members may arrange for someone to stay with the body all night. It is not uncommon for pictures to be taken of the deceased.

Floral arrangements are sent by relatives and friends as expressions of sympathy. There is an increasing trend to send flowers, for example, potted plants, to close relatives. These remain in the home so that the family may have a living memorial of the deceased. It is increasingly common among the middle class for requests to be made by family members for contributions to either the deceased's favorite charity or one of their own choice.

Following the wake, friends return to the home of a close relative. The intent of this custom, again, is to converse with family members and to offer assistance. Often socialization along with eating and talking about the deceased and the "good old days" seems to be part of the grief and mourning process.

The *funeral service* is almost always accompanied by a religious service and is usually held in church, even for the person who had no religious affiliation. Sometimes the service may be conducted at home or in a mortuary chapel. The precise type of service depends on the denomination to which the deceased belonged. The service is usually formal, with prayer, scripture, hymns, remarks, and re-viewing of the remains. The extent of the service depends on factors such as religious and organizational affiliations, prominence in the community, and family traditions. During the service, emotional outbursts are not uncommon.

Usually the *burial* immediately follows the funeral service. A previous custom was for the body to pass the home or work place on the way to the cemetery. Again, friends and acquaintances accompany the family to the grave site. This practice is particularly true in rural areas. Graveside services have traditionally been held; however, changes have been noted in this practice. Such services may now be held in a chapel at the cemetery and the body may be placed in the grave after the family leaves.

Among other evident changes is a wider use of personal clothing for burial rather than the traditional shroud for women. There seems to be some special personal meaning attached to this practice. Family plots for burial are not as widely used.

The practice of assistance from neighbors and friends is also evident the day of the funeral. Several neighborhood women may remain at the house during the time of the funeral service to prepare food. Such assistance is of great help to the family as relatives have often traveled long distances. After the burial, one of the customs is a gathering of the extended family and friends to eat. Such a gathering seems to lessen the loneliness and provides a means of support for the family.

Special visits and calls are made by relatives, friends, and neighbors for several days after the funeral. Again the purpose of such visits is to lessen the emptiness that family members may feel.

SUMMARY

This chapter has reviewed a number of problems faced by elderly blacks. In addition, various support systems that are evident were described. Varied beliefs, customs, and practices centering around illness and care were presented. Finally, materials that illustrate some of the rituals concerning death and burial were discussed.

REFERENCES

1. Anderson, M.: The pains and pleasures of old black folk, Ebony **28:**123-130, March, 1973.
2. Arth, M.: Ideals and behavior: a comment on Ibo respect patterns, Gerontologist **8:**242-244, 1968.
3. Atchley, R. C.: The social forces in later years, Belmont, Calif.: 1972, Wadsworth Publishing Co.
4. Bims, H.: The black family: a proud reappraisal, Ebony **29:**118-127, March, 1974.
5. Bowman, L.: Group behavior at funeral gathering. In The american funeral, a study in guilt, extravagance and sublimity, Washington, 1959, Public Affairs Press, pp. 16-26.
6. Brotman, H. B.: Facts and figures on older Americans, Washington, D.C., 1971, U.S. Department of Health, Education, and Welfare.
7. Butler, R. N., and Lewis, M. I.: Aging and mental health, ed. 2, St. Louis, 1977, The C. V. Mosby Co.
8. Carpenter, J. O., and Wylie, C. M.: On aging, dying and denying: delivering care to older dying persons, Public Health Reports **89:**403-407, Sept.-Oct., 1974.
9. Faulkner, A. O.: The black aged as good neighbors, Gerontologist **15:**554-559, Dec., 1975.
10. Haynes, M. A.: The gap in health status between black and white Americans. In Williams, R. A.: Textbook of black related diseases, New York, 1975, McGraw-Hill Book Co., pp. 11-30.
11. Heyman, D. K., and Jeffers, F. C.: Study of the relative influences of race and socio-economic status upon the activities and attitudes of a southern aged population, J. Gerontol. **19:**225-228, 1964.
12. Jackson, H. C.: National caucus on the black

aged: a progress report, Aging and Hum. Develop. **2:**226-231, 1971.
13. Jackson, J. J.: Aged negroes: their cultural departure from statistical stereotypes and rural-urban differences, Gerontologist **10:**140-145, 1970.
14. Jordan, W. C.: Voodoo medicine, In Williams, R. A.: Textbook of black related diseases, New York, 1975, McGraw-Hill Book Co., pp. 716-738.
15. Jeffers, F. C., Nichols, C. R., and Eisdorfer, C.: Attitudes of older persons toward death: a preliminary study, J. Gerontol. **16:**53-56, Jan., 1961.
16. Kalish, R. A.: Late adulthood: perspectives on human development, Belmont, Calif., 1975, Brooks/Cole Publishing Co.
17. Kent, D. P.: The Negro aged, Gerontologist **2:** 48-51, Spring, 1971.
18. Koenig, R.: Ideals about illness of elderly black and white in an urban hospital, Aging and Hum. Develop. **2:**217-225, 1971.
19. Lerner, M.: When, why and where people die. In Brom, O., Jr., Freeman, H., Levine, S., and Scotch, N.: editors: The dying patient, New York, 1970 Russel Sage Foundation, pp. 5-29.
20. Martin, B. J. W.: Ethnicity and health care: Afro-Americans, Ethnicity and health care, New York, 1976, National League for Nursing, pp. 47-55.
21. Messer, M.: Race differences in selected attitudinal dimensions of the elderly, Gerontologist **18:** 245-249, 1968.
22. Montagu, M. F. A.: Social problems of an aging population, J. Nat. Med. Assoc. **52:**338-342, Sept., 1960.

23. Moore, J. W.: Situational factors affecting minority aging, Gerontologist **11:**88-93, 1971.
24. Moss, B. B.: Caring for the aged, Doubleday and Co., Inc., 1966, pp. 87-89.
25. Munnichs, J. M. A.: Attitudes toward finitude (death) and the disengagement theory of aging, Proceedings of Seventh Congress of Gerontology, pp. 521-524, June 6-July 2, 1966.
26. Double jeopardy. . . . the older Negro in America today, New York, 1965, National Urban League.
27. Rubenstein, D. I.: An examination of social participation found among a national sample of black and white elderly, Aging and Hum. Develop. **2:**172-187, 1971.
28. Scott, C. S.: Health and healing practices among five ethnic groups in Miami, Florida, Public Health Reports **89:**524-532, Nov.-Dec., 1974.
29. Shelton, A. J.: Igbo child raising eldership and dependence, Gerontologist **8:**236-241, 1968.

30. Snow, L. F.: Folk medical beliefs and their implications for care of patients, Ann. of Int. Med. **81:**82-96, July, 1974.
31. United States Senate Committee on Aging: The multiple hazards of age and race: the situation of aged blacks in the United States (working paper prepared by I. B. Lindsay), Washington, D.C., 1971, U.S. Government Printing Office.
32. Vernon, G. M.: Sociology of death, New York, 1970, The Ronald Press Co.
33. Weaver, J. L.: Poverty and health in black and white. In National health policy and the underserved: ethnic minorities, women, and the elderly, St. Louis, 1976, The C. V. Mosby Co., pp. 71-90.
34. Wylie, F. M.: Attitudes toward aging and the aged among black Americans: some historical perspectives, Aging and Hum. Develop. **2:**66-70, 1971.

8 The Chicano community and its aged

FELIPE G. CASTRO
NATHANIEL N. WAGNER†

In providing health care for aged Chicanos, a broad knowledge of beliefs, customs, and practices is important. Cultural knowledge is helpful in developing a *sensitivity* to subtle cultural differences, which is necessary for understanding of the patient's needs and behaviors. The health care worker's attitude of respect and understanding and acceptance of individual and of cultural differences among aged Chicanos can improve the quality of care. This positive attitude on the part of the helping person is the result of an appreciation of the beliefs, customs, and practices of aged Chicanos. In this chapter, we attempt to develop a better understanding of such similarities and differences among aged Chicanos. Some customs, beliefs, and practices concerning aging, illness, and death that have served as a basis for the attitudes toward the life-styles of many aged Chicanos are detailed.*

AGED CHICANOS: A HETEROGENEOUS POPULATION WITH A COMMON HERITAGE

In working with aged Chicanos,‡ it is important to maintain a perspective regarding similarities and differences among members of this population. A common thread that binds aged Chicanos is their common Hispanic heritage. As a group, most aged Chicanos share a language, Spanish, a religious orientation, Catholicism, and a Mexican culture composed of a set of values, beliefs, and customs. Torres-Gil[1] indicates that according to the 1970 census there were approximately 382,000 Spanish-speaking persons over 65 years of age, of which 189,000 were Mexican American-Chicanos. Possessing a cultural orientation different from that of the dominant Anglo-American society, aged Chicanos as a group have a "world view"[2] different from that of aged Anglo-Americans.

Nevertheless the awareness of cultural commonalities existing among aged Chicanos should be balanced by a consideration of individual differences. Despite the common bond of heritage, aged Chicanos are *not* a homogenous group. Penalosa[3] cautions that in studying the Chicano it is wise to stop trying to find the "typical" or true and instead seek

---

†Dr. Wagner died on June 14, 1978.

*Appreciation is extended to Dr. Ildaura Murillo-Rohde, Associate Dean, School of Nursing, University of Washington, for her assistance in the revision of this manuscript.

‡The term "Chicano" as applied to the aged of Mexican ethnic origin is a recent form of group identification. In the past and in many present instances these individuals may instead identify themselves as Mexican Americans, Mexicans, Hispaños, or possibly as Americans, meaning that they are U.S. citizens. In this paper we will use the terms Chicano and Mexican American interchangeably.

to establish the range of variation. In fact, Penalosa adds that Chicanos may constitute one of the most heterogeneous ethnic groups.

Seward provides a useful way of looking at Chicanos. He emphasizes the need to examine the dynamics of the combined culture and personality. He states, "From such diverse learning experiences . . . there generally emerge differences in expressive styles, ego defense systems, and moral controls."[4]

Along these lines, the aged Chicano's *learning history* has been strongly influenced by two distinct cultures, the Mexican and the American. Each personality is a product of differing degrees of knowledge and values incorporated from each culture. Thus one consequence of this dual cultural exposure has been a great range of individual differences among Chicanos, as seen in their degrees of acculturation. Among aged Chicanos there are large differences in knowledge of Spanish, in degree of religious orientation, and in degree of ethnic identification. An aged Chicano may be very knowledgeable of the American culture but much less so of the Mexican culture, or vice versa. Still another aged Chicano individual may be bilingual and bicultural and therefore be able to communicate well in both English and Spanish and to participate effectively in both cultures. Thus in attempting to understand similarities and differences among aged Chicanos to meet their needs more adequately, it is essential that the helping person maintain a consideration of both the individual's Mexican culture, which he shares with other aged Chicanos, as well as the individual's personality differences.

A graphic setting in which both cultural similarities and individual differences are evident is a dance for aged Chicanos, such as a railroad union dance or a Chicano senior citizens dance. Here all respond similarly to the discriminative stimulus, the Mexican music, by dancing the traditional steps to a Mexican *corrido*. Nevertheless, large individual differences in response are observable. Some dance slowly, while others *bailan como trompos,* dance like spinning tops.

HISTORICAL ASPECTS OF CULTURE AMONG AGED CHICANOS

If Chicanos are in fact so heterogeneous, then why consider them as a group? One response to this question involves the historical dynamics of human exchange across the United States–Mexico border, an exchange occurring continually since the early years of this century. Whereas other ethnic minority groups may have experienced diminished contact with the mother country, the aged Chicanos' closeness to Mexico has facilitated continued contact with their mother country and a regeneration of cultural practices and traditions. Furthermore most aged Chicanos are heirs to the land of the Southwest,*[4] *Aztlan,* which was once a Mexican territory and was transferred to the United States on February 2, 1848, after the signing of the Treaty of Guadalupe Hidalgo at the close of the Mexican-American War. Thus many aged Chicanos are grandsons of several generations of indigenous inhabitants of the Southwest.

For other aged Chicanos, the Mexican Revolution of 1910, with its political and economic upheaval, led to their entry into the United States. Still other aged Chicanos of a younger generation immigrated into the United States as migrant workers in agriculture, in mines, or on the railroad, eventually settling here despite original intentions to save money and return to Mexico. Settling in the United States was facilitated by Mexican

---

*The *Southwest* refers to the five southwestern states of Arizona, California, Colorado, New Mexico, and Texas.

communities or *barrios,* such as those within Los Angeles. Here Mexican traditions have been maintained by families, the community, the church, Spanish language newspapers, as well as by the influx of another generation of documented and undocumented workers. In sum, many forces have combined to maintain a core Mexican culture among aged Chicanos, despite their heterogeneity.

Beginning in 1965 with the growth of the United Farm Workers movement, the term "Chicano" grew in popularity as an attempt to provide a generic term descriptive of these people—a heterogeneous people, yet a people with a common heritage. Although a greater percentage of youths identify specifically as Chicanos, this term is also applicable to the aged.

Sotomayor and Ortego[5] indicate that there exists a Chicano culture with an identity of its own. Chicano culture is the culture of people whose roots lie in Mexican traditions, yet who have been raised in the United States and have acquired a bilingual perspective. Within this culture, original Mexican customs and traditions have been modified by environmental contact with the Anglo culture. For the individual, degree of modification from tradition is dependent in part on degree of acculturation.

ACCULTURATION EFFECTS: CHANGES ON TRADITIONALISM

Degree of acculturation may be thought of as a continuum depicting degrees of orientation toward the traditional Mexican culture at one extreme, and the modern American culture at the other.[3] On this spectrum, degree of acculturation may be defined as the relative degree in which the individual has moved towards adopting as his own the values, attitudes, and behaviors of the dominant American society. In this process of cultural change, Spiro[6] has made a distinction between *acculturation* and *assimilation.* He defines acculturation as the acquisition of the culture of the dominant group (that is, adopting or identifying with the values and life-style of another culture). He defines *assimilation* as the disappearance of group identity through nondifferential association or exogamy (that is, the loss of ethnic identity by fitting into and being accepted into the dominant culture group).

Spiro's distinction is important in understanding the Chicano's access to socially valued commodities, such as lucrative employment. A Chicano individual attempting to become acculturated may not be able to assimilate into the dominant society because of nonacceptance into the group, for example, nonacceptance into higher paying jobs or professions. For the aged Chicano, assimilation may be further impaired because of negative social attitudes towards the aged, for example, the belief that they are unproductive.[7] The consequences of denied access are continuation in lower socioeconomic status and continued restriction to the Mexican culture. This correlation between low socioeconomic status and increased cultural affiliation is reflected by Grebler, Moore, and Guzman[8] who indicate that Chicanos, the second largest ethnic minority group in the nation (5.5 million people in 1970), bear a highly disproportionate share of the burden of poverty in the Southwest.

In a similar analysis of being culture-bound, Ruesch, Jacobson, and Loeb[9] speak of the individual's *cultural distance* from the American core culture, which includes the values of English-speaking, middle socioeconomic class, Protestant people. These standard values are met with difficulty by a person who is Spanish-speaking, of lower socioeconomic class, and Catholic. Increased age creates further difficulties. Thus many aged Chicanos retain traditional Mexican values and remain culture-bound, because for them acculturation in the Anglo-American core culture can be a painful psychological process. Furthermore a pride in being Mexican and a strong value for traditional Mexican customs has resulted in a sustained cultural fixedness among many aged Chicanos.

There are cases, however, in which working Chicanos have gained access into the dominant culture's work force, thus climbing in socioeconomic status, modifying life-styles, and consequently modifying attitudes and traditional practices. Bern[10] indicates that "stateways can change folkways. They do so, in part, by effecting a change in behavior; then, when behavior has been changed, attitudes often follow." These cases, however, appear to involve the younger generation of Chicanos more frequently than the older generation. It appears that in general, aged Chicanos have maintained a traditional perspective, much more so than the youth, and that the aged Chicano can be a strong source for transmission of the culture.

In clarifying the role of the aged Chicano in the transmission of cultural and traditional practices, a brief examination of the concepts of culture and tradition may be valuable. According to Keesing,[11] culture is *cultivated behavior*. Culture is "the totality of learned, socially transmitted behavior or 'custom.' "[11] Other views of culture have emphasized that culture serves as a design for living or a guide to behavior or that it involves repeating similar approved or reinforced behaviors. Skinner[12] indicates that culture is composed of social variables arranged by others, that is, parents, family, the community, and social institutions, that shape and maintain the individual's behavior usually in such a way that he, in turn, tends to perpetuate the culture. Thus a *pattern of behaviors* (that is, rituals, celebrations, or observances that are practiced because it is customary or traditional to do so) may be considered as descriptive of a culture.

Traditionalism of family organization, according to Edmonson,[13] is a potent force that has survived through centuries with little modification. Traditional practices are patterns of behavior reinforced through the years by the elders. In describing this process, Edmonson refers to the Spanish word *costumbre* (custom). Maintaining *costumbres* in Mexican tradition involves the conception of "the rightfulness of things." "The 'reason' for performing a ceremony in a particular way, or indeed, for performing it at all, is simply that it has always been; it is the custom."[13] In the Mexican culture, tradition has involved doing that which *es costumbre,* and correct, doing it because it is the way life is supposed to be.

For aged Chicanos, especially the very religious, traditional beliefs and customs are the way of life. However changes in the family structure of the modern Chicano family have disrupted the process of cultural transmission. In the traditional Mexican family, patterns of culture have been transmitted from generation to generation with the aged person holding a place of authority and reverence as the figurehead of the family. Montiel[14] states that the traditional family has been described as family centered, paternalistic, and authoritarian. In recent times these descriptions have lost accuracy because of changing family patterns. Temple-Trujillo[15] points out the traditional Mexican family, characterized by extended family relationships, *compadrazgo,* financial dependence, patriarchy, *machismo*, and the ideal child concept, is a thing of the agrarian past. To some extent, so is the role of the aged Chicano as head of the family.

Industrialization, urbanization, an emphasis on the youth culture, and other aspects of the Anglo-American society have diminished the traditionalistic role of the Chicano aged. This is a general trend, as Bengtson, et. al.[16] have indicated that the status of the aged is inversely related to the degree of modernization of the social setting. "The status of the elderly relative to that of other age groups diminishes with a shift from agricultural to an industrialized economy, or from a 'traditional' to a 'modern' social system.''[16]

Torres-Gil[1] adds that aged Chicanos, *las personas de mayor edad,* who symbolize the Chicano culture and past, bear the brunt of many problems: ''the break-up of the traditional extended family, forced assimilation, discrimination, insensitive government practices, citizenship difficulties, lack of adequate housing and transportation, low educational opportunity and language discrimination.''

Maldonado[17] has noted that in the past when the Chicano family was an agrarian system of production, Mexican traditions were maintained including an emphasis on extended family and respect for the aged. Within this system, the aged were assured of useful roles and were cared for by the family. The greater participation of Chicano youths in urbanized American society with resultant changes in family patterns has resulted in a breakdown in traditional Mexican values, customs, and practices.

Maldonado acknowledges that both generations are making adjustments to adapt to modern social and economic pressures. He emphasizes that the Chicano young will not abandon their parents merely for the sake of progress and the aged Chicano will not demand care from the young.

Given these important changes in custom and tradition, how do aged Chicanos view old age, and how do they view established institutions such as the family, the church, and the government? Crouch[18] asked these questions of 291 Chicano people 50 or more years old in western Texas.

Crouch found that as a whole, the Chicano respondents viewed old age as undesirable. The traditional value of aging as being acceptable and the will of God had been offset by the negative effects of reduced health and economic insecurity.

Although traditionally it has been the role of the young family members to care for the aged, 61% of the respondents indicated that the family did *not* have an obligation to support them, whereas 38% indicated that the family had such an obligation. The implication of this finding is that in this urban setting these respondents held less strongly to traditional views. However, a majority of respondents in a rural setting may still favor the traditional views about care for the aged.

Crouch also found that with increasing age there was a greater tendency to be satisfied with the church, although among the oldest group of respondents, 52% were dissatisfied. Respondents, in deemphasizing family support from the young, looked toward the government for aid, although many are unclear about specific services available. Also, Crouch indicates that for aged Chicanos ''the existence of a specific cultural tradition largely maintained by the predominant use of Spanish as a first language would contribute to major differences between older Mexican-Americans and other older Americans.''[18] We may tentatively conclude that despite modifications in tradition, it still exerts a significant effect on the behavior of many aged Chicanos.

SOME TRADITIONAL BELIEFS, CUSTOMS, AND PRACTICES CONCERNING ILLNESS, DEATH, FUNERALS, AND MOURNING

In our approach to beliefs, customs, and practices among Chicanos, we wish to explore the origins of present behavior and practices by exploring past traditional practices and cultural patterns. Although we acknowledge that some of the traditional behavioral patterns presented may no longer be applicable to some aged Chicanos, it is nevertheless important to examine the roots of original traditional practices that for decades have served as standards of life and living, standards from which current Chicano cultural practices have evolved.

The roots of traditional Mexican culture lie in a blend of indigenous pagan rituals of the natives who populated Mexico before the conquest with the customs and traditions imposed by their Spanish conquerors. In this process, the Spanish language replaced the indigenous *nahuatl* language, whereas the Catholic religion was easily superimposed on the indigenous religion because of the many parallels between both systems of belief.

The concept of the life cycle, time, and aging and the concept of death are paramount in shaping the attitudes towards life and living within traditional Mexican culture. The ancient Mayas believed time to be governed by the gods. Aging itself was not meaningful to them, since they were free from the notion of progress. They believed that time was nothing more than a recurring cycle of events. In this cycle, a knowledge of the future could be obtained by discovering the occurrences of the past.[19]

For the Aztecs, a preoccupation with aging appears to have been less important than the concern over the place one goes after death. Aztec texts describe the Region of the Dead, *Mictlan,* the "place-of-the-fleshless," the "common-place-where-we-lose-ourselves."[20] Other places for the dead included the paradise of Tlaloc for those chosen by this god of rain, the Heaven of the Sun, for those dying in war or sacrifice, and the "place-of-the-nursing-tree" where deceased infants were to go. There was, however, some preoccupation with aging and death, as expressed in the Aztec poem "Love and Death," in which the Aztec poet frets over the thought of parting from his beloved because of the inevitability of death. The poet questions the possibility of existence after death.[20]

Human sacrifices conducted by the Aztecs as a religious offering to the gods were a necessary part of the life cycle. Should the natives be judged by the Gods as ungrateful for their harvest, they might be punished by the gods. The practice of honoring the supernatural, which is still evident in the Mexican culture today, has led to some views that Mexican culture emphasized or was preoccupied with death.[21,22]

In views of the life cycle, there were many parallels between the pagan religion of ancient Mexicans and the Catholic religion imposed by the Spaniards. One important parallel has been the belief that the person continues to exist after death in spiritual form. Just as the Aztecs believed that the dead one traveled to a special place depending on how he died, so orthodox Catholic belief in Mexico has been that the spirit of the dead may roam the earth. In some views, the spirit must undertake a lengthy and treacherous journey before finally reaching a lake or river leading to purgatory. Because of this, old rituals of burial dictated that the dead be buried with adequate provisions, such as a new pair of sandals, with which to undertake the journey. Prayers and appropriate rituals were required, not only to expedite the deceased's journey, but also to keep his soul from falling into the power of demons. Appropriate rituals honoring the dead were also necessary to satisfy the dead, lest he return to harm those who had neglected him. The dead have also been believed to return yearly, during the Days of the Dead.

Parallel to the Aztec belief about the deaths of children, is the Catholic view in Mexico that very young children who have died are free of sin, and being *angelitos* (little angels), they go straight to Heaven.[23] A strong belief in the supernatural and its potential influences on the lives of the people has led to many rituals and holiday celebrations, such as fiestas for patron saints or the Days of the Dead, established to honor hallowed supernatural beings and the spirits of the deceased so that their good will may be won and their wrath avoided.

Customs and views of care for the ill and the aged

The issue of providing care for the aged family member is perhaps one of the most powerful issues affecting the Chicano aged and youths alike. It strikes at the core of the conflict between traditional and modernistic values and practices.

As a reflection of tradition, Clark[24] indicates that in the San Jose suburban community of Sol Si Puedes, those parents considered to be *viejitos,* elderly whose children have married, are cared for by their children as a matter of custom. The barrio community criticized young people failing to provide a home for their parents. "Mexican American people are generally horrified at the common American practice of sending aged relatives to sanitariums or nursing homes when they become ill or senile."[24]

The traditional view of youths failing to provide for aged parents is a negative one in which these youths are considered to be sinful youths or ingrates who in the future will pay for their neglect by being equally neglected by their children. One typical Mexican story tells of a middle-aged father who decided on sending his aged father to a nursing home because he was becoming a burden. As the man prepared to transport his aged father to the car for the trip to the nursing home, he told his son to bring the grandfather's blanket. The child returned with the blanket and a pair of scissors. Noticing that the child had cut the blanket in two, the father angrily questioned the child about why he had done such a thing. The child responded that half of the blanket was for the grandfather, and that the other half of the blanket was for the father for whenever he, too, would be sent to the nursing home. At this point, the father decided against sending his father to the nursing home.

For most aged Chicanos, as is probably the case in other ethnic groups, to die alone and forgotten is to suffer a painful death. Murillo-Rohde[25] indicates that to Spanish-speaking people "one of the most frightening things that may happen to them or to their loved ones is to die 'all alone,' without any of their relatives being there." For this reason, Murillo-Rohde notes, Spanish-speaking visitors insist on staying with the ill or aged person even overnight, for fear that the person may die all alone.

Another important point is that some Spanish-speaking people view illness as punishment from God. This punishment must either be suffered or atoned for. In time of grave illness, loved ones of the ill person, or the ill person himself, may bargain with God or a saint by making a *manda,* a promise or personal sacrifice such as fasting, increased religiosity, or doing penance by walking on one's knees from one sacred cathedral to another. In some cases, the penitent may walk the distance between two chapels on his or her knees, making crosses on the road with the tongue every few paces. Murillo-Rohde cautions that before nurses or other mental health workers make judgments about the mental health of such a person, they should apply the principle that "behavior is relevant to time, place, and culture."[25]

Considering the strong religious influence among Chicanos, particularly among the aged, to what extent will Chicanos seek the aid of priests or *curanderos,* spiritual healers, in times of illness or distress? In a community-based study in Los Angeles, Karno and Edgerton[26] found that the family physician, not the curandero, was the preferred source of aid for illness. This finding is corroborated by Padilla, Carlos, and Keefe[27] who obtained responses from 666 Mexican American respondents in three Southern California cities. Percentages of mental health resources used by respondents included relative or friend *(compadre),* 36%; friend, 26%; doctor, 21%; priest or minister, 16%; and curandero, 2%. Priests and ministers were among the resources most utilized by these respondents, but curanderos were not. There also appeared a dichotomy in use of mental health resources involving native (more highly acculturated) respondents and immigrant (less acculturated) respondents, with the natives exhibiting a greater use of these resources. The researchers also note, "It is only within the immigrant group, thus, that the belief in the effectiveness of curanderos is retained, and even within this group, folk curing is recommended by a minority of respondents."[27]

Although it may still be true that Chicanos, particularly the aged, accept both the scientific and religious views of illness and its alleviation, the scientific viewpoint in general appears to hold more credibility. It may be mainly in the cases of the less acculturated immigrants or the very religious natives that Madsen's viewpoint may still be significant. She states that "the godless explanation of disease produced by modern science cannot be reconciled with ancient Mexican belief that supernatural beings inflict disease as punishment for wrongdoing and restore health when amends have been made."[28]

Should the health worker encounter an aged Chicano with a strong belief in the power of the supernatural, an acceptance of this thinking may aid in understanding the person. The practitioner need not accept these views but may understand them and how they affect the aged Chicano's behavior.

Views of death

The ritual sacrifices of ancient Mexicans and the continuing Catholic emphasis on spiritual life after death have combined to emphasize death as an important part of life and living in the traditional Mexican culture. Death has been so emphasized that at times parts of the Mexican culture are referred to as a death culture.

Paz[21] emphasizes that the modern world shuns death. Its mention in modern cities "burns the lips." In contrast, the Mexican "is familiar with death, jokes about it, caresses it, sleeps with it, celebrates it; it is one of his favorite toys and his most steadfast love."[20]

Moore[22] indicates that industrialized society is apt to suppress thoughts of death because such thoughts of death, the ultimate weakness, are incompatible with success, achievement, and power, which are emphasized in American society. Thus individuals oriented toward success, achievement, and power would be more apt to resent death or see it as a painful obstruction to their progress, whereas individuals oriented toward day-to-day living would see death as a natural and inevitable part of life and living and as the will of God.

Kalish and Reynolds[29], in a community-based study of death and ethnicity, report significant information about the attitudes toward death of Mexican American (Chicano) respondents. According to the researchers, Mexican Americans indicated a strong preference for *emotional release and expressiveness* over the death of a loved one, such as by crying, by a desire to touch the body of the dead, and by a desire to express mourning for a long period of time.

Mexican Americans were more *protective of family members' feelings,* by believing that a dying person should not be told of his or her impending death, that the respondent would find it difficult to inform an ill person of that person's impending death, and that respondents would not want children under 10 years of age to visit their deathbed.

Mexican Americans exhibited a significant *religious orientation* toward death by wishing for a priest or minister to be at their deathbed. This indicated a resigned attitude that death cannot be slowed or hastened by a will to live or die but that death is in the hands of God and that people should not be allowed to die, should they want to, since it is God who gives and takes life.

Kalish and Reynolds indicate that even though Mexican Americans wish to avoid thoughts concerning death of their loved ones, death is prevalent in their everyday thoughts. They hypothesize that the Mexican American "copes with these distressing thoughts by mastering death through ritual acts, through dwelling on it until the anxiety is worked through and through integrating it meaningfully into life."[29]

The Days of the Dead

The belief in the wandering of souls after death and of their returning to visit living relatives is evident in the Days of the Dead celebration. There are two different times in which the souls of adults and children are expected. All Saints Day, November 1, is the special day for the little angels, children whose return is expected at night, whereas the adults may come anytime in the day or night of October 31. The Day of the Dead proper, *El Día de los Muertos,* is November 2, a national holiday in Mexico. On this day, bread of the dead *(pan de los muertos)* in animal forms is sold in bakeries.[30] Toor also notes, "In the markets are sold special candlesticks and censers and beautiful candles of all sizes and shades; amusing toys for children — little coffins from which a skeleton jumps when a string is pulled; funeral processions with priests carrying a coffin, their bodies and hats made of shiny black and colored paper. . . ."[23] In many respects this holiday parallels the day of Halloween, celebrated in the United States.

A different type of Halloween is celebrated in Catholic homes in which a miniature altar is constructed in the honor of dead relatives. The altar for a child contains candles, flowers, toys, candies, and the child's favorite foods, placed there so that the returning child may eat them. Similar preparations are made for adults.[30]

During this time, families also visit cemeteries taking flowers, candles, and perhaps a toy for a dead child. In the past families would also take food and alcoholic beverages to feed the dead as well as to picnic among the graves. Recently, however, Mexican public health authorities have prohibited eating in the cemeteries because such practices have been declared nonhygienic. Drinking within the cemetery has also been prohibited because of excessive drunkenness and disruptiveness.

Kalish and Reynolds[29], however, report that in East Los Angeles, they were unable to find articles of the Day of the Dead, such as bread of the dead, in bakeries or candy skeletons in Mexican shops. Only a few persons knew what they sought and these persons could not tell them where to find these items. Kalish and Reynolds state, "Whether this change in custom implies some form of acculturation or whether it foreshadows development of views and values neither Anglo-American nor Mexican cannot be predicted."[29]

FUNERAL CUSTOMS AND PRACTICES

Moore[22] indicates that a funeral is the single most important family ceremony among Mexican Americans. A funeral is an occasion for family solidarity and family members travel from great distances to attend.

Moore adds that a reason for a conservation of customs connected with death is that, in general, it is the old people who die, and that surviving young relatives seek to "do what they (the deceased) would have wanted, even if these practices go against the beliefs of the survivors."[22]

Topography of a Mexican funeral. Despite variations in funeral practices, there are some basic elements generally associated with the crisis periods following illness and death: the wake, the funeral mass, the burial, and observances of mourning after the funeral.

Death and certification. Perhaps the greatest variation in basic funeral practices depends on whether the individual has lived and died in an urban or rural setting. In the rural setting, an individual fallen ill may request that a priest or minister come to his deathbed at home. In comparison, illness in the urban setting will more likely involve illness in an institution in which the patient is visited by family members. Many Spanish-speaking families seek to be with the dying continuously, to avoid the tragedy of the ill person dying alone, particularly in an institutional setting.

Clark[24] points out that in the suburban barrio setting families follow a combination of Mexican and American funeral customs. She states that when a person is thought to be dying "the priest administers the last rights, anointing various parts of the body with holy oil."[24] A mortuary is called to handle the embalming and preparations for the wake and funeral.

In contrasting the urban with the rural, Kalish and Reynolds[29] indicated that variations in death-related attitudes and behavior extend geographically as well as temporally, with greatest changes in custom evident in modern urban settings. In comparison, "the dead in many small towns today receive the same rituals that were performed a century and more ago. Furthermore, the geographical variability in attitudes and rituals is far from universal; it is not uncommon to find communities at considerable distance from each other using almost identical ceremonies."[29]

The wake. A *velorio* or wake may be held at a church, a funeral parlor, or at a home. The deceased individual's socioeconomic status generally sets the tone for the funeral. An announcement of one East Los Angeles mortuary lists a basic cost of $600 for basic professional services that consist of (1) professional preparation of the remains, (2) minimum use of mortuary facilities, (3) automotive and other equipment, (4) conducting graveside services, and (5) one funeral escort. Many extras are offered depending on the family's income and desires.

Whereas in urban settings a wake is generally conducted in a mortuary or funeral parlor, in rural settings, in accord with Mexican tradition, the wake is conducted in the home of the deceased or possibly in the home of a close relative.

In the Mexican wake wreaths, candles, and religious symbols surround the coffin, as they do in other cultures. In a mortuary the rosary may be said in Spanish, setting the tone for the rest of the ceremony. In general the elderly Chicanos are more familiar with the *rosarios* (prayers) than are the youths.

Lloronas, or professional wailers. Lloronas have traditionally attended wakes to add to the atmosphere of tearfulness in exchange for some money. Moore[22] reports that lloronas may also be among the mourners in wakes conducted in large urban cities such as Los Angeles.

As the rosary ends, the congregation is allowed to view the body before leaving the room. A segregation by sexes is evident in Mexican wakes. Moore adds that after the wake at the mortuary, condolences are given to the bereaved family members, and the wake moves from the mortuary to the home of the deceased.

In contrast to the urban wake, the more traditional wake in the rural setting is conducted in the home of the deceased.

Osuna[31] has given a personal account of a traditional Mexican wake held for an aunt (Tia Elena) in the home of a relative in Hermosillo, Mexico. In this setting, it is customary for the family of the deceased to prepare food and drink to offer the relatives who have traveled to the wake. Black coffee, tequila, and cognac are customary drinks, served with pieces of Mexican bread called *pelucas*.

An air of respect and somberness is customary throughout the wake. Proper conduct involving respect for the dead is considered the mature and appropriate behavior and is strongly emphasized. Only the spouse of the deceased is exempt from strict observation of custom since it is believed that the spouse is too grief-stricken to observe custom. At some time during the wake, a priest is called to conduct a rosary in the room where the coffin is located. Osuna indicates that the rosary of her aunt was mostly attended by women. She reports a noticeable segregation of sexes.

The wake generally lasts all night. It is the responsibility of family members to see that the body is not left unattended. Osuna[31] reports that the sons of deceased Tia Elena had slipped out for a few hours of sleep, a behavior strongly criticized by family members who had remained in the house. "It was felt that they would at least have taken turns standing guard over the body as is customary; the fact that they were very tired was no excuse because it was their duty to watch the body."[31] Continued vigilance over the body of the deceased is expected as a symbol of continuing love and respect toward the deceased. Thus one can understand the significance of "abandoning" the body.

The burial. For the funeral procession, Osuna indicates that the wishes of her aunt were honored in that her body was transported to the church, not by automobile, but more traditionally by pallbearers. At the church a Requiem Mass was given. Here the priest sprinkled the body with holy water, then incensed it. The casket was then transported by automobile to the grave site. A last view of Aunt Elena was allowed before the coffin was lowered into the ground for burial.

In comparison, in an urban Chicano funeral at the end of the Requiem Mass, the casket was placed in a hearse for transportation to the cemetary. The mourners may form a long automobile caravan that follows the hearse with headlights on and a "funeral" sign on the upper right-hand corner of the windshield. The caravan may travel either through the city streets or on the freeway en route to the cemetery. A long caravan may also include motorcycle patrol escorts to clear traffic if the family is able to afford these extras.

Kalish and Reynolds[29] stress the significance and importance for Chicano mourners of the last few moments during and after the lowering of the casket. Many Chicano mourners are not responsive to time boundaries, such as the lowering of the casket, as marking the funeral's end. For Chicanos, funeral rituals end when the group has expiated its expression of grief. "During such periods, the stifling of the natural outpouring of feelings seems unduly cold and cruel to the Mexican American. It takes time to properly appreciate and express one's feelings of respect and loss."[29] Thus in the traditional Mexican funeral, ceremonial events are scheduled so that one can not say that the funeral event begins at a specific time and it ends at another specific time.

In conclusion, Kalish and Reynolds present five points of importance regarding the funeral behavior of Mexican Americans. According to them, such behaviors include (1) strong emotionality of Mexican American women that frequently requires the use of tranquilizers, (2) appearance of the entire family at the funeral, (3) emphasis on the wake, (4) lack of previous funeral arrangements, and (5) low interest in cremation as a method of treating the body.

Observations after the funeral. It has been noted that the lowering of the casket into the ground does not mark the end of the funeral observations. In a way, though, this marks the beginning of an extended period of mourning, the *novena,* or the 9 days of mourning. During each of these 9 days following the funeral a rosary for the deceased is said by friends and relatives. Furthermore, out of respect for the deceased, the family reduces social activities and gaiety. In some cases, daily gravesite visits are made.

Toor[23] reports that in one Mexican village in Oaxaca, Mexico, a deceased man's widow sits in the corner of the hut with her *rebozo* over her face for 9 days, without speaking to anyone. It is only on the ninth day that she may go to the river to bathe in silent mourning, thus breaking the bond with her husband. On the tenth day she burns chile seeds, purifying herself and marking the end of her mourning and a reestablishment of communications with the world.

Among the religiously devout elderly Catholic Chicanos (mainly women), going to mass at 6:00 AM to pray for the recently deceased is also a common practice. Lighting candles and chanting hundreds of thousands of Ave Marias (Hail Marys) to the Virgin de Guadalupe (the Patron Saint of Mexico), or to a personal patron saint, such as *San Martin de Porres,* are practices to ensure that the soul of the beloved is protected from evil and will safely find its way to heaven. Candle lighting and rosary rituals are also observed indefinitely during appropriate holidays, such as Mother's or Father's Day or during the anniversary date of the loved one's death.

Some modern observations of death by young Chicanos have varied significantly from tradition. As an example, about 2 weeks after the fatal automobile accident of a Los Angeles graduate student, married and with a family, a dance was organized in his honor. Midway through the dance, a ceremony honoring the deceased was conducted in which a memorial plaque was presented to his widow. A prayer and eulogy followed the ceremony. Then the dance was continued.

Although a dance celebration was in clear contrast to traditional Mexican customs stressing somberness and mourning, the modern theme emphasized the continuity of life and living as well as the idea that death need not be a somber occasion but may instead be one for celebration. The Aztec concept of the cyclical nature of man may even be reestablishing itself. This seemingly new trend in modern Chicano attitudes toward death may actually reflect the ancient Aztec attitude towards death as an occasion for the celebration of life.

Burland[32] explains, "The Mexicans (ancient natives) found death wholly acceptable. It was the way of fate, and a natural event not to be regretted. It was not so much fatalism as a true recognition of the nature of human life."

CONCLUSIONS AND RECOMMENDATIONS

Aged Chicanos are a heterogeneous group with a common Hispanic heritage; they are a group of people in which individual personality differences need to be considered against the individual's cultural background. An examination of the individual's degree of acculturation may aid the health care worker in understanding the aged Chicano's cultural perspectives. For those aged Chicanos who are more Mexican culture-bound, Mexican traditions and customs will strongly influence beliefs and behaviors. However modern, urban stresses resulting in changes in the family structure are affecting the traditional role of the aged Chicano. Traditional and perhaps romanticized views of aging are being offset by hard realities of health and economic need.

Although modern, scientific views of illness appear to predominate among aged Chicanos, their behavior may still be influenced by a belief in the power of supernatural forces. Degree of religious identification and belief appears to be an important factor affecting the behaviors of many aged Chicanos. Religious and secular practices or ''different'' behaviors need be evaluated within the individual's cultural context before a judgement regarding the appropriateness of the behavior can be made.

In working with aged Chicanos, cultural factors need to be considered. These are some basic recommendations that, if observed in conjunction with techniques specific to the health care worker's professions of nursing, social work, and public health, will improve the worker-patient relationship as well as the quality of care given the aged Chicano patient.

Learn more about the cultural background of Chicanos and other ethnic minority groups. Attending lectures, workshops, symposiums, and classes is recommended to broaden the worker's knowledge of the diversity in human cultural practices and of those practices relevant to specific ethnic minority groups. This will also increase the worker's expertise in working with ethnic minority populations.

Maintain a respectful, understanding, and acceptant attitude toward aged Chicanos. An open attitude can do much to increase communications despite cultural or linguistic barriers or differences between worker and patient. Furthermore many aged Chicanos are proud of their culture and may become personally offended by a worker's neglect of or disregard for their culture. A patient's alienation or distrust will lead to reduced cooperation despite his cordial or polite mode of communication.

Communicate clearly. Hearing loss and language barriers may impair the aged Chicano's ability to understand. Understanding may be facilitated by slow, clear speech using words understandable to the patient. Technical words or similar-sounding words, for example, close, clothes, and closet, may confuse the patient despite the context in which they are used.

Allow the patient time to express himself or herself. An aged Chicano patient struggling to speak English may become discouraged or embarrassed over a perceived inability to communicate effectively and may thus fail to express his or her needs. The worker's patience and attentiveness can serve to encourage the aged Chicano patient to attempt to fully communicate his or her needs.

Be supportive. Some aged Chicanos, having had either little exposure to or a fear of institutional settings, become anxious or confused when entering large institutional settings such as medical centers. Much of this anxiety can be alleviated by reassurance and support, such as by satisfactorily answering the patient's questions.

Consider cultural practices before imposing change. Judging a person's cultural practices to be strange or backward reflects one's own value system and a misunderstanding of or lack of appreciation for the significance of a certain belief, ritual, or practice to the aged Chicano patient. A proposed behavioral change contrary to the patient's customs should be avoided, unless the practice is clearly detrimental to the patient's physical well-being. For example, many Chicanos are accustomed to eating chile with their meals. A patient with a stomach ulcer, however, would need to be informed of the dangers of continuing this custom.

Counter anger with patience and understanding. An aged Chicano who perceives being misunderstood, neglected, or abused may become frustrated and angry. This anger may engender corresponding anger in the worker. Countering anger with anger closes communications. Although the patient may ventilate his anger, if the worker attempts to discover the reason for the angry response the patient's anger will dissipate and constructive communication will follow as the patient sees that someone is listening.

Communicate with a quiet patient. A quiet, withdrawn, and inactive aged Chicano patient may be depressed. Aging and its losses, physically, psychologically, and interpersonally, can result in reactive depression. In some aged Chicanos, a growing sense of unrealized expectations, that is, family reverence and attention as a reward for old age, may result in depression, as well as in the fear of rejection, isolation, and dying alone. The worker's attentiveness can help the aged Chicano reevaluate cultural expectations and accept modern social changes.

Reinforce the patient contingent on desired behavior. Give the aged Chicano patient attention or praise for successfully completing a task. For many aged people, praise (reinforcement) from a younger person can have much significance, contributing to increased self-esteem while countering feelings of isolation and depression. Reinforcing the patient contingently, that is, on successfully completing a target behavior, will increase the probability of such behavior and will increase activity level and morale.

Study and learn from the aged. Aged Chicanos, as well as other people, have lived through many life experiences. Much can be learned not only by listening to what the patient says, but also by examining his behavior when he speaks. Much can also be learned about culture and personality from aged Chicanos by examining what life stresses the person has endured and how he has coped with them. Many aged Chicanos enjoy the opportunity to express opinions and tell about their life experiences, given the worker's intent to listen, observe, and understand.

REFERENCES

1. Torres-Gil, F. M.: Age, health and culture; an examination of health among Spanish-speaking elderly. Los Angeles, 1976, University of Southern California, Andrus Gerontology Center.
2. Graves, T. D.: Psychological acculturation in a tri-ethnic community, Southwestern J. Anthropol. **23:**337-350, 1967.
3. Penalosa, F.: Toward an operational definition of the Mexican American, Aztlan, Chicano J. Soc. Sci. Arts **1(1):**1-12, 1970.
4. Seward, G.: Clinical studies in culture conflict, New York, 1958, The Ronald Press.
5. Sotomayor, M., and Ortego, P. D.: Chicanos and concepts of culture, Boulder, Colo., 1974, Marfel Assoc.
6. Spiro, M. E.: The acculturation of American ethnic groups. Am. Anthropol. **57:**1240-1252, 1955.
7. Butler, R. N., and Lewis, M. I.: Aging and mental health, ed. 2, St. Louis, 1977, The C. V. Mosby Co.
8. Grebler, L., Moore, J. W., and Guzman, R. C.: The Mexican American People, New York, 1970, The Free Press.
9. Reusch, J., Jacobson, A., and Loeb, M. B.: Physical and mental health in acculturation. Psychol. Monogr. **62:**1-40, 1948.
10. Bern, D. J.: Beliefs, attitudes and human affairs, Monterey, Calif., 1970, Brooks/Cole Publishing Co.
11. Keesing, F. M.: Cultural anthropology—the science of custom, New York, 1965, Holt, Rinehart & Winston.
12. Skinner, B. F.: The design of cultures, Daedalus **90(3):**534-546, Summer, 1961.
13. Edmundson, M. S.: Los Manitos, a study of institutional values. In Edmundson, M. S., Madsen, C., and Collier, J. F., editors: Contemporary Latin American culture, Tulane University, 1968, Middle American Research Institute.
14. Montiel, M.: The Chicano family: A review of research, Soc. Work **18(3):**22-31, 1973.
15. Temple-Trujillo, R. E.: Conceptions of the Chicano family, Smith College Studies in Soc. Work, **45:**1-20, 1974-1975.

16. Bengston, V. L., Dowd, J. J., Smith, D. H., and Inkeles, A.: Modernization, modernity, and perceptions of aging: a cross-cultural study, J. Gerontol. **30(6):**688-695, 1975.

17. Maldonado, D.: The Chicano aged, Soc. Work **20(3):**213-216, 1975.

18. Crouch, B. M.: Age and institutional support: perceptions of older Mexican Americans, J. Gerontol. **27(4):**524-529, 1972.

19. Patterson, F. A.: Ancient Mexico, New York, 1962, Capricorn Books.

20. Portilla, L. M.: Pre-Columbian literatures of Mexico, Norman, Okla., 1969, University of Oklahoma Press.

21. Paz, 'O.: The labyrinth of solitude—life and thought in Mexico, New York, 1961, Grove Press, Inc.

22. Moore, J.: The death culture of Mexico and Mexican Americans, Omega **1(4):**271-291, 1970.

23. Toor, F.: A treasury of Mexican folkways, New York, 1947, Crown Publishers.

24. Clark, M.: Health in the Mexican American culture, Berkeley, 1970, University of California Press.

25. Murillo-Rohde, I.: Unique needs of ethnic minority clients in a multiracial society: a socio-cultural perspective. In American Nurses Association: Affirmative action: toward quality nursing care for a multiracial society, Kansas City, 1976, American Nurses Association.

26. Karno, M., and Edgerton, R.: Perception of mental illness in a Mexican American community, Arch. Gen. Psychiatry **20:**233-238, 1969.

27. Padilla, A. M., Carlos, M. L., and Keefe, S. E.: Mental health service utilization of Mexican Americans. In Miranda, M., editor: Psychotherapy and the Spanish-speaking: issues in research and service delivery, Los Angeles, 1976, University of California Spanish Speaking Mental Health Research Center.

28. Madsen, C.: A study of change in Mexican folk medicine. In Edmondson, M. S., Madsen, C., and Collier, J. F., editors: Contemporary Latin American culture, Tulane University, 1968, Middle American Research Institute.

29. Kalish, R. A., and Reynolds, D. K.: Death and ethnicity—a psycho-cultural study, Los Angeles, 1976, University of Southern California Press.

30. Green, J. S.: The days of the dead in Oaxaca, Mexico: an historical inquiry, Omega **3(3):**245-259, 1972.

31. Osuna, P.: El funeral de mi tia Elena, Omega **1(4):**249-258, 1970.

32. Burland, C. A.: The gods of Mexico, New York, 1968, Capricorn Books.

9 Health care and the aging American Indian

MARTHA C. PRIMEAUX

There is an increasing need to recognize and understand the cultural influences of ethnic people of color since these influences hinder or help in the delivery of health care. In the past, little or no attention has been paid the culturally different people, as our nation goes about developing and delivering health care to the majority of the population.

Included in the minority group of ethnic people of color is another emerging minority group—the aged. To fully understand the aged, one must understand his background. This has a special significance in relation to the Indian aged.

According to Butler and Lewis,[1] the aged are stereotyped and discriminated against because they are old. The aged members of ethnic groups of color therefore experience double discrimination in relation to skin color and age.

The purpose of this paper is to relate the historical aspects of the American Indians' health care and their customs and rituals in relation to health care. In addition, evolution of rituals and customs involving death and burial will be discussed. Because the American Indian population does not enjoy old age in large numbers, a history of the Indian health care system is necessary in order to understand why the American Indian has a short life expectancy.

Generalities relating to Indian health care are shared in an attempt to assist the reader in understanding how cultural and social forces shape attitudes and behaviors of the elderly in the native American (Indian) population. The elderly tend to remember the past. I have found that the elderly American Indian vividly remembers his past. I will share with the reader direct quotes from the elders of three different Oklahoma tribes; they were interviewed as I prepared this paper.

HISTORICAL ASPECTS

Throughout history groups of primitive people have had individuals or groups of individuals perform certain duties that were necessary for survival. Every known human society has developed methods to deal with illness and the disease process and thereby created a medicine. Rituals related to health care among the native Americans today differ little in philosophy from those practiced 500 years ago when Europeans first came to the New World.

Vogel[2] relates that the colonist sought the services of the native American healers to employ their medicinal herbs and sought native practices to restore the health of the sick, despite the fact that they were labeled pagan, savage, and primitive. It is known that the native Americans had a precise and long history of the uses and actions of the local herbs. It is believed now that more than 200 drugs listed in the *U.S. Pharmacopoeia* were known to native Americans.

130

It is further believed that native Americans were relatively free of disease before the European invasion brought white settlers to America. The white settlers brought with them diseases to which the native American had no immunity.[3] From this very early beginning, the health of native Americans continued to deteriorate. The native Americans were forcefully removed from the traditional herbs and flora that they used in health care practices. Adding insult to injury, the few native Americans that did survive the "long walks" and "trail of tears" were forbidden to practice openly the traditional customs related to health care. Some of the practices or rituals have been lost. Others were preserved by word of mouth, but the philosophy of Indian medicine remains.

The cumulative effects of all this are evidenced today in the health level of native Americans. No one would question the statement that the health status of American Indians is the lowest of all the races of people. There is a wealth of documentation from the statistics of the Indian Health Service and Bureau of Vital Statistics.

Federal policies toward the American Indians have been fraught with difficulties, but none are more evident than those concerning the delivery of health care services. Of 400 treaties negotiated with Indian tribes from 1778 to 1871, approximately 24 provided for some kind of medical care.[4] Health care delivered by the federal government was less than desirable. It was piecemeal, inconsistent, and crisis oriented.[5]

In the early 1800s, there were meager attempts by Army physicians to deliver care to American Indians on or near military posts.[6] Stories have been told and retold for decades that these attempts were not to aid the American Indian but to protect the military, as these diseases were smallpox and other highly contagious respiratory and gastrointestinal diseases.

Native Americans have long held a special relationship with the federal government. This relationship has been created and nurtured by hundreds of treaties and laws legislated and enacted between different Indian tribes and the United States government. In exchange for specific services, of which health is only one, these tribes surrendered millions of acres of land, water, and mineral rights. It was not the giving up of a certain number of acres that mattered. It was the giving up of a total environment that the native Americans knew, valued, and loved that hurt.

A number of different federal agencies have been responsible for health care of American Indians.[7] Treaties committing the federal government were introduced in 1832 through the Department of War. In 1849 Indian health service was transferred to the Department of the Interior and then to the present agency, the Department of Health, Education, and Welfare in 1955.

INDIAN HEALTH CARE

Despite 500 years of purposeful and systematic efforts to destroy or absorb the American Indians, they show no signs of disappearing. It has been estimated that there were approximately 600,000 Indians in the New World prior to the settlement of Europeans on the Eastern shores. The 1970 census counted approximately 800,000.[8] This number is disputed by both Indians and non-Indians and it is believed that probably 1 million American Indians is the more accurate number. Of course, one of the big problems with census numbers is the confusion over who is an Indian. The past century of policies and treaties with the United States Government compounds the issue.

There is no legislative or judicial definition used to identify an individual as an Indian. For census purposes, an American Indian has been identified on a self-declaration basis.

For other purposes, one must be an enrolled member of a recognized tribe and/or living on a reservation. In additional definitions, one must be able to trace at least one-fourth "Indian blood." There are other criteria listed by various tribes and agencies.

The years of social engineering have failed to bring native Americans into the mainstream of society. Despite the fact that many items used in health care rituals were antiquated, the native Americans continued to practice and utilize Indian Medicine and managed to preserve the tradition to an amazing degree under difficult times.

Attitudes toward disease and cure vary considerably with all groups of people. This is especially true with the native Americans as a race of people. The amount of time devoted to curative ceremonies varies from tribe to tribe, but causation is central to the process.[9]

In the literature written by Anglo anthropologists and historians and in my personal contacts with a variety of Indian tribes, disease causation is not related to the germ theory in totality even today. Instead, in both traditional and not so traditional beliefs, there is still evidence that diseases are believed to be caused by natural and supernatural forces.

In Indian medicine, diagnosis and treatment are not separated. The diagnostic procedure or ceremony itself is therapeutic. In a recent interview, a modern native medicine man stated, "There is no division or distinction of the head (meaning mental) and the body disease. The whole person is sick (motioning from head to feet) and the whole person has to be treated."

In further conversation, it became clear that the process of integrating the social, mental, and physical components is Indian medicine or Indian health care. The Indian Medicine Man has an advantage over Western medical doctors in that in the majority of instances he will have a personal knowledge of the patient. If not, certainly he will possess personal knowledge of the family. The medicine man said it succinctly, "It is not the form of medicine that is important but the spiritual aspect that has meaning to our Indian people."

A 69-year-old uncle subscribes to Indian medicine because he has no trust in Western medicine. Recently he stated, "In Indian medicine you see things (which might be classified as hallucinations*). It is an experience for only a privileged few." The fear and ignorance of westernized medicine makes him cling to proven customs. The Indian medicine treatment regime is symbolic to him. This symbolism is concrete and important to his belief in a cure or certain recovery.

Since I have been in the nursing profession, I have tried to explain happenings or situations in the Indian culture scientifically. Of course, there is not always success because some things just happen and are expected to be accepted as they are. When a situation is not understood, frequently its validity is doubted. Nonetheless, lack of documentation does not mean lack of value or worth. Similarly, because a happening or situation is not recorded or written does not mean it did not happen.

Benedick states that in describing medicine from different cultures, one sometimes oversimplifies and creates anthropological monsters.[10] This has certainly been the case with Indian medicine at various times in history.

An 82-year-old hospitalized Indian patient who utilizes both westernized and Indian medicine related, "Indian medicine is not the only medicine, or Indian religion the only religion, but if we measure everything by white people standards, then we will never

---

*My own interpretation.

understand the past or the future. Both worlds have value. Our tribal ways are important to us because we can understand them. They are proven, therefore are valuable.''

Many individuals in the social and scientific disciplines have come to recognize the value of American Indian cultural life. The English word for this newfound interest is ''ecology.''

Native Americans have not been known to impose their ways on other people;[11] therefore it is difficult for the Indian person, especially the aged, to understand and accept ways forced on them by misguided health care professionals. For example, the 82-year-old hospitalized patient wanted bread, potatoes, onions, and salt to eat but was told that they were not on her diet. ''I like coffee but they brought me milk. Milk does not agree with old people — only babies.''

There is evidence that many elderly people, not just Indians, lack an enzyme necessary for digestion of lactose. Nurses working with aged Indian people have long recognized that gastrointestinal problems occur after ingestion of whole milk and that the older Indian patient has learned to avoid milk. Many such examples of conformity were given in interviews with the elders of three different tribes. When patients do not conform, whether or not they are aged, they are labeled frequently as uncooperative, difficult, and a variety of other unflattering words.

DEMOGRAPHIC DATA

Since American Indians are markedly different in demographic, social, and economic characteristics from the general population, it is helpful to reveal these differences. According to the Indian Health Trends and Services of 1974,[12] half of the American Indian population is below the age of 18. The median age is 18.4 years, which is 10 years below the general population's age of 28.1 years. Whereas 19% of the general population is 55 years old or older, only 11% of the American Indian population is in this age group. Approximately 5% of the American Indians are over 65 years old.

The average Indian life expectancy for a child born in this decade is estimated to be 64 years, compared to the non-Indian life expectancy of 72 years. The statistics of 1967, which include the present group of elderly Indians, reveal an age expectancy of only 44 years.[13]

Diseases that are almost nonexistent in other populations are still leading causes of death in the Indian population. Although the Indian health service has made great strides in reducing mortality and morbidity statistics, diseases such as tuberculosis, gastrointestinal disorders, alcoholism, and vitamin deficiencies are exceedingly common.[14]

The types and multitudes of disease processes in any given population have direct correlation to the population's environment, economic status, education level, and traditional values. These variables in turn influence the individual's health and nutritional status as well as the availability and demand for health services.

The social conditions of the Indian communities, such as impoverished socioeconomic conditions, limited educational levels, substandard housing, poor sanitation, poor nutrition, and inadequate health services, all contribute to the high incidences of deaths caused by accidents, suicide, and diseases.[15]

There is no doubt that the needs and problems of elderly American Indians are parallel to those of the 20 million elderly of the general population. However, a number of factors compound these problems for American Indians. From an economic standpoint, American Indians compare unfavorably with the total population. A great majority reside on land that is low in productivity as well as in areas of limited opportunities for employment. The average income in 1971 for half of the Indian population was at the poverty level of less than $4,000 per year. Because of the American Indian relationships with the Bureau of Indian Affairs, the majority of the Indian population did not participate in any retirement programs or the Social Security program.[16] Consequently the sole source of income for elderly American Indians is welfare. Because of poverty, the elderly Indian families live in substandard housing with poor sanitation in remote reservation or non-reservation areas with low population densities.

Geographic distance isolates Indians from health facilities and other services. In some states such as Oklahoma, where services may exist within a reasonable distance, the lack of transportation or money needed to reach these services presents a major problem. In addition, in many areas these services are in a non-Indian environment with non-Indian personnel who have different cultural norms.

Poor nutritional status is a natural consequence of the poverty and low educational levels. Statistically speaking, American Indians suffering from a chronic disease suffer to a greater degree than others because of the accumulation of various social conditions of Indian life.

THE AGED AMERICAN INDIAN

Just as in the general Indian population, there is a lack of research concerning the aging process and the American Indian. Little written documentation is available because of their short life expectancies.

Vine Deloria[17] has stated that the best method of communicating Indian values is first to find points at which issues appear to be related. Tribal society is integrated toward a circular development. View the Indian society as a circle and the non-Indian as tangent lines; the points at which they intercept can be a related issue. Aging is a common social phenomenon that is experienced differently by both societies because of the diversity in the social and cultural milieu.

American Indian individuals do not exist in isolation. Indians derive their identity, purpose, and sense of self from participation in groups, their family, and their tribe. Tribal society must be experienced directly. It is holistic. When two unacquainted Indian individuals meet for the first time, the first question after name introductions is "What is your tribe?" It is the tribe that serves as a reference group. The self-image of American Indians depends on the values and attitudes that are accepted within the tribal socialization process. I have noted that as urban Indians reach middle age they begin to talk about "going back home to live" or wanting "to be buried on the reservation." Also, urban Indians, who have lived their entire lives in the city, will refer to the location of their tribe as home.

There is concern in some circles that there is a widening of the generation gap as the younger generation accepts more of the majority culture norms and disregards the elderly's. I do not subscribe to this point of view. There is evidence in many Indian reservations and Indian communities of a return by the younger generation to tribal ways and beliefs after they have experienced years of frustration and confusion because of the conflicting values of the two distinctly different cultures. Nancy Lurie[18] calls this movement "Indian Renascence." It is based on renewed desire among American Indians for economic self-development and for increased ethnic distinctiveness.

The extended family concept of the American Indian exists, despite some claims of family disorganization. The family as an extended unit is the base for the tribe. The family and the tribe reinforce each other and are support systems for the individual.

Because the American Indian's identity and ethnic integrity are maintained through the family and tribe, the elders in the tribe have been respected throughout history. Today they are looked to for knowledge and transference of tribal culture.

There is evidence that some tribes of Indians never totally experienced a generation gap. The elderly Indians may be limited in the ways they contribute to their family or community because of circumstances of the present. In some Indian communities the value of the elderly to the Indian community is being reassessed. However, Wendel Chino has said it well: "One of the greatest values of the Indian elderly is that they represent to us a repository."[19]

I recently attended a meeting involving the construction of a nursing home in which a long, heated debate took place. After some hours, one middle-aged gentleman reminded the others, both young and old, that the Indian way was to care for the elderly in their home. There was almost immediate consensus and the topic was not pursued any further.

The provision of nursing home care on Indian reservations maintained by Indian Health Services was one of the recommendations of the 1971 White House Conference on Aging. They thought that the nursing home would not be a substitute for caring for the Indian elderly in the home environment but would serve as an extension when the elderly needed specialized services.

Probably the most characteristic feature of old age is the slowing down of activity in all realms, physical, social, biological, and psychological. As individuals grow older, regardless of race, they cannot cope with stresses of environment or social change as easily. Certainly the American Indian has experienced a great deal of social change in past years.

Perhaps the main reason that the American Indian continues to cling to certain aspects of his culture in the face of change is that there is strength in Indian ways and beliefs. Many Indians agree with Vine Deloria[20] when he states that the major problem in white America is the Christian assumption that God gave man dominion over the creatures and elements. Indian religion teaches the opposite; Man has no divine dominion over anything except himself. He is only a part of the earth's cycle, coexisting with other forms of life, and respecting the spiritual significance of each life-giving resource.

The aged Indian, especially, is reverent toward the land. In an interview, one of the elders of the Ponca tribe stated, "I and the land move as one — season to season. As we meditate in our relationship with the sun and earth, we may miss valuable knowledge that is offered by the surroundings if we are not attentive."

Jaeger and Simmons[21] write that frequent references to the individual and environment have merit in administering care, but a more encompassing and broader view of aging is considered in a threefold content: the individual in his environment, in his culture, and in his society. The culture milieu provides enough to carry a given individual through a rewarding old age. Whereas the concepts of culture may not be clearly understood, the elements of the individual's social structure are as concrete as his physical environment and can be understood in terms of an individual's expectations.

Clark and Anderson[22] lend further credence to this philosophy when they emphasize that aging is a biological event highly influenced by one's culture. The perception of the value of old age depends on the ideals of the specific culture and not on the technological development of that culture.

To the American Indian elderly, the tribal culture provides a sense of self-worth. Self-esteem in old age is a crucial factor. In discussing growing old, my mother stated, "Growing old and dying is a fact of life. Everything that lives on this earth, also, has to depart from this earth." In my experience, Indian people are not ashamed of growing old nor do they fear death since they view these as parts of the continuing life cycle.

The social conditions of the Indian community make American Indians especially vulnerable to diseases that may become chronic. Our health care system is based on the ability of the individual to pay for health services. Since the majority of American Indians are at the poverty level, they are unable to buy health services. If American Indians live near an Indian Health Service facility and are eligible for service, frequently they view the hospital as a place to die and therefore will not seek health care as a preventive measure.

Accessability and availability of health services for the Indian aged are just links of a long chain of conditions that reinforce other social conditions that have led to the American Indians' present health level.

Caring for the chronically ill person is a challenge indeed. To care for American Indians with a chronic disease such as obesity, diabetes, hypertension, tuberculosis and, alcoholism it is necessary to understand the relationships among the social conditions that have been previously discussed.

In caring for the aged Indian individual, the non-Indian must remember that he is from a distinct cultural background. The Indian individual is proud, sensitive, and desperately wants to maintain his self-worth, which is his "Indian-ness."

Attitudes cannot be legislated but health professionals caring for the Indian aged may develop a framework of care that respects differences and emphasizes humaneness. There is much strength and knowledge that can be shared if the right framework is projected in searching for answers.

DEATH AND BURIAL RITUALS

Much of the literature on death and dying contends that the naturalness of death for the aged has not been generally accepted by mankind as a whole. In the Indian culture, I believe the opposite is true. Perhaps this is directly related to the fact that Indian children have experiences with death throughout their lifetimes. They are not shielded from these experiences. Because of the short life expectancy and the high incidence of death caused by accidents and diseases, Indian children experience death before they have the capacity for full understanding. In addition, children of all ages are permitted to attend funerals. The Indian people in general look on death as a natural and inevitable part of the life cycle. The Indian aged accept it as a part of life because they understand the forces of life and the forces of nature.

There are no highly developed theories of life after death in the traditional Indian culture. Death fulfills the destiny of the American Indian and is the completion of the life cycle. There is no separation of the body and spirit. Historical evidence has been unearthed from Indian burial grounds containing items to aid the individual in changing from this world to the spirit world. The placing of items in or near the grave or in the casket exists today.

Indian religion probably has its greatest meaning in the face of death. The grief process that occurs with the loss of a loved one is not translated into feelings of guilt or sin. Perhaps the idea of the death song, which was sung when a man faced certain death, can assist in understanding the phenomenon of death among American Indians today. In the history of the death song, the individual had no sins or personal failures to confess. He became humble and sang of his deeds while facing death. Today many funerals in the Indian culture can be looked on as a celebration of the deceased individual's good life. A feast is given on the day of the burial and items such as shawls, blankets, cloth, and money are given away by relatives of the deceased. It is not unusual for the funeral service to be conducted in the home. In some Indian communities, the local Indian church or school may be utilized for the service. There are a variety of rituals and ceremonies associated with death and burial. Some are a combination of Christian beliefs and traditional Indian religion. When describing the use of cornmeal and burning of cedar at one ceremony, my mother cautioned me about giving too much information, lest it be used in opposition. There are probably as many ceremonies as there are Indian tribes.

Whether in the home or the hospital, when there seems to be evidence that life cannot be sustained the family becomes concerned for preserving the human dignity of the dying patient. Perhaps this is a carryover of the death song. The Indian family has a need to express grief as much as any other race of people. The stoicism often attributed to the American Indian people is evident under some conditions at some times. However, Indians have the same feelings as any other individuals who experience a loss and these feelings need to be expressed. The Indians prefer not to express their grief outwardly or in the presence of individuals they do not know. Instead, Indian individuals will find a time when alone or with other members of the family to display their feelings of loss.

Although the family may be lonely, they are not alone. The extended kinship system of the Indian family, as well as tribal members, serves as a strong support system in times of crisis. "What is passed and cannot be prevented should not be grieved for. It is not what you take from life but what you give to it that is important." Such a philosophy was given in 1961 to me by an elderly member of my extended family on the death of a family member.

In discussing life and death and the place of religion in American Indian life today, a 60-year-old man who is active in the native American church stated, "Religion is very important to me and my tribe. Belief in the Great Spirit sustains me in difficult times. The white man took our land, destroyed our home and part of our tribal life but he cannot take our religion. It was our religion that was important to us in survival. Had our religion been destroyed, the American Indian would have been destroyed."

Over 1,000 elderly American Indians representing 171 tribes came together to speak of needs at a conference on aging in 1976.[19] They made no extravagant demands. They asked only to live out their lives with the assurance that their basic needs would be met. They identified one other need — to remain Indian so that they may be able to pass on their cultural heritage.

REFERENCES

1. Butler, R. N., and Lewis, M. I.: Aging and mental health: positive psychosocial approaches, ed. 2, St. Louis, 1977, The C. V. Mosby Co.
2. Vogel, V. J.: American Indian medicine, Norman, Oklahoma, 1970, The University of Oklahoma Press.
3. Report on Indian health: task force six, Indian health: final report to the American Indian Policy Review Commission, Washington, D.C., 1976, U.S. Government Printing Office, p. 27.
4. Ibid, p. 28.
5. Ibid, p. 27.
6. The Indian Health Program of the U.S. Public Health Service, Washington, D.C., 1974, U.S.

Department of Health, Education, and Welfare, p. 30.

7. Report on Indian health, p. 27.

8. Public Health Service: Indian health services and trends, Washington, D.C., 1974, U.S. Department of Health, Education, and Welfare.

9. Primeaux, M.: Caring for the American Indian patient, Am. J. Nurs. 77(1):91-94, Jan., 1977.

10. Benedict, R.: Patterns of culture, Boston, 1959, Houghton Mifflin Co., p. 47.

11. Joe, J., Gallerito, C., and Pino, J.: Cultural health traditions: American Indian perspectives. In Branch, M. F., and Paxton, P. P., editors: Providing safe nursing care for ethnic people of color, New York, 1976, Appleton-Century-Crofts, p. 83.

12. Public Health Service, p. 10.

13. Summary report of National Tribal Chairman's Association, Phoenix, 1976, National Conference on Aging.

14. Public Health Service, p. 10.

15. Primeaux, M.: American Indian health care practice, Nurs. Clin. North Am. 12(1): March, 1977, p. 58.

16. Toward a national policy on aging, Washington, D.C., Nov. 28 through Dec. 2, 1971, White House Conference on Aging, p. 199.

17. Deloria, V.: We talk, you listen, New York, 1970, The MacMillan Co., p. 12.

18. Levine, S., and Lurie, N. O.: The American Indian today, Baltimore, 1968, Penguin Books, p. 295.

19. Summary report of National Tribal Chairman's Association, p. 1.

20. Deloria, V.: God is red, New York, 1973, Grosset and Dunlap Publishers, p. 96.

21. Jaeger, D., and Simmons, L. W.: The aged ill: coping with problems in geriatric care, New York, 1970, Appleton-Century-Crofts, p. 270.

22. Clark, M., and Anderson, B. G.: Culture and aging, an anthropological study of old Americans, Springfield, Ill., 1967, Charles C Thomas, Publisher, p. 3.

part IV
PSYCHOSOCIAL NEEDS OF THE AGING

The three chapters comprising this section describe and elaborate on some of the significant psychosocial needs of the elderly.

Chapter 10 by Rosemary Murray focuses on an overview of psychosocial aspects of aging. Murray's belief, not held by the general population, is that old age can indeed be "the flower of life, in full bloom."[1] Murray's positive attitude is reflected in her writing. She approaches aging in a humanistic manner and views it as the final stage of the holistic process of growing and living. She emphasizes the importance of planning for retirement in terms of financial and psychological needs. Differences between Eastern and Western cultures' philosophies regarding aging are compared and contrasted. Murray points out that the dying process is not easily accepted in our culture with its orientation toward activity and self-control. Only when we are able to acknowledge dying as a part of living can we realistically begin to appreciate life as a holistic totality of the birth, growth, and death cycle.

In Chapter 11 Nancy Woods examines the subject of sexuality and aging. Woods presents research findings of studies concerning elderly people and their need for sexual expression. Sexual taboos and the many constraints toward open expression of sexuality, which have been traditional features of our society, are explored and depicted in detail. Woods expresses the hope that the concept of sex as a natural function will be accepted as part of the aging process by gerontological nurse specialists as well as by other nurses.

Paulette Robischon and Alice Akan describe the role of the family with elderly parents in Chapter 12. Developmental tasks of the aging family are summarized and illustrated with a pertinent case vignette. Issues covered in this chapter are retirement, relocation, socialization, loss, and role change. Most helpful for the reader are the provocative questions raised. These questions provide many meaningful suggestions for the gerontological nurse who works with families with elderly parents.

It is hoped that the themes and philosophies expressed by the authors will be appreciated by the gerontological nursing practitioner. If these philosophies are acted on by nurse practitioners in their care of the aging, an enhanced quality of care and of life will result.

REFERENCE

1. Murray, R. M.: Personal communication, June, 1977.

10 Psychosocial aspects of aging

ROSEMARY MURRAY

SOCIETAL ATTITUDES TOWARD THE AGED

How a given society chooses to deal with aging and the aged depends on a variety of psychological, sociological, and economic factors. Knowledge of these factors, unfortunately, does not always offer clear explanations for specific societal attitudes toward aging.

Primitive societies

One might expect that more advanced societies, especially those characterized by advanced knowledge, technology, and affluent life-styles, would be supportive and acceptant of their aged populations. This does not seem to be the case as de Beauvoir[1] points out in her exploration of multisocial attitudes and practices toward the aged. Most of the societies studied (both advanced and primitive) seemed to reflect extremely negative attitudes toward aging, such as reduced social status and input, discrimination, and, at the extreme, annihilation. However, a few primitive societies, for example, the Aranda tribe of Australia, the Zanda tribe of the Sudan, and the Ojibway tribe of North America, perceived old age as virtuous, mystical, or magical and tended to treat the aged with deference and respect. Primitive cultures relied heavily on the preservation of tradition, spoken history, and the belief in supernatural causation for basic social structures and practices. Since the tribal elders had roles as leaders and law or code enforcers, historians, and close communicants with "spiritual influences," this may have accounted for their relatively favorable position.

Powerful or prestigious positions for the aged in primitive or nomadic societies were, however, a rarity. Usually the aged were disposed of intentionally by murder, with or without the benefit of tribal ceremony, or by forced suicide. The aged were also disposed of "unintentionally" through abandonment as tribes migrated or through starvation when the aged were purposely ignored in food rationing as supplies fell short.

It should be remembered that in primitive societies the primary force governing most social behavior was survival, and in most cases, survival of the fittest. It is not surprising then, that both extremes of the age spectrum, the very young and the very old, were not likely candidates for survival. The plight of female infants, the sick, the weak, and the deformed was equally bad. These societies could not and would not nurture unproductive and abnormal members. Social status and life itself were based on the ability of the individual to contribute to the tribe's maintenance and perpetuation. "Life insurance" in such societies could only be guaranteed to productive men and reproductive women.

Agricultural societies

The aged fared considerably better in the more stable agricultural societies. With the acquisition of land, the development of animal husbandry, and increased stores of food surpluses, migration in search of food became unnecessary. In addition, these same factors helped to ensure the support of the elderly since maximum productivity by every member was not a necessity in agrarian societies. The aged could still perform lighter but necessary tasks that contributed to the general welfare. The aged became the collective repository for a wealth of knowledge, experience, and skills necessary for the growth and development of a culture based on tradition, verbal history, and strong, common bonds between family and community groups.

The aged retained power by virtue of their knowledge, accumulated property, and ability to make good judgments based on a lifetime of practical experiences. The role of family or community elder carried with it the respect of all community members. Deference to and status of the aged in agricultural societies marked a high point for the aged in our social evolution. Some of this status is retained today in European and American farming communities. Deference to the aged may also be seen in rural, highly traditional, and religious communities.

Technological societies

In industrial and highly technological societies, the status of the elderly has declined. It seems ironic that those people who have experienced and survived more major social changes than any other group should now be considered obsolete by the society that emerged only through their creative, resourceful, and adaptive participation in social progress. Nevertheless the aged in Western societies have yet to achieve the preferred social status and degree of life satisfaction enjoyed by the majority of the aged in agricultural societies.

WESTERN AND EASTERN CULTURAL ATTITUDES TOWARD THE AGED

At this point it is also necessary to draw some distinctions between Western and Eastern cultures regarding the status of the aged. Whereas Eastern cultures generally have a lower economic standard of living, the aged of most Eastern cultures enjoy greater social status than do their Western counterparts.

There are two major reasons for this apparent cultural discrepancy between the East and the West. In Eastern cultures, life is viewed as a holistic process. Every aspect of the life process is experienced and accepted as a natural event. Therefore old age and death receive the same respect and appreciation as any other part of the life process. Some Eastern cultures venerate old age as a holy state of great religious significance and offer the aged considerable respect. In other Eastern cultures, death is not considered a terminal event, but rather a transitional period in which the individual progresses from a lesser to a higher plane of existence. Reincarnation is not so much a rebirth as a renewal of life. Viewed in this context, old age is but a phase in the continuous flow of life.

Western cultures hold a different concept of the life process. Their tendency is to perceive life less holistically and more as a series of stages or periods of development in which each stage is viewed according to its own relative social worth. The life process is not seen as a whole.

In our technological society, positive attitudes are shown toward youth, physical beauty, and economically rewarded productivity. Since childhood and young adulthood are directly related to one or more of these characteristics, they are considered optimum periods in the life cycle. Late adulthood and old age show marked decrements in these characteristics and receive proportionately less of our social esteem. Those individuals no longer young, no longer physically beautiful according to "youthful norms," and no longer the recipients of large economic rewards for productivity are viewed negatively by our society.

Whereas we have intellectual awareness of death, the dying process is not accepted as a natural event in the life process. Throughout history we have failed to accept the reality of death. In early life death appears distant and does not seem to be a real part of one's life. As we age death is thought to be something that happens only to others. In old age talk centers around the proximity of or even the wish for death, yet the elderly tenaciously cling to life.

Chronic illness and old age are considered negative states, often found in association, that confront the individual and society with the unavoidable reality of death. Because of the negative value attached to death and all events associated with it, we isolate or ignore the chronically ill and the aged. Long-term care facilities, old age homes, and retirement villages are excellent examples of how our society avoids this confrontation with old age and death. The expression "out of sight, out of mind" is perhaps enacted through these social institutions. The unfortunate consequences of such negative social values are denial of and destruction of many opportunities for self-fulfillment and dignified death, which are bound to the final years of life for each of us.

Everyone, but especially those in the health care professions, should become familiar with Kubler-Ross' approach to death and dying.[2] She believes that accepting death is not easy for our culture but that acceptance is necessary if we are to assist those who are dying and allow them to do so with dignity. Whether one accepts her five stages of dying (from denial to acceptance) is not particularly important. It is important to acknowledge death, deal with it, and prepare for it; but it is most important to incorporate it into our concept of living. Only then can we begin to appreciate life, including death, as a total process. The aged may then receive the respect due those who are living to the fullest measure the complete life cycle.

Another reason for the cultural discrepancy between East and West is the strong and persistent ideology of familism[3] fundamental to many Eastern cultures. Familism describes a kinship system in which the patriarch or family elder and his wife exercise complete authority over all family members (that is, anyone related to the patriarch or his wife by birth, marriage, or adoption). This authority extends to household activities, jobs, money, property, and, throughout most of history, marriage. This ideology of familism is reinforced by reciprocal paternalism and filial piety. Additional support for familism is derived from reverence for ancestors.

In varying degrees the pattern of familism is being broken down as more and more Asian countries undergo rapid westernization, mechanization, and urbanization. To the extent that this patriarchal kinship system remains operative, the aged enjoy status, self-respect, and considerable assurance of maintaining their social welfare and support systems.

Traditionally China, Japan, India, and the Philippines have demonstrated great respect for the aged. Their social complex provides for the aged who would not necessarily fall under the kinship system. The Chinese model of "vegetarian halls" offers refuge for the aged without relatives who might otherwise be relegated to weak and poorly run government welfare systems. Vegetarian halls are institutions of worship that willingly accept aged without kin, provide for their material needs, and offer them self-respect. In return the aged perform duties necessary for the maintenance of the spiritual sanctuary. In addition, these vegetarian halls, so named for their compulsory vegetarian diet, provide the aged with a quasi-family structure that incorporates family roles, status, fellowship, and support. The obvious benefits of such institutions are that the aged retain their self-respect, are aware that they are making a social contribution, and derive considerable social security.

Other institutions, such as those related to neighborhoods, guilds, and trades, provide similar benefits for those people outside the kinship system. The Philippines utilize the extended family concept whereas Eastern and Far Eastern countries practice adoption of young and old to provide support and security for the aged. The idea of family is pervasive throughout most of the social structuring that respects and supports the aged. Familism and family-like institutions are found predominately in those Eastern cultures that preserve the social complex of patriarchy and filial piety.

Contrary to popular belief, Western cultures do have family patterns that can be supportive of the aged. We do not have patterns distinctive of either the nuclear family (mother, father, and unmarried children) or of the extended family (all persons related by blood, marriage, or adoption). What we see is a complex network of relationships that might best be termed a modified extended family.

The modified extended family assigns the aged peripheral or secondary status as opposed to the primary status of the family patriarch in Eastern cultures. Because of the secondary status of our family elders, respect and material support for them depends on the younger individual's degree of affection for and willingness and ability to voluntarily assist elderly parents financially. The elderly in our society may hope for filial respect and support, but they can not be assured of it as family elders of the patriarchal system can be.

Western cultures are more mobile and equate living alone or in nuclear family settings with personal independence. Even the aged express this type of independence by remaining in their own homes, independent of their children, as long as possible. Less than 10% of three generational families live together under the same roof. If they do live in this fashion it is usually because the older person is either too sick or poor to live alone.[5] For many of the aged, home ownership represents the greatest portion of their capital investment, especially when income is based only on pensions and social security benefits. Many people over 65 years of age (58%) do own their own homes. Even though the elderly enjoy owning their own homes and the sense of familiarity, security, and independence it brings, property taxes and home maintenance represent unusual financial burdens for those on fixed incomes.[6]

Separation from parents who maintain homes in inner city areas becomes inevitable as their children move to the more socially attractive suburbs or are forced to relocate because of employment. Also, many of the elderly are beginning to relocate to areas where the climate is more temperate. California, Florida, and the Southwestern states have shown a proliferation of elderly populations and retirement communities. Elderly from Northeastern states frequently migrate to Florida for the winter and return to their homes during the warmer summer months. This practice of temporary relocation obviously exists only for those elderly of sufficient financial means.

Because of the ease, accessibility, and relatively low cost of transportation and telephones, communication between the generations is at a fairly high level. Holidays and special occasions usually bring the generations together periodically throughout the year. Although grandparents are not seen as patriarchs, there is a reciprocal fondness between grandparents and grandchildren. Visiting grandparents is a frequent and pleasant experience for children in Western cultures. These practices encourage communication and intergenerational mixing.

The difference between family patterns of East and West may be more attitudinal than anything else. This difference in the Western culture is, more often than not, translated into a lack of esteem and role significance for the elderly.

SOCIOCULTURAL CHANGE

As the youngest and most technologically advanced of all western societies, the United States prominently demonstrates the problems of rapid sociocultural change. Although rapid change affects every age group, the elderly are required to make the most marked adaptations. Their cultural precedents frequently came from rural communities, from foreign countries, and from a time when social change was considerably less dynamic. Whereas we were once concerned with "generation gaps" we are now seeing "intrageneration gaps" resulting from constant social flux. Children of the 1960s have different social values from children of the 1970s, even though they may be siblings from the same family group. The degree of life satisfaction of both young and old adults depends on their ability to adapt to rapidly changing social attitudes, practices, and environmental influences.

The aged are somewhat disadvantaged in this rapid social and technological evolution because there are no historical role models for them to draw on for social reference. They must carve out a role for themselves in a culture that has ambiguous attitudes toward aging. The roles that the elderly recognize from their own youth and young adulthood no longer fit comfortably into the current social structure. Roles for the elderly and their corresponding social interactions that were appropriate in the first half of the century are no longer appropriate in the second half. The disparity between obsolete role expectations and current cultural demands of the aged creates considerable psychosocial conflict in the American culture.

This type of role conflict is even more pronounced for the foreign-born. Many difficulties arise from acculturation. Clark[4] offers testimony from elderly subjects of subcultural and ethnic communities. These elderly could exhibit only personal characteristics that they deemed appropriate to the role of the aged person in their own parent cultures. Even though these aged persons were acculturated, they were unable to emulate the aged role as defined and prescribed by the American culture. Because of this conflict with society, psychopathology became extreme and institutional psychotherapy was necessary for resolution of this conflict. Of course these represent extreme cases, but neither role conflict in the aged nor the emotional distress it causes is unusual.

PROBLEMS CONCERNING THE AGED

In the past the aged were not considered to be a problem of social concern because by the time an individual became physically old and could no longer work he was also very close to death. Today the aged live longer, are generally healthier, and "retire" from the work force at about 65 years of age. The aged, by virtue of their growing numbers and visibility, have become a social problem. I have labeled aging as a problem and defined "problem" as a perplexing situation or a question proposed for solution. The growing number of active, relatively healthy, and potentially productive retired persons has created the need to identify and give meaning to a new phase of considerable duration in the life cycle. Consequently we have turned to our scientific resources for solutions to this problem.

Aging, as the life process, is a holistic process. Gerontology, as should any other life-science study, should attempt to utilize a holistic approach in its investigations. In the past, studies of the aging process concentrated primarily on disease states found in the aged. Such a pathological orientation did little to encourage positive social attitudes toward aging. If research on aging is to be of real value, it must examine health as well as disease. We have a tremendous need for knowledge about normal aging. We must also establish a positive social climate that will nourish and utilize research concerning theories of normal aging. According to Busse, "attempts to prolong life which fail to also improve the lot of the aged [are of] limited value. In fact, the mere prolongation of life may be more of a detriment than an asset for all concerned."[7] The concept that old age and death are normal processes in the life process must be incorporated into our social awareness. If future studies result in knowledge that can prevent or retard the pathology frequently associated with aging or old age, such information will probably do little to prevent the normal consequences of eventual aging, which appear at this time to be inescapable and universal. Even in the best of all future worlds, concludes Butler,[8] where negative environmental, genetic, and disease entities are removed so that life may be lengthened and enhanced, we must still accept that old age and death are part of the human experience.

The acceptance of human mortality need not predispose us to think of old age as a disease state. Although 85% of the aged have some form of chronic disease,[9] most of the aged need little assistance from others in their daily lives. It must be remembered that many items are included in this chronic disease category that do not alter appreciably the quality of life. Hypertension is considered a chronic disease but it may be controlled with medication and thus may minimally affect the individual's ability to function. The same may be true for senile diabetes controlled by medication, diet, or exercise. Decreases in vision and hearing are often termed "chronic diseases" that frequently affect the aged, yet with glasses and hearing aids the individual may have minimal loss of sensory input. When "chronic disease" is a term used to describe all types of decreased or altered physical functions, it is easy to see why so few of the aged are truly incapacited by "chronic disease." In fact, only about 4 of every 100 aged men and women in the United States live in institutions.[10] Many aged living in institutions are there because they are homeless rather than chronically ill.

INDIVIDUAL DIFFERENCES IN THE AGED

Every phase of the life cycle is characterized by constant change along a continuum of psychological, sociological, and biological interactions with the environment. These interrelationships become more complex with age since they are influenced by a lifetime of interchange and adaptations. As we mature, human development, especially from the psychosocial aspect, becomes highly differentiated. The aged develop personality traits and patterns of psychosocial interactions unique to the individual. According to Neugarten, "we can expect differences between individuals to be accentuated with time as educational, vocational, and social events accumulate one after another to create more and more differentiated sets of experiences from one person to the next."[11] A high school class, for example, may be more alike at graduation in terms of life patterns, interests, and abilities than they will be at age 25, 40, or 60 years.[12]

Too frequently we have tried to cluster all older people into a group termed "aged" with the expectation that predictions about the group will have applicability to each individual. In general there are some characteristics that do apply to all aged but, more often than not, we see exceptions rather than conformity. Many have personal experience with people who are "old" at 40 and "young" at 80. Certainly Madame Alexandra Baldina-Kosloff, former prima ballerina with the Bolshoi Theater Ballet of Moscow, is a striking example of this incongruity. At age 91, she still conducts and participates in dancing classes held in her Southern California studio. Jack LaLanne, physical fitness expert, recently celebrated his sixty-second birthday by swimming a mile in Long Beach Harbor, pulling 76 children in 13 boats behind him. Howard Rusk, M.D., at age 76 continues to expand his vision of rehabilitation for all the disabled as founder and director of the Institute of Rehabilitation Medicine in New York City. Picasso continued painting his masterpieces into his 90s. Winston Churchill remained politically active in his 80s. These represent but a few of the notable exceptions to the stereotype of old age. Similar exceptions are to be found in many of our own active parents, grandparents, and great grandparents.

DISENGAGEMENT THEORY

Such active and involved older persons would not appear to support the theory of disengagement proposed by Cumming and Henry in 1961. This theory maintains that as people age there is an inevitable, gradual, and mutually satisfying process of disengagement from society.[13] Disengagement, according to the theorists, is a universal process whereby the individual and society gradually withdraw from each other so that when death of the individual occurs there is minimal functional social disruption.

From the beginning the disengagement theory has been opposed, especially by those in the psychological and sociological sciences. Henry has modified her theoretical approach to recognize those elderly who persist in life-styles of engagement and those who engage in other activities after they have disengaged from their former social roles. Cumming has adhered closely to the basic outlines of the theory of disengagement. Rose describes Cumming as a functionalist who, he says, extends the universal "functional prerequisites of culture to include the necessity of society to pre-adjust to death." Rose contends that functionalists assume "that whatever is, must be" and that they invalidate observations by exaggerating them. They also ignore historical trends and minimize cross-cultural variations. Rose identifies certain new trends that he believes are counteracting forces that promote disengagement of the elderly. Briefly summarized, these trends are as follows:

1. Larger numbers of people over 65 years old are more vigorous and less likely to disengage because of disease and frailty.
2. Increased economic security of the elderly may allow them greater opportunity to engage in more costly leisure activities.
3. The aged are more socially involved in activities to raise their status and privileges.
4. Earlier retirement may allow the elderly to form new reengagements that may extend into late life.
5. The types of engagements available to older people have increased in number and openness.[14]

Some authorities do not consider total disengagement inevitable, except shortly before death. For those who perceive that death is near, some form of generalized disengagement may become evident. Elias et al.[15] indicate that there is "some indirect evidence that young children, as well as elderly adults, who are dying exhibit disengagement behavior."

ACTIVITY THEORY

There are probably more proponents of the activity theory than there ever will be for the disengagement theory. The activity theory is based on the assumption that the degree of life satisfaction or morale is related to the degree of social involvement or role activity of the aged individual. In reviewing past studies on the aged, Palmore found that most evidence supports the activity theory, showing a positive relationship between activity or social interaction and life satisfaction. For the majority of normal aging persons, continued engagement in some form of social activity seems to be typical. Furthermore the amount of activity is strongly related to past life-styles and external factors.[16] Past life-styles, external factors, and personality patterns probably hold the key to the particular pattern of adaptation for each individual as he ages.

RETIREMENT

Retirement is a critical changing point in the aging process. Several factors are of major concern at retirement. Most Americans have a work orientation. From work we derive role identification, job-related social interactions, achievement, and financial rewards. In addition, leisure time and activities are justified as a relief from work. Presently retirement represents a loss or at least a decrease in work-related roles, social interactions, and money and a feeling of guilt related to protracted leisure time.

Retirement does not need to represent absolute role loss. It can mean role change to an equally satisfying role. Aged individuals whose careers have involved creativity and intellectual challenge, such as artists and academicians, have continued in these or similar role activities beyond the retirement period and maintained a relatively high degree of life satisfaction. In fact, persons who have chosen art as a second career after retirement were just as "engaged" as those who chose art as a first career.[17] What is needed is to abandon forced retirement and institute voluntary retirement. Thus those people still physically and intellectually capable and involved can maintain their productive social roles until they voluntarily relinquish them. Such a practice will then result in a gradual blend of social involvement and aging rather than in the crisis retirement creates today. Furthermore intellectual and creative aspects should be utilized in role change after retirement. Perhaps role activities for the aged could include work that draws on the individual's creative capacities that have lain dormant during years of work in productive but noncreative areas. Gerard, for example, believes that "the dominant challenge of aging at the human level is at the higher reaches of organization where the integrative functioning of the nervous system permits a rich and labile behavior, and that the social organization of men uses and rewards such behaviors."[18]

It is necessary that the individual plan for retirement. Financial planning is essential if the years after retirement are to offer any type of financial security. Retirement is usually not an event considered in depth by the young adult. Perhaps this relates to our avoidance of the thought of our personal old age and our concerns with contemporary problems related to jobs, children, and the like. Financial planning can help provide some of the resources necessary to maintain some degree of one's acquired life-style and allow the individual a broader range of leisure activities.

Finally, we must develop a pattern of leisure activities that has personal meaning that can be adapted or expanded to fit the postretirement period. We must learn to seek out and cultivate those leisure activities that contribute to our sense of self-worth and social value. In this way a life-long positive attitude toward leisure activities can assist the aged in substituting meaningful leisure activities for job activities following retirement.

STUDIES OF AGING

The results of the Bonn Longitudinal Study of Aging should be significant in the orientation of future research in aging. The investigators conclude that gerontology should be defined as a "science of different forms or 'patterns' of aging and their biological, social and ecological correlates. Patterns of aging would then be defined in terms of biological, social and perceptual-motivational processes."[19] Theories related to psychological development and social roles and interactions should be used as instruments for the assessment of the individual's life course in late adulthood. The investigators conclude by stating that "any kind of prediction of adjustment to aging or planning services and support for the aged would require a systematic assessment of the different 'subsystems' which define the aging process in a given individual-environment interaction." These subsystems represent a host of factors including personality, intellect, life satisfaction, social competence, health, and economics that constitute a total personal complex. They seem to be advocating a holistic approach in which the outcome of these multiple interrelationships are evaluated as one ages according to each individual's unique personal interaction with the environment. Therefore there does not exist any one way to successfully age against which all individuals are measured. Rather, each individual should be supported according to the strengths and limits of his own aging pattern's potential as determined by the dimensions of his individual and environmental interactions.

Normal aging will probably be characterized by contrasting periods of disengagement and activity in accordance with the internal state of the individual and the external forces or situations with which he interacts. Certainly the individual must be supported by those measures that will best evoke harmony between the individual and his environment. Harmonious individual-environmental interaction is probably the most significant sign of "successful aging."

Studies of aging should be concerned with the individual, and self-fulfillment should be the goal of human behavior. How each individual may perceive this, work toward it, and achieve it remains part of that elusive complexity found in all human beings. What should be recognized in every stage of human development is the enormous potential for self-fulfillment residing in each of us. "Self-fulfillment," states Laszlo, "is the actualization of potentials in all of us. It is the pattern of what can be, traced in actuality."[20] From the time of conception until death, the developmental process represents a blending of potential patterns with actualized patterns. This patterning of self-expression and self-expansion unfolds in time as one ages. Self-fulfillment cannot be achieved maximally until the final phase of old age. In this respect, old age is truly the flower of life in full bloom. Whereas we may never fully understand its complexity, this should not mar our appreciation of its beauty or destroy our sense of wonder in its creation.

REFERENCES

1. de Beauvoir, S.: The coming of age, New York, 1973, Warner Paperback Library.
2. Kubler-Ross, E.: On death and dying, New York, 1969, The Macmillan Co.
3. Tibbits, C., and Donahue, W., editors: Social and psychological aspects of aging, New York, 1962, Columbia University Press, pp. 442-458.
4. Clark, M.: The anthropology of aging. In Neugarten, B. L., editor: Middle age and aging, Chicago, 1968, The University of Chicago Press, pp. 436-439.
5. Butler, R. N., and Lewis, M. L.: Aging and mental health, ed. 2, St. Louis, 1977, The C. V. Mosby Co., p. 121.
6. Tedrow, J. L.: Emotional, physical, and legal aspects of aging. In Reinhardt, A. M., and Quinn, M. D., editors: Current practice in family-cen-

tered community nursing, St. Louis, 1977, The
C. V. Mosby Co., p. 277.

7. Busse, E. W.: Theories of aging. In Busse, E.
W., and Pfeiffer, E., editors: Behavior and adap-
tation in late life, Boston, 1969, Little, Brown &
Co., p. 11.

8. Butler and Lewis, p. 19.

9. Butler and Lewis, p. 101.

10. Shanas, E.: Living arrangements and housing of
old people. In Busse, E. W., and Pfeiffer, E.,
editors: Behavior and adaptation in late life, Boston, 1969, Little, Brown & Co., p. 132.

11. Neugarten, B.: A developmental view of adult
personality. In Neugarten, B., editor: Relations
of development and aging, Springfield, Ill.,
1964, Charles C Thomas, Publisher, p. 189.

12. Neugarten, p. 190.

13. Cumming, E., and Henry, W.: Growing old,
New York, 1961, Basic Books, Inc., Publishers.

14. Rose, A. M.: A current theoretical issue. In

Neugarten, B. L., editor: Middle age and aging,
Chicago, 1968, The University of Chicago Press,
pp. 184-189.

15. Elias, M. F., Elias, P. K., and Elias, J. W.:
Basic processes in adult developmental psychology, St. Louis, 1977, The C. V. Mosby Co.,
p. 142.

16. Palmore, E.: Sociological aspects of aging. In
Busse, E. W., and Pfeiffer, E., editors: Behavior
and adaptation in late life, Boston, 1969, Little,
Brown & Co., pp. 57-60.

17. Elias et al., pp. 133-135.

18. Gerard, R. W.: Aging and organization. In
Birren, J. E., editor: Handbook of aging and the
individual, Chicago, 1959, University of Chicago Press, p. 273.

19. Thomae, H., editor: Patterns of aging, Basal,
1976, S Karger, pp. 160-161.

20. Laszlo, E.: The systems view of the world, New
York, 1972, George Brazillar, Inc., p. 109.

11 Sexuality and aging

NANCY FUGATE WOODS

nonexistent
impossible
normal
infrequent
healthy
slower
discouraged by society
difficult to imagine

Recently a group of health professionals used the above phrases to characterize sex for older people. Their responses reflect the wide range of contemporary attitudes about sexuality and aging in this country. Professionals at one end of the continuum believe that older people are either incapable of or no longer desirous of sexual activity or perhaps both. Health professionals at the opposite end of the continuum contend that sexual expression is both healthy and normal for the older population. Others note a social milieu that is intolerant of sexual expression in aging persons. These viewpoints reveal that health professionals are not divorced from sociocultural forces and are not granted immunity from myth and misconception.

This chapter will explore sexuality for aging persons. First some research findings describing the effects of the aging process on sexual functioning will be explored. Next the sexual behavior of aging persons will be examined. Finally barriers to the full experience and expression of sexuality will be analyzed from both biological and psychosocial perspectives.

EFFECTS OF AGING ON SEXUAL FUNCTIONING

Little basic research has been conducted on the effects of aging on sexual functioning, with the notable exception of the efforts of Masters and Johnson (1966). It might be posited that lack of such research reflects (1) a denial that aging shall come for each of us, (2) the societal prohibitions against sex among the aging that precludes such study, and (3) the fact that research in the area of sexual functioning is still not "acceptable" to funding agencies. Nevertheless Masters and Johnson pioneered in this area, exploring biologic changes in sexual functioning for both aging women and men.

Women

Masters and Johnson[10] noted changes in sexual functioning in their study population of 61 aging women. Involutionary changes involved the breast tissue as well as the genitalia. The postmenopausal women had steroid-starved vaginal walls, which were thin as tissue paper and no longer possessed the corrugated look characteristic of the younger woman's vagina. The color of the vaginal walls had changed from the reddish purple

151

associated with youth to a light pink color. Diminution of vaginal length as well as width and loss of the elasticity of the vaginal wall were noted. Some atrophy of the breast tissue was also noted. Masters and Johnson[10] also described phase-specific changes that were evident among aging women during the sexual response cycle.

Excitement. During the excitement phase the rate of production and amount of vaginal lubrication diminished. Among the women 60 years of age and older, between 1 and 3 minutes were required for adequate lubrication. However three women who were consistently sexually active, that is, continued to have intercourse once or twice weekly, had no such interference with lubrication. In addition, flattening, separation, and elevation of the labia majora disappeared among women after age 50 and vasocongestion of the labia minora diminished. Expansion of the vaginal breadth and depth decreased. Uterine elevation and tenting developed more slowly and were less marked. The degree of myotonia or muscle tension also appeared to decrease with aging.

Plateau. During the plateau phase further evidence of diminished vasocongestive capacity was apparent. Areolar engorgement of the breast was less intense, labial color change was observed less frequently among women 60 years of age or older, and the swelling of the orgasmic platform appeared reduced in intensity. Secretions from Bartholin's glands had also diminished among the postmenopausal women.

Orgasm. With orgasm, fewer contractions of the orgasmic platform were seen in postmenopausal women, with some women actually experiencing discomfort caused by uterine contractions. Contraction of the rectal sphincter only occurred with severe levels of sexual tension in this population.

Resolution. During the resolution phase, nipple erection became apparent more slowly in older than younger women, and congestion of both the clitoris and the orgasmic platform subsided quickly.

The aging women's response is similar to that of the younger women's. Many of the changes described result from steroid starvation accompanying the menopause. However these do not make cessation of sexual activity imperative. As the woman ages, both the duration and intensity of her physiologic responses to sexual stimulation diminish gradually. The phases of the sexual response cycle can still be observed, however, and orgasmic experience is not precluded by the aging process. Thus there is evidence that sexual function can persist far into later life provided the woman is in reasonably good health and has an interested and interesting partner.

Men

Masters and Johnson[10] also investigated sexual function among aging men by studying 39 men. As the men aged, the physiologic changes in sexual response paralleled those described earlier for the women. An increase in the time involved in each phase of the sexual response cycle was the most characteristic change with increasing age. The ways in which sexual response of aging men differs from that of their younger counterparts will be described for each phase of sexual response.

Excitement and plateau. During the excitement phase, vasocongestive changes either appeared more slowly or were less intense for aging men than their younger counterparts. Although aging men needed more time to attain an erection, they could maintain their erections for extended periods of time without ejaculation. Thus with aging, these men actually gained improved ejaculatory control. When erection was lost, a lengthy refractory period sometimes followed, during which further stimulation could not elevate the man's sexual tension level.

Vasocongestion in the scrotal sac was less evident during these phases and the scrotum appeared less tense in older than in younger men. Testicular elevation and vasocongestion of the testes in aging men was not as pronounced as among their younger counterparts. Nipple erection and the sexual flush did not occur as frequently in aging men. The degree of muscle tension appeared less in aging men. The only other difference among older men was that during the plateau phase the color change at the coronal ridge of the penis was not observed.

Orgasm. Fewer contractions of the penis and rectal sphincter were observed with orgasm, and the force of ejaculation was decreased. The reduced force of expulsion at ejaculation may explain why older men may not perceive ejaculatory inevitability as do younger counterparts. If the aging man maintained his erection for a long period of time, seepage of semen took the place of a more forceful ejaculation. Psychosexual satisfaction was not noted by men who experienced seepage of semen rather than ejaculation.

Resolution. The resolution period occurred more rapidly in aging than in younger men. Loss of erection and testicular descent followed shortly after ejaculation. Only vasocongestion of the scrotum and nipple erection disappeared slowly. The refractory period, that period of time during which further sexual stimulation could not increase sexual tension levels, tended to increase with the man's age.

The aging man actually has certain advantages over younger men. He gains improved ejaculatory control and simultaneously experiences a reduced ejaculatory demand; that is, he may be satisfied to ejaculate during every second or third intercourse, rather than with each attempt. Thus there are reasons to be optimistic about the aging man's ability to enjoy a full and satisfying sexual relationship, provided that he is in relatively good health and has an interested and interesting partner.

Implications for health care providers

For aging persons there is no universal point in the life cycle at which sexual function reaches an obligatory halt. Given good general health and a sanctioned and interesting partner, the biologic functions might persist into the last decades of life. Practitioners who recognize that sexual function is possible for aging persons may foster healthy sexuality among them in several ways. First clinicians can include a sexual assessment as a valid part of the aging person's health appraisal. Next the practitioner can provide anticipatory guidance regarding some of the age-linked physiologic changes in sexual functioning. Clinicians may also be able to interpret the changes in sexual functioning that clients are experiencing, for example, decreased vaginal lubrication or decreased ejaculatory demand. Finally nurses may institute interventions designed to foster sexual health. For example, the woman with a steroid-starved vagina may have comfortable vaginal intercourse by using a water-soluble lubricant; the aging male who has concerns about his decreased ejaculatory demand can probably benefit from reassurance that this is not a sign of impending impotence.

SEXUAL BEHAVIOR AMONG AGING PERSONS

The work of Masters and Johnson[10] established that in healthy elderly persons the biophysiologic components of sexual response persist, though with some changes. With this ''potential'' capability in mind, let us explore the actual incidence of sexual expression among aging persons.

The literature in this area is difficult to compare and contrast since different investigators have neither studied the same variables nor have they incorporated similar statistics. However an attempt will be made to summarize the general trends observed by several investigators.

The Kinsey studies

Some of the earliest studies in the area of sexual behavior were conducted by Kinsey and his associates. We shall consider these findings while recognizing that only a small proportion of the total sample was comprised of elderly persons. Kinsey, et al.,[7] interviewed 126 men who were 60 years of age and older; approximately 75% were white. The mean frequency of intercourse per week decreased with age for the white men. Kinsey also found that the percentage of men who were impotent tended to increase with age. Whereas 20% of the men were impotent at age 60, 75% reported impotence at age 80.

In the volume devoted to sexual behavior of women, Kinsey et al.[8] present data regarding the sexual behavior of 431 women ranging from 46 to 60 years of age. Mean frequency of intercourse per week also decreased with age for women. Although frequency of masturbation decreased with age among married and previously married women, it remained nearly constant among single women in this age range. Similar data were not discussed with regard to those women over 60 years old because of their small numbers.

Studies of aging women

Christenson and Gagnon[2] explored the histories of 241 single white women, 50 years of age or older. Never-married females were selected to ensure some uniformity of their social experiences. For women 50 to 70 years of age, an aging effect in relation to sexual behavior was observed. Marital status also influenced women's patterns of behavior. Incidence of coitus appeared to decrease with age for married women, as did masturbatory behavior and the experience of sexual dreams to orgasm. Among the women who were no longer married, there existed considerably different patterns of behavior. About 40% of the women who were 50 to 59 years old still reported they were having intercourse. This figure dropped to about 12% in the 60-year age group and disappeared entirely from subsequent age groups. The incidence of masturbation was nearly double that of the married women, with about 60% of the women reporting that they masturbated at age 50 years and 25% of the women at age 70 years. Sexual dreams leading to orgasm never entirely disappeared in this group of women, even among those who were 70 years old or older.

Christenson and Gagnon[2] also reported that sexual activity levels of women before age 30 did not seem to be related to marital sexual activity after age 50 but did seem to be positively associated with postmarital coitus. Thus the sexual activity patterns established early in life did not have as great an effect in later life on marital sex as they did on nonmarital sex. Religiosity as determined by church attendance seemed to influence sexual behavior patterns in later life, with those who were more religious being less sexually active. As might be expected, women with younger spouses tended to have higher coital rates than those with older spouses.

Christenson and Johnson[3] examined data similar to that just described in relation to 71 never-married white women. About one third had never experienced intercourse. Among these women, incidence of intercourse, masturbation, and dreaming to orgasm decreased with age. An abrupt decline in all these activities was evident by age 55 years. Those women who had a high level of activity in early life were still very active in later life. Some of the women reported having multiple orgasms into their 50s and 60s. Eight of the women who had homosexual relationships demonstrated an aging pattern similar to the sexually active women in the rest of the sample. Menopause was not directly related to change in erotic levels for women.

Studies of aging men

Finkle et al.[4] interviewed 101 randomly selected clinic patients ranging in age from the middle 50s to the middle 80s. Those with genitourinary problems were excluded. Potency was defined as having copulated at least once within the past year. Ability to have intercourse declined with age, with 65% of the men under 70 years old retaining their potency as opposed to only 34% of those over 70 years old. The percentage of sexually active men decreased with age, as did the frequency of intercourse. It is important to note that men gave several reasons, in addition to impotence, for discontinuing intercourse. These included lack of desire for sexual activity, absence of a partner, and refusal of the partner to be involved in sexual activity.

Freeman[5] distributed a questionnaire to an unspecified number of men who were volunteers or were from organizations and physicians' private practices, or who were persons named by physicians and social workers. He received returns from 74 of these. The average age of the sample was 71 years with a range from 64 to 91 years old. These aging men reported that their desire for sexual activity exceeded the persistence of their ability.

Rubin[18] also reports data about the sexual activity of aging men. He distributed questionnaires to 6,000 men listed in *Who's Who in America* who were over the age of 65 years. Eight hundred thirty-two replies were received. Seventy percent of the married respondents engaged in intercourse on a regular basis and about half of those 75 years of age and older reported that intercourse was still satisfactory. Most men reported they still had morning erections, but 30% of this group indicated that they were impotent. About one fourth of the group currently masturbated or had done so after they were 60 years old.

The Duke studies

The most extensive survey research done in the area of sexuality and healthy aging has been conducted by investigators from the Duke Center for the Study of Aging and Human Development. Since 1953, a study involving aging subjects residing in the central portion of North Carolina has been conducted by an interdisciplinary team. None of these subjects is a resident of a nursing home or hospital, and as a group they represent a generally successful adaptation to aging.

In 1960 Newman and Nichols reported results of an investigation of the sexual activities and attitudes in 250 men and women between the ages of 60 and 93 years old. Of the 149 persons who were still married and living with their spouses, 54% indicated they were sexually active, in contrast to 7% of the nonmarried. Those who were older than 75 years reported a significantly lower level of sexual activity. The respondents often attributed this to loss of the spouse or to debilitating illnesses. Women in the sample reported less sexual activity than men, whites reported less than blacks, and those of high socioeconomic status reported less than those of low socioeconomic status. Each person rated strength of sexual drives as lower in their old age than in earlier life. However, the strength of sexual interest persisted throughout the life cycle: those who had relatively strong sexual urges in youth were more likely than those who had weaker urges to maintain at least moderate levels of sexual interest as they aged.

Pfeiffer, et al.[16] reported results of a longitudinal investigation that included data obtained at 3- to 4-year intervals. The subjects numbered 254 for the first data collection period but were subsequently reduced to 190 and 126 respectively during the last two periods. At the first interview the average age of the subjects was 70.93 years. Intraindividual changes in sexual activity were observed over two interviews for 160 subjects. Although the most prevalent pattern was not to be sexually active at either occasion, 30% of these subjects indicated that their sexual activity had remained the same as or had increased from the time of the first interview. Fourteen percent of the subjects reported rising patterns of sexual interest. A third finding of great importance was the report of congruence between spouse pairs. Among the 31 spouse pairs in the larger sample, there was 91% agreement in the reporting of sexual data.

Those persons who had discontinued sexual intercourse prior to completion of the entire study were asked to describe their reasons for doing so. Death of the spouse was the single most common reason, followed by illness of the spouse, loss of potency, and finally loss of interest. When death of the spouse was eliminated, in most instances both husbands and wives attributed cessation of intercourse to the male partner. Data were also available with regard to the age at which intercourse was discontinued. For men and women, respectively, the median ages were 68 and 60 years.[16]

A later report by these same investigators focused on 39 subjects who had survived throughout all four data collection periods. These individuals reported sexual behavior patterns that may be generalized to all elderly who are in optimum health.[17] The average age of these subjects was 67.23 years at the first interview, and 76.89 years at the last. The proportion of men who continued to be interested in sex remained high during the entire 10-year period, but a much lower proportion of women declared continued sexual interest. Both men and women experienced a decline in sexual activity with age. The investigators note that an interest and activity gap was apparent for men and increased in magnitude with age. In contrast, interest and activity for the women remained low throughout the study.

The Duke program later explored sexual interest and activity during the middle years.[15] Two hundred sixty-one white men and 241 white women between the ages of 46 and 69 years from middle and upper socioeconomic levels were interviewed regarding their sexual behaviors. Whereas these findings paralleled the sex differences described previously, there was strong evidence that sex continued to be a very important aspect of middle life. Only 6% of the men and 33% of the women in this age group no longer expressed an interest in sex, and only 12% of the women were no longer sexually active. A noticeable decline in sexual interest and activity was reported during the decade from age 45 to 55 years.

A later study of these same subjects[14] indicated that the level of sexual functioning in younger years, present age, present health status, social class, antihypertensive drug therapy, present life satisfaction, physical function rating, and excess worry over physical examination findings all influenced the level of current sexual functioning among the middle-aged men. For women, marital status and age were the most significant determinants in addition to past sexual enjoyment. Those persons who had enjoyed sexual functioning during their youth were more likely to continue to do so during middle age. Presence of a capable and socially acceptable partner seemed to be a more significant variable for women than for men. It is suggested that the middle-aged woman may be inhibiting her sexual interests in the absence of an acceptable partner.

Note on the aging homosexual

Weinberg and Williams[19] surveyed 3,667 persons from various locations in the United States and received 1,057 returns from homosexual men. (Additional homosexuals from the Netherlands and Denmark were included in the study.) These investigators found that older homosexuals were less involved in the homosexual world and had homosexual sex less frequently. However older homosexuals rated themselves as ''no worse off'' on selected measures of psychological dimensions than the younger homosexuals, and in some instances as ''better off.'' Thus the stereotype that portrays the homosexual man as declining in psychological health as he ages probably results from attributing meaning to the social and sexual situations of the older homosexual, which are inaccurate. There are no studies that parallel this investigation for homosexual women.

BARRIERS TO SEXUAL EXPRESSION FOR AGING PERSONS

So far we have established that the changes in sexual functioning of men and women may reflect biologic alteration and, perhaps more significantly, emotional and social influences. We have noted that there is no single point at which sexual functioning reaches an obligatory halt and that sexual interest persists into the latest decades. Whereas biologic changes in human sexual response do parallel age, they do not preclude orgasm or sexual satisfaction. Men actually achieve increased ejaculatory control and women who have been sexually active throughout life do not exhibit some of the interference with vaginal lubrication that was thought to be age related. Thus for the healthy elderly documentation supports their ability to experience and give sexual pleasure far into old age.

Why, then, do we frequently encounter the assumptions that sexual expression for aging persons is impossible, unnatural, or nonexistent? I contend that these barriers are attitudinal and stem from basic assumptions about the aging population. The first assumption is that aging can be equated with infirmity. Whereas some pathological conditions do interfere with sexual functioning and do need to be considered in caring for aging persons, all elderly persons are not infirm, particularly as demonstrated in the Duke studies.

The second assumption that creates barriers for elderly persons' sexual expressions is that the elderly are asexual. As the foregoing literature demonstrates, this assumption is not well grounded in fact and parallels some of the assumptions held about children's sexuality. Thus in our society we are on the brink of accepting sex as a natural function but *only* for those *not* at far extremes of the life cycle. The following pages will examine how biologic and psychosocial factors influence sexual expression among elderly persons.

Biologic barriers

Several mechanisms can limit sexual expression. Whereas most sexual difficulties probably arise from the cranium and not the genitals, there are some pathological conditions that have been associated with sexual difficulties. Usually these physiologic functions are thought to be necessary to support sexual response: (1) adequate circulatory supply to the genitals to support vasocongestion, (2) functional neural pathways to conduct sensory, motor, and reflex impulses, (3) appropriate hormonal milieu, inasmuch as it influences genital structure and function, and (4) intact genitalia. Interference with any or all of these may preclude some aspects of sexual experience.

One may encounter several examples of physiologic interference in clinical practice with aging persons. Obstruction of circulation to the genitals may result in sexual dysfunction in men; this may be seen in men with Leriche's syndrome who are impotent. Neurological deficits may interfere with sexual potency, as in men who have had radical prostatic surgery or surgical procedures in which the pelvic nerves are disrupted. Some women may find that steroid starvation of menopause induces vaginal changes that may interfere with intercourse. Surgical trauma or removal of the genitals may interfere with sexual expression. Often men who have had transurethral prostatectomies experience retrograde ejaculation into the bladder. Whereas this "dry ejaculation" may alter the man's perception of his potency, it does not necessarily preclude intercourse or sexual satisfaction.*

Although these problems may interfere with sexual expression, it should be noted that they are not common *only* to aging persons or to *all* aging persons. These same phenomena may interfere with the sexual expression of younger persons. It should also be noted that these difficulties interfere with only two sexual options, intercourse and masturbation to orgasm. The extent to which these phenomena preclude sexual functioning will depend on the number of options seen as acceptable forms of sexual expression by each person.

Other forms of sexual expression, for example, caressing, kissing, and hugging, are not interfered with by genital dysfunction. The cultural definition of acceptable sexual practices may unnecessarily limit the outlets available to the elderly and to other age groups as well. Clinicians need to assess their personal biases before counseling aging persons about their sexuality. Lack of acceptance may be conveyed through the clinician's nonverbal behavior; this, in turn, may cause the aging person to feel that concerns about sexuality are ludicrous and not a legitimate topic for discussion with the health professionals.

Psychosocial barriers

Although certain biologic interferences do exist, the most pervasive barriers to sexual expression among the elderly seem to be those barriers created by thoughts, feelings, and values of the aging person and our society as a whole. First we will discuss some of the psychosocial barriers aging persons have identified. Finally we will explore some of the barriers in this society.

Aging women are confronted with barriers related to their partners. Often women are widowed and lack a socially sanctioned partner. Other women may be married to a partner who can no longer function sexually. Lacking the opportunity for sexual expression, the woman may inhibit her interest. This is likely to be reinforced by attitudes that equate sexual expression with "penis-in-vagina" intercourse. Unless options other than vaginal intercourse with a spouse are available, these women find their sexual expression very restricted. Some women see menopause as the end of their sexual relationships.

Masters and Johnson[10] found that some women who received relatively little satisfaction from their sexual relationships or found them repugnant used their age or menopause as a culturally acceptable way to free themselves from their "marital duty." Also Masters and Johnson[10] found that some women actually believed that intercourse was unsuitable for the aged and consequently were no longer sexually active. Other researchers noted that some postmenopausal women linked their decreased interest in sex to the fact that procreation was no longer possible, whereas others felt an upsurge in interest since pregnancy was no longer a threat.[11]

Aging men are not immune to the belief that sex for the aging person is not socially acceptable. In Masters' and Johnson's sample,[10] cessation of sexual intercourse was also associated with monotony in the relationship, usually caused by boredom with the partner. Although some men attributed their inactivity to preoccupation with their careers or

---

*Both Kaplan[6] and Masters and Johnson[9] discuss these phenomena in much greater detail.

financial affairs, others blamed either physical or psychological fatigue. Overindulgence in food or drink also was cited as an interference with sexual expression. Finally fear of failure interfered with sexual expression for men; having failed once at intercourse, some men withdrew from their regular sexual activity rather than risk embarrassment on another occasion.[10]

The problems with sexual expression cited by aging women and men often reflect some broader sociocultural proscriptions that they have internalized. The first barrier springs from the belief that sexual expression exists primarily for procreation, not recreation. This effectively establishes age boundaries for sexual expression dependent on fertility. Pfeiffer[13] sees a parallel between this belief and the incest taboo: children's anxieties about their parents' sexual activity spill over into adulthood, and consequently the younger generation discourages sexuality among the aging.

Portrayal of the elderly as an asexual group may be responsible for the interpretations assigned to sexual expression in this age group. What is defined as a healthy, normal expression of sexual interest for a man in his 30s is labeled lechery for a man in his 70s. It should be noted that similar epithets exist for aging women, especially those involved with younger partners.

Clinicians can institute consciousness-raising activities for the elderly as well as for the younger generations. However, that is merely a beginning. Knowledge about sexual functioning in aging persons must be supplemented by an examination of attitudes and values. Value clarification strategies can be instituted preventively with adolescents and young adults. Models of acceptance may help foster the same in the elderly and their families.

Another sociocultural phenomenon perhaps responsible for limiting sexual expression in the elderly is our tendency to isolate young and old. By removing older persons from the general milieu, we remove the reminders of our own aging. This may result in a distorted view of aging persons and a tendency to think of ''them'' as very different from ''us,'' especially in the area of sexual expression. Nursing care for the aging in *their own homes* may reduce the necessity for isolating the elderly and may simultaneously foster a better understanding between generations.

Finally if we conceive of the elderly as infirm, we assume a need to protect them, therefore we have sex-segregated areas in nursing homes. One might ask ''for whom does this protective environment exist?'' Are we ''protecting'' the elderly from some injury likely to result from expressions of caring? Are we protecting the elderly from their desires for companionship and love that may lead to late-life marriages? Are we protecting the children of the elderly from their feelings about their aged parents as sexual beings? Are we protecting institutional staff from confrontation of their own value systems?

Fortunately we have seen that the aging have the capacity for creativity and adaptation. An important example is the cohabitation of elderly men and women, a phenomenon created out of the necessity of our social welfare programs that render marriage a less desirable economic state!

SUMMARY

This chapter has explored some of the research findings describing sexual potential among aging persons, the need for sexual expression into the final decades of human existence, and the barriers that our society, rather than our biology, has instituted. As the milieu becomes more tolerant of sex as a natural function, there is hope that this acceptance will be extended to the aged. If not, we will have legislated a premature death to a very important facet of our humanity.

REFERENCES

1. Bussee, E., and Eisdorfer, C.: Two thousand years of married life. In Palmore, E., editor: Normal aging: reports from the Duke longitudinal study, 1955-1969, Durham, N.C., Duke University Press, 1970.
2. Christenson, C. V., and Gagnon, J. H.: Sexual behavior in a group of older women, J. Gerontol. **20:**351-356, 1965.
3. Christenson, C. V., and Johnson, A. B.: Sexual patterns in a group of older never-married women, J. Geriatr. Psychiatr. **7**(1):88-98, 1973.
4. Finkle, A., Moyers, T., Tobenkin, M., and Karg, S.: Sexual potency in aging males: frequency of coitus among clinic patients, J.A.M.A. **170** (12):1391-1393, 1959.
5. Freeman, J.: Sexual capacities in the aging male, Geriatrics **16:**37-43, Jan., 1961.
6. Kaplan, H.: The new sex therapy, New York, 1974, Brunner/Mazel, Inc.
7. Kinsey, A., Pomeroy, W., and Martin, C.: Sexual behavior in the human male, Philadelphia, 1948, W. B. Saunders Co.
8. Kinsey, A., Pomeroy, W., Martin, C., and Gelhard, P.: Sexual behavior in the human female, Philadelphia, 1953, W. B. Saunders Co.
9. Masters, W., and Johnson, V.: Human sexual inadequacy, Boston, 1970, Little, Brown & Co.
10. Masters, W., and Johnson, V.: Human sexual response, Boston, 1966, Little, Brown & Co.
11. Neugarten, B., Wood, V., Kraines, R., and Loomis, B.: Women's attitudes toward the menopause, Vita Humana **6:**140-151, 1963.
12. Newman, G., and Nichols, C. R.: Sexual activities and attitudes in older persons, J. Am. Med. Assoc. **173:**33-35, 1960.
13. Pfeiffer, E.: Sexual behavior in old age. In Busse, E. W., and Pfeiffer, E., editors: Behavior and adaption in late life, Boston, 1969, Little, Brown & Co., pp. 1951-1962.
14. Pfeiffer, E., and Davis, G. C.: Determinants of sexual behavior in middle and old age, J. Am. Geriatr. Soc. **20:**151-158, 1972.
15. Pfeiffer, E., Verwoerdt, A., and Davis, G. C.: Sexual behavior in middle life, Am. J. Psychiatry **128:**1262-1267, 1972.
16. Pfeiffer, E., Verwoerdt, A., and Wang, H. S.: Sexual behavior in aged men and women: 1. observation on 254 community volunteers, Arch. Gen. Psychiatr. **19:**753-758, 1968.
17. Pfeiffer, E., Verwoerdt, A., and Wang, H. S.: The natural history of sexual behavior in a biologically advantaged group of aged individuals, J. Gerontol. **24:**193-198, 1969.
18. Rubin, I.: Sexual life after sixty, New York, 1965, Basic Books, Inc., Publishers.
19. Weinberg, M., and Williams, C.: Male homosexuals: their problems and adaptations, New York, 1974, Oxford University Press.

12 The family and its role with the elderly parent

PAULETTE ROBISCHON
ALICE M. AKAN

This chapter is concerned with the final stage of the family life cycle. As parents age, new generations emerge — the children grow to adulthood and have families of their own, and with time these grandchildren, too, establish homes and have children. Earlier marriages, earlier assumption of parental responsibilities, and increased life expectancy have resulted in larger proportions of aged individuals in our society and a significant increase in the number of multigenerational families. Three- and four-generation families are no longer uncommon. As families grow and expand, roles and responsibilities evolve and change, but most older people retain a significant place in the family structure.

The structure and functions of the nuclear family have been clearly identified and are probably well understood by most readers. Aging families, too, serve special functions, and the aging husband and wife face crucial developmental tasks through the later years.[1] The developmental tasks of the aging family can be summarized as follows:

1. Finding a satisfying home for the later years
2. Adjusting to retirement income
3. Establishing comfortable household routines
4. Nurturing each other as husband and wife
5. Facing bereavement and widowhood
6. Maintaining contact with children and grandchildren
7. Caring for elderly relatives
8. Keeping an interest in people outside the family
9. Finding meanings in life[2]

Aging is a continuous process that incorporates previous experiences, life-styles, patterns, and personality traits. The subjective experiences of age are highly individualized as a result of cultural and psychological variables as well as of the observable physiological changes that occur with the passing of time. The cumulative effect of the physiological, psychological, and social factors can be viewed as a positive, new dimension in the life process with new opportunities for growth and achievement, but this does not deny the problems and challenges of age. Indeed, every family is eventually confronted with crisis situations as a result of the aging of one or more of its members.

The following case study is typical of many aging families and illustrates some of the common problems confronted by aging parents and their children. It begins with the father's retirement, is followed by his death some years later, and ends many more years later at the approaching end of the mother's life. In this family the time span is 30 years — a lengthy aging family stage, but not unusual when one of the parents has extreme longevity. The study has three parts: first, the year when the parents and then the mother alone were independent; second, the period during which the mother lived with a son and his family; and third, the period during which the mother was institutionalized. Following each part of the narrative is a discussion of several prominent themes appearing in each phase of Mrs. Forte's story. The themes are relocation, socialization, loss, and role change. A discussion of retirement follows part one.

PART 1

Mrs. Forte sat proudly next to her husband, sharing his pleasure at a large banquet honoring his mandatory retirement after many years of municipal service in a suburban town. He was 65 years old; she was 63. They had raised two sons, both married and living nearby with their families. Armed with retirement gifts of a new camera and a check, they set out on a car trip across the country. On their return they sold their home and spent a winter in a warmer climate where they thought they would retire. They did not like being surrounded by "old people" so they returned and bought a smaller home in a semirural area. Feeling too distant from family and friends, they moved back to town and rented one of the numerous apartments they were to occupy over the next several years. Finally they settled in a garden apartment near the home of one of their sons. Meanwhile the other son had been transferred to a distant state. The next 20 years were active ones for Mrs. Forte, but less active for her husband, who was content to sit and read, becoming increasingly an observer of people and events around him. However, he remained mentally alert and in touch with current events. One by one the Forte's siblings, their spouses, and dear friends died. The next generation took their parents' place in maintaining contact with the Fortes.

Mrs. Forte's husband nursed her through an episode following a hip fracture. Then a few years later Mr. Forte suffered a devastating stroke. He spent some time in the county long-term facility, then in several nursing homes. He was miserably unhappy away from home and made little progress. Mrs. Forte insisted on bringing him home, against medical and family advice. She had a visiting nurse a few times and quickly learned to manage his care. For the next 5 years her energies were devoted almost solely to the care of her husband who was confined to a wheelchair. They celebrated their 60th wedding anniversary during this period. Mrs. Forte was most ingenious in devising ways to care for her husband, and although she was somewhat disabled by her old hip fracture and increasing arthritic and cardiovascular problems, she did a remarkable job of caring for him until he had another cerebrovascular accident and died.

Mrs. Forte remained in her apartment. She flew, for the first time, to visit her youngest son and family across the country. When she returned home, her eldest son, who was now retired, and his wife kept in daily telephone contact, did the shopping when Mrs. Forte could not do so, and helped her with laundry and heavy house cleaning. They worried about her going out alone; she insisted on walking to nearby stores for small items and to the mailbox. Her vision and hearing were diminishing. She tried a number of hearing aids but with little success. She had eye surgery and later had spinal surgery and recovered rapidly from both. One of her old friends went to live in a church-operated retirement home and Mrs. Forte sometimes talked of wanting to apply for admission there. One son supported her in this, but the other did not. Mrs. Forte was ambivalent about it, still fiercely independent and proud of her capabilities. Furthermore she was reluctant to consider the requirement of turning over her dwindling assets to the home.

The elder son who lived nearby, who had not wanted his mother to enter the church home, died suddenly of coronary heart disease. This posed a problem for Mrs. Forte. It was not realistic for her to depend on her son's widow, her married granddaughter, and an aging niece to look after her. Other family members lived at great distances. She refused "outside" help. She walked with a cane or walker, suffered almost continual pain in her back, had difficulty with stairs, and had spells of weakness. Despite this, she was almost always in good spirits. She reconsidered entering the church home after her son's death but there was now a long waiting list for admission. Her surviving son and his wife persuaded her to move to their home in another state. She was then 89 years old.

During the 26 years described above, the Fortes confronted and dealt with a number of the crises of aging. The following material examines some of the crisis events and raises questions to be considered in working toward resolution.

Retirement

Retirement, whether elective or forced, precipitates many changes that require adaptive and creative responses in the aging individual and his family. For many it is a major crisis of aging; although one is freed from the obligations and responsibilities of work, a personal identity crisis may result because of loss of occupational identity, economic loss, loss of work-related socialization, and large amounts of unstructured free time.

It is more important at this time to look at what one is retiring "to" than at what one is retiring "from." The Fortes looked forward to retirement with anticipation, for to them it provided an opportunity for new satisfactions and activities — more time to spend with the children and grandchildren, freedom to travel, and the possibility of a move to a new community.

The transition to retirement status can be eased somewhat by advance planning and development of multiple interests and skills throughout the earlier years. Creative use of leisure time and motivation toward activity that has personal meaning prevents energy from being dissipated by boredom, inactivity, and frustration.

Consideration of the following questions prior to retirement might be helpful in planning for the transition to a more leisurely life-style:

1. What meaningful activities will continue after retirement?
2. What changes in life-style are imposed by retirement?
3. What personal and family resources can be used to cope with these changes?
4. What new opportunities does retirement make possible?

Relocation

Moving is a disruptive event at any age. It means separation from familiar surroundings, disruption of social relations, and possible changes in life-style. In the early years a move is usually a deliberate choice that most frequently represents a form of upward mobility and results in more favorable living conditions. However for the aging family, a move may be necessitated by declining income, increasing physical disabilities, or the desire to reestablish close contact with family members in distant locations.

The elderly frequently move to apartments, retirement villages, nursing homes, or to the homes of family or children. The move, whether by choice or necessity, may require drastic changes in life-style, climate, and social relations, and it may perhaps result in increasing dependency. Their adjustment to the new surroundings is frequently complicated by disruption of long-established patterns at a time when increasing physical impairment and sensory loss make adaptation more difficult.

Older persons need to be actively involved in decisions involving their living conditions, with their personal wishes and needs taking priority over those of other family members whenever economically and physically possible. When it is not possible, the transition will be even more difficult and may result in increasing disability, depression, and even morbidity.[3]

The need for advance planning and deliberation prior to relocation is aptly demonstrated by the Fortes. They sold their home immediately on retirement in anticipation of moving to a retirement community in a warmer climate. They had clearly identified the advantages of such a move, but had not anticipated the disadvantages, which included geographical separation from family and life-long friends. The result was a number of moves over a short period of time and many regrets over their decision to sell their home.

In planning for relocation, one can consider the following:

1. How does the older person feel about it?
2. Will it enhance his ability to maintain independence?
3. Will it enable social relations to be maintained or provide opportunities for new social contacts?
4. Will the number and frequency of family contacts be increased or decreased?
5. Will the environment be safe in view of the person's physical condition?
6. In what ways will the new environment be different from the old?
7. In what ways can "sameness" be maintained?
8. Are family and/or community resources readily available?

Socialization

In the case of the Fortes, old satisfactions and activities continued after retirement. Mrs. Forte still managed the household tasks, but on a smaller scale. Mr. Forte was less active than before but had more time to read. Contact with the children, grandchildren, and great-grandchildren became increasingly important as old friends and siblings died, but it also became more difficult because of the mobility of the family and the need for the children to accomplish their own tasks asssociated with middle age. However the children worked at maintaining close and meaningful relations with the parents. Continuing social interaction among family members in this case was relatively easy because there was general mutual concern and the family had always been fairly close-knit and mutually supportive. For aging parents in families where there are preexisting hostilities and dissension based on earlier experiences, social contact will be more difficult.

Peer contacts become increasingly difficult to maintain in old age because of separation by death and by decreasing mobility resulting from increasing physical disability. In these cases families can be helpful in seeking out community social agencies and in encouraging establishment of new relationships where these are desired. Opportunities for cross-generational contact may prove to be stimulating and educational for young and old alike and may help to compensate for the decreasing number of age peers.

Life expectancy for women has increased more rapidly than for men and has resulted in women far outnumbering men in the later years, which reduces the opportunities for heterosexual social relationships and results in large numbers of widows among the aged. This group can serve as a mutually supportive peer group but it requires some reorientation to new social roles.

Loss

It is relatively easy to recognize and empathize with the grief and mourning the aged person suffers as a result of the loss of siblings, spouse, and friends through geographical separation and death. It is more difficult to recognize and understand that there may be similar reactions of grief and mourning over the loss of familiar and treasured objects and possessions, and even over change itself.

The resistance to change that is frequently seen in the elderly may result from more than patterns, habits, and attitudes developed over the years. It is probably a resistance to loss at a time in their lives when loss is almost an everyday occurrence. As there is less energy to cope with change, decreased tolerance for deviations and newness is commonly observed.

Selling a home and furnishings to move into an apartment or nursing home requires giving up a part of one's beloved memories as well as a life-style that may have represented a significant part of one's life. This loss might very well precipitate a grieving process that, unless satisfactorily resolved, can interfere with adjustment to the new environment.

Role changes

Individual and family roles evolve and change as time and life progress. New roles that are assumed can compensate for the loss of previous roles if they are viewed as worthwhile positions in the family and social structure.

The crisis of retirement has already been identified. For men and women who have defined themselves primarily in terms of their occupational identity, the role changes with retirement will be particularly difficult. For these individuals it might be useful to maintain ties to their previous occupation through continued membership in professional organizations, unions, or job-related volunteer work and consultation.

In the case of the Fortes, the husband and wife roles remained central in their lives after retirement. Their children were grown and had families of their own and, although they retained their positions as parents and grandparents, most of their time and energy was now spent nurturing each other. Mrs. Forte continued with the traditional responsibilities of managing a home, but with the crisis of illness these responsibilities were readily assumed by the more healthy spouse. The ease with which this role reversal occurs is dependent upon the strength of the relationship, the health of the spouse, and the degree to which the required tasks were previously learned and shared. After Mrs. Forte's recovery, she subsequently nursed her husband for an extended period of time following his stroke. During this time she became increasingly independent and self-sufficient and assumed almost total responsibility for the management of their affairs. Continued family contact and support were important during these years because the demands of her husband's care made other social contacts virtually impossible.

Eventually she was widowed, as are most aging women, and after more than 60 years of defining her role as primarily wife and mother she was faced with the task of making a meaningful life for herself alone. The transition was eased somewhat by the close availability of family, but many are not so fortunate and must rely primarily on inner resources and social agencies in dealing with the problems and loneliness of widowhood.

Meanwhile the children had become parents and grandparents themselves. The family remained mutually interdependent but family structure and relationships became increasingly complex with the emergence of each succeeding generation.

PART 2

She waved and had tears in her eyes as she was helped into the plane that was taking her to live with her son and daughter-in-law about two months after her son's death. She had protested about this change in her life, insisting that she could continue to live alone. Her physicians, friends, and family believed that her desires and perception of her abilities were unrealistic and were relieved that she would now have the close attention she needed. A pleasant, newly decorated second floor room with easy access to a bathroom awaited her arrival. She settled in, got reacquainted with the family, learned their habits and patterns of living and they hers, made contact with the local church, and began to know the neighbors. She took short daily walks by herself. She helped with household tasks. However, her physical condition gradually declined and she became confined to the house. Her vision and hearing further diminished. She continued to be an avid letter writer and was disappointed if she did not receive some piece of mail daily. Her main occupations were crocheting and listening to recorded books obtained from the state library. She said that she had "read" more books in a few months than in her whole lifetime. She reminisced a lot, fixed old photo albums, and puttered around her room, which contained her own furniture and mementos. She would have liked to busy herself in the kitchen, too, but this did not work out, for she was too slow compared to the faster pace of the rest of the family. Her appetite was becoming a problem and she could no longer distinguish among many foods. She began to eat meals in her room. She was up several times during the night. Her care became a severe emotional strain on her family as they needed to provide constant supervision. They worried that they would find her fallen one day, and this did happen. Her daughter-in-law found her crumpled at the foot of her chair with a fractured hip. She was hospitalized, had a hip replacement, and with only mild protest was placed in a nursing home to recuperate. She was then 92 years old.

Relocation

It is not uncommon for the aging parent to make a number of moves after retirement. Sometimes moves are planned in a deliberate attempt to find more suitable accommodations or are necessitated by changing needs and circumstances. Frequently, however, the number of moves is a reflection of a lack of planning and indicates a general dissatisfaction with living conditions and discontent with the life-style necessitated by increasing age. At some point in his or her life, an aging parent may move in with an adult child, usually at the child's insistence because he is concerned over the parent's ability to continue to manage safely alone. For the parent this may represent the first step in a progressive loss of authority and a relinquishing of power.

The success of multigenerational households depends on a number of factors: the degree to which the parent was included in the decision to move; the attitude of the adult children toward the parent, which may be condescending, respectful, or resentful; the ability of the family to tolerate unusual behavior; the degree of privacy afforded each member of the household; the extent to which the parent is able to maintain a degree of independence; the extent to which the older person is included as a family member; and the ability of the family members to adapt to the mutual role changes and identify useful and meaningful roles for each family member.

Socialization

If the move to an adult child's home requires a geographic relocation, there will be further disruption of social relations and possible separation from surviving friends. Socialization with age peers usually becomes more difficult at this point because of decreasing mobility and increasing sensory loss. If the family lives in an age-segregated community, opportunities to establish relationships with age peers are further diminished and boredom, resentment, and depression may result.

On the other hand, a sensitive and adaptable family provides opportunities for multigeneration communication and interaction that may not have existed previously. The family provides an audience for the older person's reminiscing that may result in an increased interest in family history or increased respect on the part of grandchildren for past accomplishments.

In the case of Mrs. Forte, the children were able to create an emotional climate in which she could grow and develop new satisfactions and interests. Her pastimes of knitting and crocheting became meaningful and useful activities since she prepared items for the church bazaar and family gifts, and the talking books provided intellectual stimulation and growth. Socialization and privacy needs were mutually respected, but the different pace and life-style of the younger family made adjustment difficult.

A concerned and devoted family can help to make the adjustment of an aging parent easier when it becomes necessary for the parent to share the household with a grown child. In any case, the following questions need to be considered:

1. How can the family help the older parent maintain ego integrity in the face of loss of power and authority?
2. What opportunities are there for socialization and privacy?
3. What safety features need to be considered for the aged parent?
4. What roles and tasks can be shared that provide meaning and a sense of usefulness?
5. How does each person involved feel about living in a multigenerational family?
6. What are the family attitudes toward aging?
7. How can earlier family conflicts be resolved or minimized?

Loss

With each subsequent move, the aging person tends to experience increasing dependence and loss of authority. When a move is necessitated by declining health and an increasing need for assistance, there tends to be an idealization of the lost environment that can make the adjustment more difficult. It is helpful at this time if the older person can be surrounded by familiar and treasured objects from the past, as in Mrs. Forte's case. Also some kind of sustained contact with the previous environment might be helpful when feasible.

Loss of friends and spouse generally occurs at the same time as loss of physical abilities and requires concurrent reorientation of self-concept and adaptation to new life-styles. Diminishing sight, hearing, and taste threaten safety and nutritional status but, equally important, they decrease opportunities for experiencing previous pleasures and finding fulfillment in activities that were common in earlier years. Creative adaptations in activity and opportunities are required to overcome the effects of cumulative physical impairment and separation from old friends.

Role changes

The aging parent in a multigenerational household plays many roles. It is a difficult position at best to be parent and grandparent in the home of an adult child on whom the parent may be becoming increasingly dependent. Different generations have differing needs and priorities and different developmental tasks to be achieved. The success of such an arrangement depends on the extent to which competing needs can be identified and dealt with realistically and openly.

The position of the adult child is also not an easy one. He is in some ways caught in the middle by being both parent and child. It can be a difficult physical task and also a great emotional strain to care for a parent who is declining when one remembers that parent as a strong, healthy, and independent individual on whom the child was dependent for so many years.

The mutual dependence, competing needs, and complex role relationships in a multigenerational family challenge the family to identify meaningful and mutually satisfying roles for each family member. The following are some of the questions that need to be re-solved:

1. What roles can an aging parent perform?
2. How much role diversity can the family tolerate?
3. How are overlapping roles dealt with (for example, the existence of two parent-child relationships)?

PART 3

She lies in bed a lot in the nursing home these days. She is thin as a wisp, bent, and full of arthritic pain; she has further diminished vision, she is almost totally deaf, her legs are edematous, and her appetite is markedly decreased. She is mentally alert and well-oriented most of the time. She is still immaculately groomed, has her hair fixed by the residence hairdresser, and is always neatly dressed. Her main objections to being in the nursing home are "nothing is mine" and "I need to share my bathroom with my roommate." She no longer seems to worry about the ex-penses for her care; she realizes that her cash reserves are long gone, and that her son, with govern-mental help, is managing costs. She participates little in nursing home activities except for religious services occasionally and then sits off by herself. She has made few friends among the residents. One friend, whom she visited often in her room, died recently and her roommate has just been taken to the hospital. She finds most of the other residents depressing. Most do not speak to each other; they sit quietly in their wheelchairs in the lounge. She cannot crochet anymore. She needs help with dressing, bathing, and transfers to wheelchair. Her daughter-in-law still visits every morning, her son almost every day on the way home from work, and her grandson and his wife stop in at least once a week. Her son is 62 years old and looking forward to retirement in a few years. The family brings her food treats from home, which she enjoys. On her last birthday her family brought in a party lunch for her to share with her dining table companions. It is becoming increas-ingly difficult to transport her, so she goes home only on holidays now and returns to the nursing home a few hours later. She is feeble and no longer speaks of the future in terms of going home. She says that she has lived long enough and can be heard praying aloud to die. Yet she seems to hold on tenaciously to life. She is 94 years old now.

Relocation

Often major environmental and social changes occur simultaneously with an aged per-son's decreased ability to cope with such changes. The need for institutionalization forces the aged person to confront his or her decreasing physical abilities and increasing dependency on others. At the same time it requires adaptation to a new environment, new social contacts, and a new routine. The move to a hospital or nursing home may precipi-tate grief, anger, a sense of helplessness, and depression. However persons who have de-veloped successful coping patterns in the past will probably continue to do so if they are able to appraise the stress situation realistically.

How individuals react to the prospect of institutionalization and their adjustment to the move seems to be related to the type and degree of orientation prior to the move and the extent to which they were included in the decision, as well as to personality factors.[3] The fear of institutionalization that is common among the aged needs to be acknowledged and the individual needs to be encouraged to express his anxieties and doubts. Previously successful coping patterns need to be identified and supported. It is particularly important at this time that the family be supportive, understanding, and reassuring so that the aged member will not feel alone and abandoned. Continuing and consistent contact with family before, during, and after the move will help to reduce the fear of the unknown and the feelings of aloneness.

In recognizing the impact of nursing home placement on the aged individual, one must not minimize the effect on the other family members when placement becomes necessary. They too may suffer from fear, guilt, and a sense of powerlessness. Even when the move was anticipated and planned for, there are many decisions to be made and uncertainties to be dealt with. Family members may need help in realistically appraising the strengths, weaknesses, and needs of the older person and in dealing with their own emotional responses to the separation. The goal is to facilitate the development of a support system in the family.

The patterns of socialization among the aged are probably far more complex than can be readily comprehended. Consider, for instance, that the aging adult has functioned in a variety of social situations for approximately 6 to 10 decades and has developed social skills and adaptive behaviors that have enabled him to cope with change over time and in new environments.

A number of theories have been proposed to explain the social behavior of the aged, such as the disengagement theory, the activity theory, the developmental theory, and others. Whereas it is possible to cite studies that tend to support one or another of these theories, it is probably most important in the case of a particular aging individual to identify previous patterns of socialization and sources of satisfaction that can be drawn on to facilitate the adjustment when institutionalization becomes necessary.

Some may view community living as a welcome alternative to the loneliness of a small apartment or rented room, whereas others see it as loss of privacy and opportunities for solitude. In either case, the choice of friends is limited by the population of the institution. It is also important in evaluating the opportunities for socialization to consider that the resident population may come from different social, economic, and cultural backgrounds and may have few shared experiences. It is also well to remember that the group we call the ''aged'' easily includes two generations, and a 70-year-old may have little in common with a 90-year-old.

The family is an important structure to provide stability and familiarity during the period of adjustment to institutional living, but the increasing age of the children may make their availability as primary social contacts for the aging parent very difficult.

Role change

. As age and infirmity increase, there is a need for finding new ways for the aged to achieve self-fulfillment and maintain dignity. Role flexibility helps to make this possible by intensifying involvement in some roles while discontinuing others and by continuing to create new roles that fulfill new or changing needs.

Loss

Loss of health is a serious problem for the aged, but loss of control over one's immediate environment may pose an even greater threat. An abrupt change in long-established habits and patterns of living is extremely disruptive and the aging parent needs continued family support and affection. During this final phase in the life cycle, loss is nearly an everyday occurrence — loss of health and physical abilities, loss of control and authority, loss of friends and family by death, and possibly loss of familiarity in the environment as a result of relocation.

During this time, the family, too, needs to cope with existing and impending loss. The physical and emotional distress of an aging parent causes stress on the children and other family members. There is a need for supportive services for the adult children if they are to deal successfully with the effects of continued interaction with the parent. There is also the need for the family to cope with the impending death of the aging member.

Because of the multitude and magnitude of the real and potential losses at this point in the life cycle, the persons involved may need help and support from outside the family system. Nursing, medical, pastoral, and social services might be used as community resources capable of providing specific types of support.

SUMMARY

This chapter has identified some of the common problems associated with the aging process and has suggested ways in which family interactions and support can be helpful in confronting these problems and dealing with them effectively. Healthy, successful aging is possible and is achieved by many through the development of inner strengths and through the understanding, support, and encouragement of family members. It is obvious that a single case history can not deal with all the types of situations and family patterns that may exist in other multigenerational families of various cultures. It is hoped, though, that the questions raised and the readings suggested will stimulate the pursuit of creative solutions to a wide range of situations and problems confronted by families that include aging members.

REFERENCES

1. Duvall, E. M.: Family development, Philadelphia, 1971, J. B. Lippincott Co., pp. 438-440.
2. Duvall, p. 441.
3. Yawney, B. A., and Slover, D. L.: Relocation of the elderly, Social Work, **18:**86-95, May, 1973.

SUGGESTED READINGS

Adamson, M., and Holley, M.: Implications for nursing in social disengagement theory. In Reinhardt, A. M., and Quinn, M. D., editors: Family-centered community nursing, St. Louis, 1973, The C. V. Mosby Co., pp. 237-244.

Beverly, E. V.: Nursing homes: matching the facility to the patient's needs, Geriatrics **31:**100-110, April, 1976.

Beverly, E. V.: Helping your patient choose and adjust to a nursing home, Geriatrics **31:**115-126, May, 1976.

Butler, R. M., and Lewis, M. I.: Aging and mental health; positive psychosocial approaches, ed. 2, St. Louis, 1977, The C. V. Mosby Co.

de Beauvoir, S.: The coming of age, New York, 1972, G. P. Putnam's Sons.

Duvall, E. M.: Family development, Philadelphia, 1971, J. B. Lippincott Co.

Fandetti, D. V., and Gelfand, D. E.: Care of the aged: attitudes of white ethnic families, The Gerontologist **16:**544-549, Dec., 1976.

Glick, P. C.: Updating the life cycle of the family, J. Marriage Fam. **39:**5-13, Feb., 1977.

Kellett, A.: Update on aging: its problems, its promises, Image, **7:**10-21, 1975.

Morgan, L. A.: A re-examination of widowhood and morale, J. Gerontol. **31:**687-695, Nov., 1976.

Otto, H. A.: A framework for assessing family strengths. In Reinhardt, A. M., and Quinn, M. D., editors: Family-centered community nursing, St. Louis, 1973, The C. V. Mosby Co., pp. 87-94.

Robertson, J. F.: Grandmotherhood: a study of role conceptions, J. Marriage Fam. **39:**165-174, Feb., 1977.

Robischon, P., and Smith, J. A.: Family assessment. In Reinhardt, A. M., and Quinn, M. D., editors: Current practice in family-centered community nursing, St. Louis, 1977, The C. V. Mosby Co., pp. 85-100.

Saul, S.: Aging: an album of people growing old, New York, 1974, John Wiley & Sons, Inc.

Schvaneveldt, J. D.: The interactional framework in the study of the family. In Reinhardt, A. M., and Quinn, M. D., editors: Family-centered community nursing, St. Louis, 1973, The C. V. Mosby Co., pp. 119-138.

Silverman, A., et. al.: A model for working with multigenerational families, Soc. Casework, **58:**131-135, March, 1977.

Simos, B. G.: Adult children and their aging parents, Soc. Work, **18:**78-85, May, 1973.

Sobol, E. G., and Robischon, P.: Family nursing: a study guide, ed. 2, St. Louis, 1975, The C. V. Mosby Co., pp. 158-182.

Tedrow, J. L.: Emotional, physical, and legal aspects of aging. In Reinhardt, A. M., and Quinn, M. D., editors: Current practice in family-centered community nursing, St. Louis, 1977, The C. V. Mosby Co., pp. 261-281.

Yawney, B. A., and Slover, D. L.: Relocation of the elderly, Soc. Work, **18:**86-95, May, 1973.

part V

ACTION AND SERVICE FOR THE ELDERLY: NURSING EDUCATION AND AGENCY COLLABORATION

Dr. Edward O. Moe, a nationally recognized community sociologist and health services planner, is the author of Chapter 13. This chapter is a detailed review of past and present achievements in building an array of specialized organizations and agencies on the community level to deliver both health and social services. Moe points out that what is needed now are new ways of building comprehensive programs to deliver health and social services for specific groups, especially the aging. This will require increased collaboration and coordination between community agencies. Moe describes and documents the need for interorganizational collaboration that focuses on the formation of agency networks addressed particularly to the provision of health care services for the elderly.

Moe defines and provides examples of three service levels: basic, supplementary, and facilitating. The chapter includes an informative guide for area planners on program resources for the aging. Also identifying linkages between existing service providers in a community are illustrated in diagram form.

Moe states that through such arrangements as those described and reviewed in the chapter, agencies are being linked in more effective ways for efficient service delivery to the elderly. Community health planners, agency directors, and community health nurses serving the elderly are more able now than at any previous time to study the emerging networks linking agencies that serve the aging. Also they can now determine alternative cost-effective ways of strengthening these networks as one way of improving the delivery of health services to the elderly. The content of this chapter is of extreme importance to nurses serving the elderly because often community nurses' roles become effective linkages between various aging services located in different community agencies.

In Chapter 14 an experienced gerontological nurse, Dr. Thelma J. Wells, sets forth a comprehensive and detailed overview of the historical development of gerontological nursing. She traces the history of gerontological nursing to its beginnings in the workhouses for the poor and infirm in England during the nineteenth century.

Most nursing of the elderly occurs in the homes of aging patient-clients in community settings and is provided by nurse practitioners. For the most part, community health nurses that serve the elderly have had only limited educational preparation in gerontological nursing. Wells points out that continuing education programs now provide the opportunity for practicing community health nurses to upgrade their knowledge and skills in the care of the elderly. Also emphasized is the fact that graduate education in gerontological nursing is just now being developed. Wells further stresses that gerontological content must become a more significant component of all basic nursing education. Nursing must be committd to quality care for the elderly. Wells emphasizes the pressing need for clinical nursing research concerned with significant nursing problems of the elderly. Her chapter should be of immeasurable assistance to all basic and graduate nursing students as well as those in continuing education programs and inservice educational programs.

In Chapter 15 Charlotte Eliopoulos describes in detail the role and function of the gerontological nurse in an institutional or community setting. She provides explicit examples of how the nurse can translate biopsychosocial concepts and problems of the aging into nursing practice. She discusses a number of strategies that the nurse can use to teach other nursing personnel in nursing homes. Also emphasized are numerous ways in which the gerontological nurse can function as an advocate in bringing about improved care for the elderly through service collaboration with other health team members. This chapter provides a guide for today's community health nurse who serves elderly patients in developing and implementing effective technologies in caring for aging persons as a health team member.

13 Agency collaboration in planning and service: the emerging network on aging

*issues and conditions—some underlying principles**

EDWARD O. MOE

Over the past several decades deliberate attempts have been made to coalesce agencies, organizations, informal natural support groups, and individuals into loosely linked service networks. What has been happening may be viewed as a process of building a new service system or new patterns in a renewing system. Strengthening cooperation and collaboration among those involved in planning and delivery of services has been seen as one way or the best way to overcome fragmentation and to improve the quality of services people receive.

Emerging networks or loosely linked systems now exist in various service fields. One such network exists in the field of aging. Significant initiatives both at the local level and the federal level have been made to build and/or strengthen the emerging systems. At the local level, health and welfare councils, community services councils, councils on aging, and other groups have attempted over the years to strengthen cooperation and collaboration in planning and delivery of service. Federal initiatives through the Older Americans Act and the creation of the area agencies on aging have provided additional resources and a new mechanism to strengthen collaboration and provide services where they were not available previously.

Whereas there is a great deal of information on the emerging networks, including the one on aging, much of what is known is imprecise and incomplete. Harder and firmer information is needed about the present status of the networks and the steps that might be taken to strengthen them. The present climate at the beginning of a new political administration is particularly appropriate for looking back at what we have done and looking forward to where we are going, for probing our achievements, and for clarifying the task confronting communities and society in improving human well-being and human services.

In keeping with this perspective, I explore agency collaboration through the following "sets" of ideas: (1) past and present achievements in organization — the setting for the "issues on collaboration," (2) some assumptions about organizations and collaboration among organizations, (3) some selected research findings, and (4) organizational alterna-

---

*Paper presented by Dr. Edward O. Moe at a workshop on Rural Gerontology Research, Pennsylvania State University, University Park, Pennsylvania, May 24 to 27, 1977.

tives—levels of cooperation and collaboration and some ways of achieving collaboration.

PAST AND PRESENT ACHIEVEMENTS IN ORGANIZATION— THE SETTING FOR THE ISSUES ON COLLABORATION

To put contemporary society and the human community in perspective, one must keep in mind that our society benefits from and suffers from a tremendous explosion in knowledge, particularly scientific knowledge and related technologies. This knowledge explosion is the basis for the industrial, urban, and bureaucratic revolutions in the modern world. It is these three revolutionary forces that have produced a new society and the communities of today and tomorrow. These forces also provide the context in which attempts to deal with the problems of society, the community, and human services must be conceived. The effects of these forces pervade every aspect of life.

A way of conceptualizing problems in communities

It is now evident that one of the significant achievements of American society and American communities has become a substantial weakness, that is, specialized competence and the placing of this competence in specialized organizations and agencies. This came about in a natural and seemingly ordered way in both the public and private sectors. What has not been recognized until recently is that the development and provision of specialized competence has led to three classical forms of isolation and estrangement.

1. Separation and isolation of agencies from each other
2. Separation and isolation of agencies from the community
3. Estrangement of agencies from the people they serve and those they might potentially serve

Many factors have contributed to this isolation. Once agencies were established they became possessive of programs and areas of work. These were their "property" and they were defensive about any intrusion by other agencies or by the community. At the same time, the community and various "coordinating" groups more or less assigned responsibility for particular programs to an agency. Frequently the community was pleased to be rid of programs as a general responsibility.

The isolation of agencies from each other and from the community, together with specialization and professionalization of agency staffs, led to an estrangement from the people served and those that might be served. This estrangement was further increased by conceptions of the helping function that tended to force people receiving help into a paralyzing passivity.

What has emerged within each community therefore is an enormously complex array of specialized organizations, programs, and services with a built-in dilemma of major proportions. On one hand, there is the array of public and private services with interconnections between the local and national levels. Conversely, at both the community and national levels, there is difficulty in relating these services to each other in such a way that an effective attack can be made on significant problems. These problems may be aging, rehabilitation, alcoholism, poverty, drug abuse, unemployment, and education or youth services or they may be the composite difficulties confronting neighborhoods or communities. In either case, the problems usually transcend the services of any specific organization and demand the cooperation and articulation of many services and the work of many agencies.

Not only is this a major difficulty for individuals and communities, it is also a problem for the agencies offering services. Under present conditions it is impossible for an agency working alone to achieve its own program objectives, however great its resources may be. To be effective, each must actively relate what it does to the work of other agencies and organizations. The dynamic properties of the situation "arise not simply from the interaction of the component organizations, but also from the field itself. The ground is in motion."[11]

Whereas it is quite clear that this is what is needed, or even demanded, if constructive efforts at improving the quality of human services are to be made, agencies and their staffs find themselves trapped. Agency executives and staff members talk eloquently of cooperation and coordination, but efforts to achieve these conditions are frequently weak to the point of futility.

National, state, and local relationships: a systems view of organization

Let us turn our attention for a moment to that aspect of the problem complicated by national, state, and local relationships. We cannot consider action at the local level apart from the relationships and mechanisms through which the functions and services of national parts of organizations are delivered to their local counterparts. A complicated yet simple and promising way of viewing organization at various levels is to view each level as a system. At the local level, for example, a unit of a national organization, whether public or private, is in many respects a system in its own right. It develops out of its purposes, the interaction of the people who compose it, the things these people have built around themselves, and the character of their interrelation to the community, to the state and region, and to the national organization of which they are a part.

A local unit of a national organization is not only a system in its own right, it is also a subsystem, or unit, of a community and of a national organization. Research and experience in national-local and organization-community relationships point out the subtleties, intricacies, and nuances in these relationships. Local units accept assistance and funds from the community and their national counterparts and maneuver to preserve their autonomy and to meet their own goals. At the same time they attempt to function as a subunit of the community and of their national organization. Requirements that are imposed tend to become additional forces in the field of action. There are long-established patterns of how to play one relationship against the other. Occasionally there is also the kind of cooperation that brings great credit to our pluralistic, federal system approach.

Some restraining forces and blocks to collaboration

There is substantial concurrence between research and experience concerning the major restraining forces and blocks to collaboration. The following are some of the major ones.

1. The organizational setting itself
   a. Climate of competition, conflict, distrust, and suspicion
   b. Continuing competition for funds, people, leadership, and position
   c. Concern about survival or loss of organizational identity with high involvement and commitment of one's own organization
2. Lack of clarity in the goals of collaborative ventures
   a. Failure to clarify the field or the problem on which there is to be collaboration
   b. Confusion over who is to be served

3. Concern over authority and control
4. Concern as to whether gains for ''our'' organization and for the people to be served will be as great as the costs
5. Inadequate, outdated, or ignored informal and formal agreements among organizations
6. Lack of organizational commitment including lack of concern about collaboration as a high-risk venture, an invitation to share failure
7. Poor communications practices
8. Lack of skill in working out and implementing collaborative relationships and agreements and lack of sensitivity and skill in implementing such relationships
9. Greater than anticipated time demands
10. Unwise use of ''pressure'' or ''clout'' to force collaboration
11. Tendency for collaborative or umbrella groups to take over member organizations' responsibilities
12. Inadequate means of assessing impact of collaborative activities

This is an imposing list of restraints and blocks. Criticism of agencies and services over the past decade has tended to stress the constraints and restraints. It is likely that researchers and practitioners have overlooked or failed to identify many of the linking and collaborative relationships between and among organizations. Lists such as this one do not tell the whole story.

SOME ASSUMPTIONS ABOUT ORGANIZATIONS AND COLLABORATION AMONG ORGANIZATIONS

One of the major difficulties in interpreting and assessing research and experience on interorganizational relationships is determining the assumptions that are made. Aldrich[2] identified three assumptions that tend to encourage such study. The first is that cooperative relations are ''good'' for two specific reasons: performance is higher and resources are used more efficiently when there is nonduplication of services, which is an outcome of cooperative relations. A second major assumption is that innovations are developed when organizations attempt to cooperate.[1] The third assumption is that agreements, overlapping boards, and joint actions by organizations are the best ways to deal with the changing organizational, community, state, and federal relationships. In many respects these assumptions attempt to answer questions for which research is undertaken.

Klonglan et al.[24] at Iowa State University made explicit another level of assumptions. They attempt to clarify the conditions and limitations confronted in collaboration. They identify a number of studies that illustrate each of the following assumptions.

1. Organizations are faced with a situation of limited resources.
2. Organizations must obtain resources from other units in their task environment.
3. Drawing on outside resources reduces an organization's authority.
4. Organizations prefer autonomy and engage in interaction only when resource needs cannot be met within the unit.
5. Organizations prefer low level interorganizational relations and will engage in higher level relations only after lower levels have failed to fulfill their resource needs.
6. Different levels of interorganizational relations can be ordered in terms of form and intensity of interactions.

This set of assumptions is helpful in understanding the state of the art and state of research in interorganizational relationships.

SOME SELECTED RESEARCH FINDINGS

It was more or less inevitable that the increase in research on organizations and organizational processes over the past quarter of a century would identify interorganizational fields and interorganizational relationships as significant areas of study. These areas have emerged as major concerns of practitioners.

Research and scholarly writing on organizations have clarified two perspectives in which collaboration can be examined. In one perspective collaboration is a dependent variable. It is the outcome of action and interaction among other variables. A second perspective views collaboration as an independent variable that has impact on the following:
1. Availability and quality of services to various populations
2. Recipients of services — their behavior, attitudes, and knowledge
3. Organizations and their internal structures and processes
4. Relationships with other organizations — changes in the form, content, and quantity of such relations
5. Communities — the interorganizational fields — and the changes in structure and processes, such as the determination of priorities, decision making, the allocation of resources, and the formalization of collaborative activities

The very brief review of research findings centers on the impact questions. Klonglan et al.[21] studied the outcomes or effects on 400 persons in alcohol programs in four communities and related outcomes to the amount of collaboration among the organizations involved. The findings were mixed. In three communities, the greater the amount of interorganizational relations, the greater the client outcome. However, the community with the highest score on interorganizational relations had the lowest client outcome score.

Richards and Goudy[34] studied residents' perceptions of the effect of a model cities program on coordination among agencies. Residents saw no increase in coordination.

Aiken and Hage[1] assessed the effects of interdependence among organizations on intraorganizational structure. Interdependence tended to increase complexity in organizational structure, to increase organizational innovations, to develop more internal communication channels, and to decentralize decision making. Price[33] studied the effects of one organization's co-opting members from other organizations to serve on advisory boards. Organizations that followed this practice were found to be more effective than those that did not do so. Sriram[41] found a significant positive relationship in more than 300 organizations between strong interorganizational relationships and organizational effectiveness. Form and Nosow[15] found somewhat the opposite in their study "Community in Disaster," in which organizations that were autonomous tended to be most effective. Hall[18-19] found that external pressures on organizations for interaction with other organizations have beneficial effects. External pressure increased communication and interaction among members, produced greater commitment, resulted in more exercise of authority at various levels, and increased cohesiveness among members.

Studies by Griffen et al.[16] and Dynes and Quarantelli[10] found that the more cooperation and collaboration among organizations, the more effective the recovery of a community after a disaster. These findings are very different from the Form-Nosow findings mentioned previously. It is likely that the difference in years in which the studies occurred may be significant. Under today's conditions there is much evidence to support the conclusion that no organization, however many resources it may have at its disposal, can achieve its objectives by working solely on its own. Achievement of significant ends, viewed from both the perspective of organizations and that of the community, requires collaboration.

ORGANIZATIONAL ALTERNATIVES—LEVELS OF COOPERATION AND COLLABORATION AND SOME WAYS OF ACHIEVING COLLABORATION

The present high interest in relationships among organizations and agencies as units or parts of the community is influenced by two significant insights. The first concerns the nature of the problems people confront. The second concerns the nature of the response of organizations and agencies and whether or not the responses are sufficiently comprehensive and specific to make a difference. Communities are the least reduceable units in which to see problems whole and to relate education and services in the attempt to resolve them.

Piecemeal approaches in attempting either to produce an environment of quality or to set the conditions for quality living have had limited success. Some significant gains have been made in setting up comprehensive physical planning programs, health programs, rehabilitation programs, and other programs. What is needed now is comprehensiveness on a more inclusive basis, a basis that would:

> encompass the life of people in a limited area—a community, or in some cases, a neighborhood—as it is actually lived and which would see problems as wholes, the way they are experienced, as well as in parts, the way services usually work at resolving them; adequately recognize the interrelationships among the social, physical, economic and political-governmental factors in problems and solutions; involve the residents of neighborhoods with professionals and specialists in public and private agencies in both clarifying problems and developing ways of attacking them.[29]

In this sense, agencies, their staffs, and the people are trapped and victimized. Despite the basic separation and estrangement between agencies and the people and the existence of fantastically complex problems in cooperation and coordination, building the array of specialized organizations and agencies is still a major achievement. The question is what we will do with the organizations now that we have them. Imaginative, new ways of relating an agency and what it does to the work of others are needed. What we urgently need are new ways of building comprehensive programs and implementing them, utilizing the best ways that we know. This leads to a look at alternatives.

Alternatives in organizational patterns

Over time there has emerged in the American community a large number of "community decision organizations."[46-47] Examples of community decision organizations are community councils, health and welfare councils, community services councils, councils on aging, area agencies on aging, urban renewal organizations, antipoverty organizations, civil defense and disaster relief alliances, housing authorities, youth bureaus and authorities, model cities and model neighborhood organizations, federations of churches, and city and county health and welfare departments; the list is very long. In varying degrees, these community decision organizations have become the legitimate means to carry out policy decisions and programs in various areas.

Each of the decision organizations has sought and won the support of influential people. Each has a director or executive director who has earned a varying amount of influence and respect. Counterparts of most of the community decision organizations exist at the national level. It is now clear that neither at the community nor at the national level have we attained the kind of joint decision making and joint action needed to deal realistically with the problems we confront.

Despite all of the efforts at cooperation to date and the growing body of evidence as to its effectiveness, the actions of a single organization or unitary organization, incomplete as they may be, are still seen by many to be more satisfying than joint actions. The time demanded to work through the trade-offs, the compromises, and the achievement of consensus in a joint action seems an invitation to failure. A major reason for this is that if an agency thinks it knows what and how to do something, it will do it. Whether or not it makes any sense to the community is another question. When agencies jointly tackle a big and important problem because they know they cannot do it alone, they frequently find themselves unprepared or poorly prepared to invest the effort and the time that the planning and action require.

It is essential to clarify the choices open to us in basic organizational strategy before considering the new or different ways of working. An analysis of the choices suggests four basic approaches:

1. *Single organization of unitary action by an organization to achieve its own goals.* This is the old pattern; it is effective within limits.
2. *Federative organizations — cooperative action through membership in a federation to achieve inclusive goals with member organizations free to set their own goals.* This, too, is an old pattern but one with more promise than has yet been realized.
3. *The formation of coalitions — informal cooperative arrangements among organizations to set inclusive goals, but with individual organizations being free to set their own specific goals.* These are usually short-term arrangements that emerge to meet a problem or a crisis and then dissolve.
4. *The building and/or strengthening of emerging networks. These are informal and some formalized cooperative arrangements among agencies, organizations, and constituencies to improve planning and service delivery in specific fields such as aging.* These networks are somewhat like coalitions. They tend, however, to be both emergent and to have some continuity over time. Single organizations, federations, and coalitions become part of the network.

For survival in today's system, an agency's basic strategy in the community must combine all four approaches. Greater emphasis than ever needs to be placed on the emerging networks and on initiating collaborative mechanisms through which the networks can become more effective. The network, with its informality and specificity, may well be the means of strengthening local natural support systems, for example, in aging and in enhancing what older people are able to do for themselves.

Emphasis on network membership should not be interpreted as, nor should it lead to, neglect of the internal structure or the capability for unitary action on the part of the agency. An agency must be strong internally if it is to have anything to contribute to the community. For an organization to help solve problems and take a significant role in the community, it must be strong in its own right, take an active role in federation, and seize the initiative in helping form and in responding to coalitions. Such actions strengthen the emerging networks and tend to increase their effectiveness.

Interaction among organizations at the community and national levels is not predetermined. Interaction emerges out of their relationships with each other in the community. Uncertainty, lack of clarity, and other problems in the community can be reduced by organizations relating to each other in more deliberate ways to attain both limited specific objectives as well as the major goal of improving the levels of human well-being.

Levels of cooperation

In the context of these organizational alternatives we can examine specific means, specific activities, and specific kinds of interaction, cooperation, or collaboration. Counting, measuring, and scaling these activities provide a basis for determining the level of cooperation among organizations. Some recent research has centered attention on the question of interaction. Aiken and Hage[1] approached level and intensity of interaction among agencies somewhat as practitioners have done by counting the number of joint programs. In 1969 Finley[12] identified 17 activities with which the level of intensity of cooperation could be measured and that would distinguish low, middle, or high level cooperation. He found the items to be scalable, using Gutman scaling techniques (which simply means that if you reached item 10 on the scale of 17 items, you would also have done items 1 through 9).

Others following Finley, notably Klonglan et al.,[23-24] found also that activities could be categorized as indicating low, medium, and high levels of collaboration. The list below draws on and summarizes both research and experience.

Low levels of collaboration
  1. Awareness of the existence of other organization(s) to which the agency should be related
  2. Acquaintance with director(s), staff, and counterparts in other organizations to which the agency should be related
  3. Acquaintance with programs and activities of organizations to which the agency should be related
  4. Unplanned, unscheduled communication between and among staffs and board members
  5. Unplanned, unscheduled personal interaction
  6. Limited exchange of program information as to needs, trends, emphases, and projections
  7. Membership on interagency councils with general planning, coordination, and evaluation responsibilities

Middle levels of collaboration
  8. Planned, specific provisions of sharing of information on policy changes, programs, and impact of programs
  9. Deliberate, planned exchange and interaction among staffs
  10. Exchange of personnel, resources and materials, and technical assistance
  11. Planned participation in programs initiated by other organizations; participation in coalitions initiated by other organizations; and an invitation or expectation that other organization(s) will participate in projects or coalitions you initiate
  12. Providing funds, source of funds, and sponsorship

High levels of collaboration
  13. Joint planning and joint initiation of projects and coalitions
  14. Joint use of staff and joint staff training and development
  15. Joint development of budgets and use of funds
  16. Planned overlapping of boards and joint setting of policies
  17. Planned continuing collaboration supported by jointly determined policies and agreements
  18. Joint development and implementation of a plan for comprehensive services

Among other things, this list provides a perspective on the range of collaboration from low levels to high levels. It may be used to determine the levels an agency has reached and its relationships with other agencies and organizations at a given time. By helping to define where an agency is, the list can be used to formulate specific guidelines for raising the existing level or for achieving the level of collaboration that is seen to be appropriate in working with other organizations. Also it is useful in helping to think about and define the abilities and the skills of an agency staff at a given time and what the staff needs to do to establish relationships that will enable the agency to be effective in achieving its own goals.

Services, planning, and delivery in the emerging aging networks

The attempt over the years to conceptualize a system of services has emphasized a number of ideas and sets of ideas that help give meaning and character to the emerging networks. Three are of particular relevance in the context of this paper: (1) the concept of services in the way they are used as basic, supplementary or facilitating services, (2) the qualities social planners have come to regard as essential in an arrangement of services such as availability, accessibility, integration or coordination, responsiveness, effectiveness, and efficiency, and (3) the linking mechanisms service providers may use in getting resources and program supports from other service providers or other community agencies in the planning and delivery of services. The interplay among these ideas and others is basic to the patterns that emerge in networks in different localities, and it tends to give the networks an enduring quality over time.

Basic, supplementary, and facilitating services

The push for functioning networks is rooted in the inherent relationships among services. Viewing services as basic, supplementary, and facilitating illustrates the effects of fragmentation and suggests some ways of overcoming it. Basic and supplementary services are those that are of direct benefit to the recipients in overcoming problems or conditions about which they are concerned. Facilitating services are those that enable people to find and use the basic and supplementary services.

In another sense basic services are those services thought to be essential, for example, to assure older people of a socially acceptable quality of life. As indicated in the listing below, these include items such as a minimal income, health and medical care, adequate housing, legal protection, and educational services.

Supplementary services are those that complement, extend, and make effective the basic services. They have value in their own right. Their value is maximized, however, by the way they complement the basic services and by the total contribution both types of services make to those who receive them. The following are some examples of supplementary services.

1. Making the most productive use of benefits gained from basic services, for example, consumer education designed to increase purchasing power through comparative shopping
2. Reducing unnecessary reliance on basic services, for example, a day care center that permits an earlier release of hospitalized patients
3. Enhancing an older person's sense of worth and usefulness, for example, opportunities for volunteering in various community organizations and programs or participation in a continuing education course

Table 5. An example of a service*

	Health	Nutrition	Home help	Community participation	Education	Income maintenance	Employment	Housing	Protective services
Basic services	Medicare Medicaid Nursing homes Hospitals Neighborhood health centers Health maintenance organizations Extended care facilities Mental hospitals	Title VII programs Meals-on-Wheels	Homemaker service Telephone reassurance Friendly visiting programs	Religious programs Senior center activities RSVP	Adult Education Remedial education Continuing education	Social Security SSI Private pension programs Veteran's benefits Tax relief	Public employment agency services Private employment agency services Vocational rehabilitation training programs	Public housing programs Retirement hotels Homes for the aged Retirement villages Adult foster homes	Protective services Legal aid
Supplemental services	Visiting nurses Home health aides Health screening programs Day care	Nutrition education	Handyman service	SCORE Senior citizen clubs and organizations Recreation programs offered by various community groups and organizations	Library services Preretirement education Hobby or special interest programs Mobile library Mail-a-book services	Senior discounts Coops Food stamp program Consumer protection services	Foster grandparents Green thumb Employment for senior citizens as teacher aides, library assistants, etc.	Tenant councils	Lawyer referral services
Facilitating services	——— Transportation ——— Information and referral ——— Community awareness ——— Outreach ——— Follow-up ——— Escort ——— Counseling				——— Transportation ——— Information and referral ——— Community awareness ——— Outreach ——— Follow-up ——— Escort ——— Counseling				

*From Guide to Program Resources for Area Planners In Aging. A Publication of Project Tap. The Institute of Gerontology, The University of Michigan—Wayne State University, and The School of Social Work Continuing Education Program, The University of Michigan, 1974.

4. Reducing states of loneliness and social isolation, for example, telephone reassurance and friendly visitors services
5. Expanding opportunities for personal pleasure and enjoyment, for example, recreational programs and other forms of leisure time activity

Facilitating services derive their importance from their instrumental value. They enable people to know about, to get to, and to use the basic and supplementary services. Information, counseling, and transportation thus become a facilitating and integral part of any service system or network.

Table 5 illustrates the relationships among services. The categorization of services may differ by community, state, or region of the country or by the theoretical views of researchers or practitioners. The relationship between services and the interrelationships between agencies providing services is basic to an understanding of the emerging networks in aging.

Such a table may be used in a number of ways. It shows the services that exist in a community or area. Given the conditions, it can be used also by the agencies and institutions and the resources of a community or area to construct a model services arrangement. The model arrangement could then be used to guide planning and action in developing an improved service system or network.

Linkages between existing services and service providers

Sociologists, gerontologists, and practitioners in the field of aging have been and are concerned about linkages between services and agencies in the emerging aging networks. Levels of collaboration discussed previously are one way of measuring linkage, at least in general terms. The service matrix provides another perspective on the inherent relationship among services. Still another and more specific view is gained by examining the mechanisms service providers use to obtain needed program supports from other agencies. Suppose, for example, that a senior center in a community had determined and documented the need for a Title VII congregate meals program. It had proposed such a program and received support for it. In both planning and implementing the program it would need assistance from other service providers.

The following list identified some 23 possible linking mechanisms or types of assistance that might be needed:

1. Purchase of services
2. Information processing, dissemination, and exchange
3. Technical assistance
4. Joint program or project evaluation
5. Standards and guidelines
6. Loaner staff
7. Outstationing
8. Liaison teams and joint use of staff
9. Staff training and development
10. Screening, employment, counseling, and placement
11. Volunteers
12. Ombudsman
13. Outreach
14. Intake
15. Diagnosis
16. Referral

17. Follow-up
18. Case management
19. Ad hoc case coordination
20. Case conferences
21. Joint program development
22. Joint projects
23. Multiservice centers

Fig. 1 shows the agencies involved in the congregate meals program and the types of assistance provided. The linking mechanism or type of assistance is identified by the number in the block. The Welfare Department is linked through purchase of services, the community action program through referral, and the Welfare Council through information processing, dissemination, and exchange. Other service providers are linked in other ways.

The direct links are between the senior center and various service providers. Existence of the direct links creates or can create in some sense relationships among all the agencies involved in the congregate meals programs.

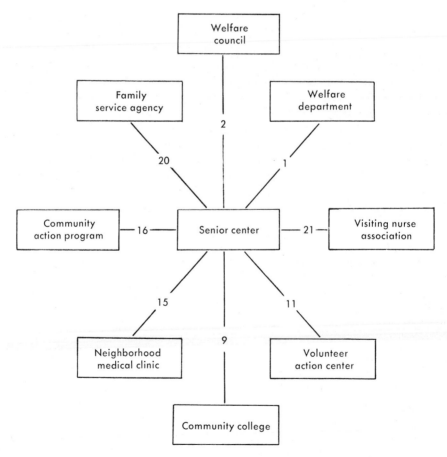

Fig. 1. Linkage diagram for Title VII congregate meals.

Through such arrangements as these, agencies are being linked. Out of all the activities that have occurred and those that are now in process, loosely linked networks are being created. Theoretically and methodologically we are more able now than at any previous time to study the emerging networks and to determine alternative cost effective ways of strengthening them as a way of improving social services.

REFERENCES

1. Aiken, M., and Hage, J.: Organizational interdependence and intra-organizational structure, Am. Sociol. Rev. **33**(6):912-930, 1968.
2. Aldrich, B. C.: Relations between organizations: a critical review of the literature, (paper presented at the annual meeting of the American Sociological Association, Washington, D.C.), Minneapolis, 1970, University of Minnesota Press.
3. Aldrich, H.: Organizational boundaries and interorganizational conflict, Hum. Relations **24**:279-293, August, 1971.
4. Blau, P. M.: Exchange and power in social life, New York, 1964, John Wiley & Sons, Inc.
5. Blau, P. M., and Scott, W. R.: Formal organizations, San Francisco, Chandler Publishing Co., 1962.
6. Chiamcharoen, A.: Cooperative interaction and goal attainment among rural development organizations: a study in interorganizational relations, Ph.D. dissertation, Ames, Iowa, 1974, Iowa State University Press.
7. Clark, B. R.: Interorganizational patterns in education, Administr. Sci. Q. **10**:224-237, Sept. 1964.
8. Dahl, R., and Lindblom, C.: Politics, economics and welfare, New York, 1953, Harper & Row, Publishers.
9. Dynes, R. R.: Community conflict: an explanation of its absence in natural disasters, Columbus, Ohio, 1969, Disaster Research Center, Working Paper No. 41, Ohio State University Press.
10. Dynes, R. R., and Quarantelli, E. L.: Interorganizational relations in communities under stress, Columbus, Ohio, 1969, Ohio State University Press, Disaster Research Center, Working Paper No. 19.
11. Emery, S. E., and Trist, E. L.: The causal texture of organizational environment, Hum. Relations **18**:21-32, Feb., 1965.
12. Finley, J. R.: Relations between development organizations: a preliminary report of scaling interorganizational relations, Ithaca, New York, 1969, Cornell University Press.
13. Finley, J. R.: A study of interorganizational relationships, unpublished Ph.D. dissertation, Ithaca, New York, 1970, Cornell University Press.
14. Finley, J. R., and Capener, H. R.: Interorganizational relations: concepts and methodological considerations, (paper presented at the annual meeting of the Rural Sociological Society, San Francisco), Ithaca, New York, 1967, Cornell University Press.
15. Form, W. H., and Nosow, S.: Community in disaster, New York, 1958, Harper & Row, Publishers.
16. Griffin, C. T.: A causal model analysis of role performance of coordinators in the operating system following a disaster, unpublished Ph.D. dissertation, Ames, Iowa, 1972, Iowa State University Press.
17. Hage, J., and Aiken, M.: Organizational permeability, boundary spanners and organizational structure, (paper presented at the annual meeting of the American Sociological Association, New Orleans, La.), Madison, Wisc., 1972, University of Wisconsin Press.
18. Hall, R. H.: Organizations, structure and process. Englewood Cliffs, N.J., 1972, Prentice-Hall, Inc.
19. Hall, R. H.: Perspectives from outside medical sociology: research on large scale organizations, (paper presented at the annual meeting of the American Sociological Association, New Orleans, La.), Minneapolis, 1972, University of Minnesota Press.
20. Klonglan, G. E.: Coordination among agencies for rural development: some current research and policy needs, (paper presented at the National Conference on Non-Metropolitan Community Services Research), Columbus, Ohio, 1977, Ohio State University Press.
21. Klonglan, G. E., Dillman, D. A., Wright, J. S., and Beal, G. M.: Agency interaction and patterns and community alcoholism services, Ames, Iowa, 1969, Sociology Report No. 73, Department of Sociology, Iowa State University Press.
22. Klonglan, G. E., Warren, R. D., Winkelpleck, J. M., and Paulson, S. K.: Interorganizational measurement in the social services sector: differences by hierarchical level, Administr. Sci. Q. **21**:675-687, Dec., 1976.
23. Klonglan, G. E., and Yep, B.: Theory and practice of interorganizational relations, Ames, Iowa, 1972, Iowa State University Press.

24. Klonglan, G. E., Yep, B., Mulford, C. L., and Dillman, D.: The nature and impact of interorganizational relations, Ames, Iowa, 1972, Iowa State University Press.

25. Leadley, S. M.: An integrative model: cooperative relations among organizations, (paper presented at the annual meeting of the Rural Sociological Society, San Francisco), University Park, Pennsylvania, 1969, Pennsylvania State University Press.

26. Levine, S., and White, P. E.: Comments on: exchange as a conceptual framework for the study of interorganizational relationships, Amer. Sociol. Q. March, 1961.

27. Levine, S., and White, P. E.: The community of health organizations. In Freeman, H., Levine, S., and Reeder, L., editors: Handbook of medical sociology, Englewood Cliffs, N.J., 1963, Prentice-Hall, Inc.

28. Moe, E. O.: Community services planning: a new approach, Bureau of Community Development, Salt Lake City, 1965, University of Utah Press.

29. Moe, E. O.: Principles in the model cities concept, Division of Community and Urban Development, Salt Lake City, 1969, University of Utah.

30. Moe, E. O.: Agency collaboration in planning and service, (paper presented at the National Conference on Social Welfare, Centennial Forum, Atlantic City, N.J., 1973).

31. Moe, E. O.: The nature of today's community. In Reinhardt, A. M., and Quinn, M. D., editors: Family centered community nursing: a sociocultural framework, St. Louis, 1973, The C. V. Mosby Co.

32. Mulford, C., and Klonglan, G. E.: Developing coalitions for social action (paper read at the National Conference on Voluntarism and America's Future: Prologue to the third century, Washington, D.C.), Ames, Iowa, 1972, Iowa State University.

33. Price, J. L.: Organizational effectiveness: an inventory of propositions, Homewood, Ill., 1968, R. D. Irwin, Publisher.

34. Richards, R. O., and Goudy, W. J.: Evaluations of citizen participation and interagency cooperation in the Des Moines model city program, Ames, Iowa, 1971, Sociology Report No. 96, Iowa State University Press.

35. Rogers, D. L.: Costs and benefits of alternative strategies for interagency coordination. In Rogers, D. L., and Whiting, L. R., editors: Aspects of planning for public services in rural areas, Ames, Iowa, 1969, NCRCRD.

36. Rogers, D. L.: Organizational coordination in rural development: a research proposal. Ames, Iowa, 1971, Department of Sociology, Iowa State University.

37. Rogers, D. L.: Towards a scale of interorganizational relations among public agencies, Sociol. Soc. Research **59:**61-70, 1974.

38. Rogers, D. L.: Sociometric analysis of interorganizational relations: application of theory and method, Rural Soc. **39:**487-503, 1974.

39. Rogers, D. L., and Glick, E. L.: Planning for interagency cooperation in rural development, Ames, Iowa, 1973, Center for Agricultural and Rural Development Report 45, Iowa State University.

40. Rogers, D. L., and Molnar, J.: Interorganizational relations among development organizations: empirical assessment and implications for interagency systems, Ames, Iowa, 1975, Center for Agricultural and Rural Development Report 62, Iowa State University Press.

41. Sriram, C. M.: Towards a theory of organizational—environmental relationships, M. S. Thesis, Houston, 1969, University of Houston.

42. Thompson, J. D.: Organizations and output transactions, Am. J. Sociol. **68**(3):309-321, 1962.

43. Thompson, J. D.: Organizations in action, New York, 1967, McGraw-Hill Book Co.

44. Thompson, J. D.: Thoughts of interorganizational relations: a conclusion, Interorganizational research in health: conference proceedings, Baltimore, Md., 1970, The Johns Hopkins University Press.

45. Thompson, J. D., and McEwen, W. J.: Organizational goals and environment: goal setting as an interaction process, Am. Sociol. Rev. **23:**23-31, Feb., 1958.

46. Warren, R. L.: The interaction of community decision organizations: some basic concepts and needed research, Soc. Serv. Rev. **41**(3):261-270, Sept., 1967a.

47. Warren, R. L.: The interorganizational field as a focus for investigation, Administr. Sci. Q. **12:**396-419, Dec., 1967b.

48. White, P. E.: Intra- and inter-organizational studies: do they require separate conceptualizations? Administr. Soc. **6:**107-152, 1974.

49. White, P. E., Levine, S., and Vlasak, G. J.: Exchange as a conceptual framework for understanding interorganizational relationships: application to non-profit organizations, Baltimore, Md., 1971, The Johns Hopkins University Press.

50. White, P. E., and Vlasak, G. J.: A selected bibliography focusing on interorganizational research on health, 1960-1970, Baltimore, Md., 1971, The Johns Hopkins University Press.

51. White, P. E., and Vlasak, G. J.: Interorganizational research in health, Baltimore, Md., 1970, The Johns Hopkins University Press.

14 Nursing committed to the elderly

THELMA J. WELLS

HISTORICAL DEVELOPMENT

Care of the sick and frail elderly has always been entrusted to those individuals who occupy a nursing role in society. Prior to the development of modern nursing, care of ill elders was probably the responsibility of the dominant woman in a family unit. Those elderly people who were without family and needed care became the responsibility of designated social institutions, usually the religious community. Thus in preindustrial societies, in which few people survived to old age and the family was a cohesive economic and social unit, care of the elderly was not a societal problem.

Controversy did arise during the industrial revolution in England when social and economic pressures led to the development of the Poor Law. Workhouses were built as part of a system designed "to discourage the able-bodied from seeking support from public funds."[1] Although these institutions were not created to care for the frail and sick aged, such individuals who were without other resources had no choice but to become workhouse inhabitants. Their care was provided by fellow inmates called pauper nurses. These "nurses" were uneducated, unsupervised, often ill, and sometimes alcoholics; the "care" was deplorable.[2]

It was in such a setting that modern gerontological nursing can be said to have begun. Agnes Jones, an intelligent, attractive, and wealthy Nightingale-trained nurse, pioneered the improvement of nursing care for the ill, poor, and socially neglected elderly in Britain. In 1864 she was "called by God as well as sent by Miss Nightingale to work in the Liverpool Infirmary," a large Poor Law institution in northwestern England.[3] In the first months she dismissed 35 pauper nurses for drunkenness and wrote that she found "men wore the same shirts for seven weeks. Bed-clothes were sometimes not washed for months. The diet was hopelessly meagre compared to a hospital standard."[4]

Miss Jones, with 12 nurses under her direction and Miss Nightingale as her ally and mentor, not only improved the standards of care in that institution but demonstrated that such improvements decreased the cost of maintaining the sick.[5]

Early nursing history in the United States, while characterized by outstanding leaders, fails to reveal any particular nurse leader primarily focused on work with the elderly. This may reflect the limited impact of a relatively small proportion of aged patients in a young country or it may reflect a lack of interest in gerontological nursing by American nursing history researchers.

In the more than 100 years since Miss Jones, gerontological nursing has been evolving into a creditable specialty area. Peplau[6] identified three trends in the evolutionary pattern of a specialty, which can be discerned in the history of gerontological nursing: (1) increased knowledge about phenomena relevant to a particular field, (2) advances in technology stemming from development in basic and applied sciences, and (3) the public's attention on needy and neglected areas.

Knowledge growth

Although study of the aging process is probably as ancient as civilization, it was not until the mid-1940s that gerontology became an area of organized scientific interest.[7] Birren and Clayton[8] surveyed literature in the field and noted an exponential growth pattern. Gerontological literature generated between 1950 and 1960 equalled all the field's literature produced in the prior 115 years.

Medical interest in aging stems from Hippocrates, but modern study is usually dated from 1909 when Nasher coined the term "geriatrics" (*geron,* old man; *iatrikos,* medical treatment).[9] Medical textbooks focused on the specialty began to appear in 1914.[10] However, true expansion of medical study in aging was also a mid-1940s development, noted by the founding of the American Geriatrics Society in 1942.[11]

The first nursing textbook for care of the elderly appeared in 1950—*Geriatric Nursing* by Kathleen Newton, a nurse in ambulatory care.[12] A review of nursing literature from 1955 to 1965 showed an almost steady increase in gerontological nursing care and health service publications from 18 articles produced in 1955 to 71 in 1965.[13]

During those 10 years the first gerontological nursing research was published. In Britain, Doreen Norton, with a nurse and physician colleague, initiated a systematic exploration directed "to improve nursing techniques in the management and care of the elderly sick."[14] Assessment based on the elderly person's functional level in activities of daily living, suitable clothing, therapeutic chairs, and pressure sore prevention are examples of studies reported in this classic work. The initial research, focused on the institutionalized elderly, was followed in 2 years by the historic American study, *The Elderly Ambulatory Patient.*[15] Doris Schwartz and her colleagues explored a series of questions about the care of elderly, chronically ill outpatients. The study included patient health care knowledge, medication errors, food patterns, ambulation, and travel profiles.

Nursing research in the field of aging has steadily increased. Robinson[16] surveyed the nursing literature produced between 1966 and 1975 to identify gerontological nursing studies. She found 48 published research reports on aging and the aged that were directed by nurses.

Technological advances

Advances in public health and postnatal infant care over the last 100 years contributed greatly to the gain in life expectancy for Americans.[17] The impact of technological growth is acknowledged by Cutler and Harootyan: "It took only 70 years to increase average life expectancy by 40 percent of the total gain achieved during the last three millennia of human existence."[18] The fact that the number of Americans 65 years of age and older has increased more than sixfold since 1900 is due in part to technological advances.[19]

The significant growth of the elderly population and advances in medical care have brought a corresponding increase in nurses' contact with older people. Most nursing of the elderly occurs in the home, as attested by the increasing older client caseloads of nurses working in the community. Census data reveal that of the noninstitutionalized elderly 5% are homebound and about 85% have one or more chronic diseases that may result in physical care problems.[19] Nurses in acute care settings are also frequent providers of care to the elderly. Persons over 65 years of age are twice as likely to be hospitalized during the year than are individuals under 65. Furthermore, older people stay in the hospital twice as long as younger people and are more likely to be rehospitalized during the year.[19] Long-term institutional care of the elderly has been expanding rapidly, with more than 1 million nursing home beds provided in 1971.[20]

Public attention

In recent years a number of public hearings and publications have focused attention on the quality of care provided to the approximate 5% of the aged population who are institutionalized.[21-23] Investigations have revealed numerous abuses, such as "negligence leading to death and injury; unsanitary conditions; poor food or poor preparation; hazards to life or limb; misappropriation and theft; inadequate control of drugs; reprisals against those who complain; and assault on human dignity."[24] The publicity generated has initiated a wide variety of reform measures.

Less dramatic, but equally important, discussion of the elderly as a minority group has focused attention on negative stereotyping, segregation, and discrimination as factors of age alone. Consciousness raising of the aged has been a feature of the 1970's with the proliferation of such organizations as the Gray Panthers, the American Association of Retired Persons, and the National Caucus of the Black Aged.

Gerontological nursing: a specialty

These factors of knowledge growth, technological advances, and public attention led to the development of gerontological nursing as a specialty area. The American Nurses Association established a national practice division, Geriatric Nursing, in 1966.[25] Ten years later, the division's name was changed to Gerontological Nursing Practice, reflecting knowledge and attitude growth within the specialty. At the same time the division's standards of nursing practice were revised to incorporate the nursing process and the increasing scope of practice in care of the elderly.[26]

The first master's program to prepare nurses as clinical specialists in gerontological nursing was developed in 1966 by Virginia Stone at Duke University School of Nursing. This pioneer program was offered for 7 years and produced the first 12 specialists in this field.[27] However, at the time of the Senate Subcommittee on Long-term Care hearings on trends in long-term care (1969 to 1973) there were no graduate level programs for gerontological nursing.[28] A major growth in master's level specialization has occurred subsequent to, and perhaps as a result of, the Senate hearings and the consequent increased federal and professional committment to the elderly.

Significant advances have occurred in gerontological nursing literature. The first journal exclusively focused on this field, the *Journal of Gerontological Nursing,* began publication in the spring of 1975. The first nursing textbook in the field since Newton's format from the 1950s appeared in 1976. Irene Burnside's *Nursing and the Aged* led the field in a vast array of new publications focused on the elderly person and his health care.[29]

Gerontological nursing is a young, often little understood specialty in nursing. Few nurses have been academically prepared in the field, which has slowed dissemination of applied knowledge of aging into nursing as a whole. Because there is little awareness of the breadth and depth of modern gerontological nursing, many nurses believe it to be simply a kindly attention to the bedfast old. In their ignorance they foster a passive acceptance of some of the most complex care problems in nursing, such as mental disorientation, incontinence, and pressure sores. Modern gerontological nursing draws from a large body of knowledge and seeks new knowledge to promote health, prevent illness, treat disease, and provide rehabilitation for elderly people. It is a nursing specialty characterized by dynamic, pragmatic actions aimed at helping the older person achieve and maintain the level of physical and social functioning appropriate to his individual life-style and environmental needs. The emphasis is on positive care dimensions: wellness, mobility, independence, and interdependence. Such an emphasis does not negate the underpinnings of nursing, comfort and support.

Basic to gerontological nursing is the belief that the elderly individual has the right and freedom to choose his individual level of physical functioning, social role, and, when the time comes, a death with dignity and comfort. To facilitate these rights and assist the elderly individual with choices, the nurse in gerontology must demonstrate excellence in nursing care, communicate knowledge and methods to help other nurses achieve such excellence, become a change agent in the health care system for the improvement of services to the elderly, and become an active participant in scientific inquiry, interdisciplinary professional care teams, and community affairs related to the needs of elderly people.

Modern gerontological nursing is just beginning. In the years ahead it must spread its knowledge base throughout all of nursing and substantially enlarge its care dimensions through research focused on positive elderly patient/client outcomes. A key to the future is education.

EDUCATION IN GERONTOLOGICAL NURSING
Preprofessional education

There have been four major surveys of gerontological content in basic nursing programs.[30-33] The most recent survey was conducted by the Division on Gerontological Nursing Practice of the American Nurses Association. Questionnaires seeking information about gerontological nursing content were sent to all 1,374 basic nursing education programs in 1975. Eighty-three percent of the schools responded. However, the returned data were characterized by inconsistencies, generalizations, difficulties in interpretation, and incomplete responses. This interesting finding, not noted in other surveys, may indicate a period of dynamic growth difficult to document in a complex questionnaire. Within the constraints imposed by such data some indication of progress in gerontological nursing education and its current status can be discerned.

Fourteen percent of the reporting schools indicated that they offered specialized courses in gerontological nursing; the majority required them for students. Earlier surveys had reported a range of only 5% to 12% of schools that taught such a course. Thus there is evidence of growth in the number of specialized courses on aging offered in basic nursing preparation. However, as in earlier surveys, the majority of responding schools stated that they incorporated principles of gerontological nursing into some aspect of course work.

These surveys illustrate the major debate concerning gerontological nursing in basic nursing preparation: integration or specialization. Those who adhere to an integration philosophy tend to be proponents of curriculum framed within growth and development concepts. They believe that specialization in gerontological nursing is a type of segregation that fosters a negative attitude toward aging and promotes disinterest in the field. Those who adhere to a specialization in gerontological nursing philosophy present the need for differentiation of content areas before integration is possible. They believe that current integration of gerontological nursing content into basic curriculum is both superficial and inadequate.

A great deal of the argument is related to the scarcity of nurse educators with specialized knowledge and clinical practice in gerontological nursing. If every school of nursing desired or were required to have specified content in the care of the aged, there presently are not enough teachers in the field with either appropriate academic specialization or self-taught knowledge and skill to assume such a task. With few prepared individuals to differentiate and teach content in gerontological nursing, the case for integration is not only more easily accepted but may be the only approach possible for some schools. The merit of either integration or specialization of gerontological nursing content in basic preparation will not be solved until there are enough adequately prepared nurse educators in the field of aging who can teach from both curriculum perspectives.

Within the gerontological nursing specialization viewpoint there is concern about when and how to teach specific content directed toward nursing the elderly. Gunter taught a two-credit course entitled "Nursing Function in Gerontology" to 162 undergraduate senior students.[34] She evaluated the students' attitudes toward old people (Tuckman-Lorge stereotype scale) and work preference before and after the course. The results indicated that although misconceptions about aging decreased, so did the number of students who expressed a strong interest in working with the aged. Gunter concluded that courses on aging should be given earlier in the student nurse's learning process.

Kayser and Minnigerode[35] reported a study of 311 baccalaureate nursing students, some of whom were taking or had completed a sophomore two-semester human development course with gerontology contact.[35] Their findings reflected that such a course had little effect on student attitude improvement (Tuckman-Lorge stereotype scale) or work preference in aging. However, the cross-sectional design and the unspecified extent and depth of specific gerontology content in the designated course weaken the finding.

Using an experimental design, Heller and Walsh[36] studied the effects of a 45-hour course, "Basic Concepts in Nursing The Aged," on 110 second year associate degree nursing students' attitudes toward old people (Kogan scale) and work preferences for the aged. Course content and laboratory experience were developed within the context of Festinger's cognitive dissonance theory and were focused on positive experiences with the well elderly. Prior to the special course, all the students demonstrated similar attitudes toward old people. Testing after the course revealed that students who had taken the course had a highly significant change toward more positive attitudes. Further, those students increased their preferences for work with the aged.

It is evident that more research is needed before specific conclusions can be drawn concerning the when and how of gerontological content in basic curriculum. The problem remains significant as a potential key to recruitment into gerontological nursing specialty practice areas. Although the population 65 years and older is increasing and the birth rate is decreasing, one study of baccalaureate nursing students revealed that work in geriatrics was least preferred and work in obstetrics and pediatrics was most preferred.[37] Not surprisingly the study results indicated that students gave geriatrics the highest scores for being "depressing, dull, and slow." Enlightening and motivating gerontological nursing input at appropriate education points might reverse such negative viewpoints.

Other countries

There are no published data concerning gerontological nursing content in the basic preparation of nurses in other countries. However, informal contact with nurses in western European nations suggests that gerontological nursing education is a growing area of interest and concern. In 1970 the World Health Organization Regional Office for Europe convened a working group to discuss education and training in long-term and geriatric care.[38] Their report endorsed the need for such nurse training and implied that European nursing schools needed to develop more fully this aspect of their curricula. There has been considerable discussion in England concerning a proposal to require a 3-month specialized study in geriatric nursing at the basic level of nurse preparation. Currently, geriatric nursing is both integrated in curriculum and available as a 3-month special study option in that country.

Continuing education

During 1972 to 1973 the American Nurses Association presented a nationwide continuing education program, sponsored by the Department of Health, Education and Welfare, for nursing home nurses to update knowledge and skill in gerontological nursing.[39] Approximately 3,000 nurses, nearly 10% of those employed in nursing homes, attended the 3-day sessions held in 42 regional areas. The majority of those attending currently worked in nursing homes, were in administrative positions as head nurse or higher, and had their basic preparation in nursing in a hospital diploma school of nursing. Seventy-six percent of these nurses stated that they had not had any formal geriatric nursing content in their basic education and had not attended a previous conference related to geriatric nursing or nursing home care. Additional background data on these nursing home nurses revealed that they were not markedly different from nurses employed in other settings.[40]

The deficiencies in preparation in gerontological nursing will need to be remedied in continuing education programs long after nursing schools have learned to adequately prepare nurses in the care of the old. Not only is continuing education in gerontological nursing necessary to address preparation deficiencies, it should also be a significant component in the newly developing formal continuing education programs across the country. While controversy surrounds such programs (for example, questions of whether they should be mandatory or voluntary, method of credit approval, appropriate content, and funding) there is no doubt that the concept is well grounded, well accepted, and a major thrust of nursing in the 1970s.

Continuing education programs differ from formal academic study in that they are directed to specific rather than general content, usually extend over a shorter period of time, and provide a certificate of completion rather than an academic degree.[41] Such programs differ from inservice education in that they are designed to enlarge knowledge or skills in specific aspects of nursing, not to impart knowledge necessary to function in a particular agency. Undoubtedly some inservice education programs have well-developed continuing education components.

Because continuing education programs are available in a variety of formal and informal patterns of varying length and depth, it is difficult to determine the quantity and quality of such programs in gerontological nursing. However, Buseck[42] identified three priorities for both continuing education and inservice education programs for nursing home nurses that can be generalized to all nurses who care for the elderly. These were (1) to promote positive, dynamic nurse attitudes toward the elderly, (2) to provide a scientific knowledge base in gerontology and gerontological nursing, and (3) to increase nurse management and teaching skills.

Preparation of the gerontological nurse practitioner has been an area of growth in continuing education. The American Nurses Association defines the nurse practitioner or clinician as a registered nurse with special preparation, which can be obtained in continuing education as well as formal academic programs.[43] The nurse so prepared is described as a primary care provider able to assess physical and psychological status of clients, interpret data, develop and implement therapeutic plans, and follow the client through the continuum of care. Guidelines are available for short-term continuing education programs,[44] and eight such programs are listed in the most recent Directory of Programs Preparing Registered Nurses for Expanded Roles.[45]

Continuing education in geriatrics: England

Continuing nursing education in geriatrics has been available in England for some years, but the quality of programs varies widely. The Joint Board of Clinical Nursing Studies (Adam House, 1 Fitzroy Square, London W1P 6DS, England) was set up in 1970 to develop standards and coordinate and supervise postregistration nursing education.[46] There is an approved geriatric nursing syllabus, and a small number of hospitals have developed 6-month courses under the guidance of the Joint Board.

Inservice education

One of the needs evident from the nursing home scandals is for inservice education programs focused on care of the elderly. Such programs are distinguished from other types of advanced study in that they are administered by an employer and are directed to upgrading knowledge and skills necessary to function within a specific agency.[47] The Department of Health, Education and Welfare Long-Term Care Facility Improvement Study supported the need for inservice training and equity in the financial burden such training would create.[48] The suggestion has been to make the cost of such education a reimbursable item under publically funded programs.[49]

Graduate-level education

Since the early 1970s Master's specialization in gerontological nursing has shown significant growth. Seven programs were listed in the American Nurses' Association's Directory of Programs Preparing Registered Nurses for Expanded Roles.[50] Three additional programs are in existence (University of California, Los Angeles; University of Cincinnati, and University of Rochester). In addition, several other programs are in developmental stages (for example, Kansas University and University of Maryland). Although it is difficult to monitor the extent of graduate education in gerontological nursing, it would appear to be in a period of major expansion.

During such a period diversity can be expected; this is confirmed by an examination of descriptions of current programs. Graduate programs in gerontological nursing appear to be more dissimilar than similar; they vary in program title, entrance requirements, and length. More important, they vary in the percentage of curriculum directly focused on gerontology and gerontological nursing, range and extent of clinical experience with the elderly, and research content and practice directed toward clinical nursing issues in gerontology.

It is logical that a beginning specialty would struggle with unclarified objectives, poorly differentiated content, and diverse educational methodologies. Such a specialty suffers from a scarcity of qualified teachers and an inadequate pool of knowledge to address the array of complex problems with which it is faced. However, it is well to advise prudence and to urge increased discussion during expansion periods.

Prior to curriculum building in gerontological nursing it is expedient to delineate a philosophy of nursing, aging, and the health-illness continuum. Thus a framework for subsequent course content is set. Conceptual models from nurse theorists and individual nursing schools are helpful but at this point are not definitive for gerontological nursing.

Once a philosophy and framework are identified, specific curriculum facets emerge. One approach to the teaching of gerontological nursing at the graduate level is that of promoting health and providing care to the elderly in terms of function and dysfunction in life processes. This frame rests on a social definition of health and illness. That is, one is well when he can do those things that are necessary and meaningful in his life even though he has one or more pathological conditions. A function-dysfunction framework avoids an emphasis on disease and relates to the elderly person's identification of needs and problems. From this perspective relevant concepts for specific content arise, for example, mobility, energy, sexuality. Furthermore, such an approach necessitates a continuum of wellness to illness, that is, content progressing from the essentially well elderly living in the community to the acutely and chronically ill elderly living at home or in institutions.

Specific knowledge and skills taught within a program, again, are dependent on underlying philosophy. However, there is no doubt that all nurses, especially clinical specialists, need "expanded skills." These skills are as much observation and interviewing as they are the fuller use of traditional instruments such as the stethoscope and the use of nontraditional instruments such as the otoscope. It is possible to teach these skills in a function-dysfunction framework throughout the program and to integrate skills within selected dynamic concepts. However, curriculum development in this area is hindered by a lack of gerontological nursing faculty with "expanded skills" and few teaching materials that concentrate explicitly on the elderly person.

There are key gerontological nursing graduate education issues in the years ahead: delineation of theory, development of core curriculum, and the focus of research. It would seem appropriate that these and other issues be addressed not only within the various forums available for gerontology and higher education but within the American Nurses Association Practice Division in Gerontological Nursing.

Doctoral preparation

The first doctoral study in nursing was established in the 1920s at Teachers' College, Columbia University. Currently there are 12 doctoral programs in schools of nursing and several more are being developed. Nurses have been able to pursue doctoral study in nursing for one of five types of degrees: Doctor of Nursing Science (D.N.S. or D.N.Sc.), Doctor of Nursing (D.N.), Doctor of Public Health Nursing (D.P.H.N.), Doctor of Nursing Education (D.N.Ed.), and Doctor of Philosophy (Ph.D.).[51] Eight of the current doctoral programs offer a Doctor of Philosophy in Nursing degree, with the most recently developed emphasizing clinical nursing research.

The focus on clinical nursing research, which is evident in doctoral programs developed within the last 2 years, is a significant evolution in nursing. Nurses with doctoral degrees prior to 1960 were usually nurse educators holding doctorates in education. For the next 10 to 15 years doctoral study for nurses was frequently directed toward acquiring a Ph.D. degree in another discipline. With a growing number of nurses with doctoral degrees for guidance (1,539 in 1972)[52] and recognition that nursing has not conducted sufficient research into its own practice, the development of doctoral study directed toward clinical nursing seems appropriate and commendable.

There is an urgent need for nurses prepared in gerontological nursing at the doctoral level. Research into the diverse, complex, and extensive care issues and problems relevant to nursing elderly people needs the leadership and guidance of well-prepared nurses and there are few doctorally prepared nurses with an interest in aging. Robinson[53] noted that a perusal of nurses' dissertation subjects up to 1973 revealed only 13 that dealt with aging, the aged, or geriatric nursing. Nursing education and practice rest on research; gerontological nursing will be encumbered until doctoral preparation in this field is given priority.

SUMMARY

Gerontological nursing is a specialty field for research, practice, and education and has developed under the guidance of many nurse leaders, notably Jones, Newton, Norton, Schwartz, and Stone. These gerontological nurse pioneers are positive role models: women of intelligence, vision, courage, and conviction. As a young and growing nursing specialty in a time of great need and social change, we would do well to be guided by their examples.

In the years ahead gerontological nursing must become a significant component of all preprofessional nursing education. Deficiencies in basic knowledge and gains in advanced knowledge in nursing care of the elderly must be addressed by well-planned, competently taught continuing education programs. Graduate level gerontological nursing programs must move toward a common philosophy and identifiable content core. Doctoral study in this field must be a top educational priority.

Nursing is committed to the elderly; past and current advances in gerontological nursing document this view. But commitment represents neither a single feeling state nor a simple set of behaviors. It is not just being kind to the elderly and remembering that one does not need to shout to old people because all are not deaf. Commitment is recognizing that there is little known about effective nursing of the old and searching to find new knowledge. It is believing enough in the value of one's cause and those elderly people in one's charge to try. It is not easy but, as a potential key to quality nursing for all age groups and an indicator of nursing's role in the health care system, it is both exciting and worthwhile.

REFERENCES

1. Abel-Smith, B., editor: A history of the nursing profession in Great Britain, New York, 1960, Springer Publishing Co., Inc., p. 3.
2. Cobbe, F. P.: The workhouse as a hospital, London, 1861. In Abel-Smith, B., editor: A history of the nursing profession in Great Britain, New York, 1960, Springer Publishing Co., Inc., pp. 12-13.
3. Abel-Smith, p. 48.
4. Cook, E.: The life of Florence Nightingale, vol. 2, London, 1913, Macmillan & Co., Ltd., p. 128.
5. Woodham-Smith, C.: Florence Nightingale 1820-1910, New York, 1951, McGraw-Hill Book Co., Inc., p. 299.
6. Peplau, H.: Specialization in professional nursing. In Riehl, J., and McVay, J., editors: The clinical nurse specialist: interpretations, New York, 1973, Appleton-Century-Crofts, pp. 19-31.
7. Beattie, W. M.: Concepts, knowledge, and commitment: the education of a practicing gerontologist, Gerontologist **10:**5-11, Winter, 1970.
8. Birren, J. E., and Clayton, V.: History of gerontology. In Woodruff, D., and Birren, J., editors: Aging, scientific perspectives and social issues, New York, 1975, D. Van Nostrand Co., pp. 15-27.
9. Lively, B.: Historical aspects of aging and disease, Mod. Geriatr. **4:**204-212, 1974.
10. Nasher, I. L.: Geriatrics, Philadelphia, 1914, P. Blakiston & Sons.
11. Lawton, A. H.: The historical developments in the biological aspects of aging and the aged, Gerontologist **5:**25-32, 1965.
12. Newton, K.: Geriatric nursing, St. Louis, 1950, The C. V. Mosby Co.
13. Basson, P. H.: The gerontological nursing literature: search, study, and results, Nurs. Res. 16: 267-272, Summer, 1967.
14. Norton, D., McLaren, R., and Exton-Smith, A. N.: An investigation of geriatric nursing problems in hospital, London, 1962, The National Corporation for the Care of Old People (Republished by Churchill Livingstone, 1975), p. 8.
15. Schwartz, D., Henley, D., and Zeitz, L.: The elderly ambulatory patient, New York, 1964, The Macmillan Co.
16. Robinson, L. D.: Gerontological nursing research. In Burnside, I., editor: Nursing and the aged, New York, 1976, McGraw-Hill Book Co., pp. 586-597.
17. Cutler, N. E., and Harootyan, R. A.: Demography of the aged. In Woodruff, D., and Birren, J., editors: Aging, scientific perspectives and social issues, New York, 1975, D. Van Nostrand Co., pp. 31-69.

18. Ibid, p. 33.
19. U.S. Department of Health, Education, and Welfare: New facts about older Americans, Washington, D.C., 1973, U.S. Government Printing Office.
20. Burnside, I.: Gerontology and gerontological nursing. In Burnside, I., editor: Nursing and the aged, New York, 1976, McGraw-Hill Book Co., pp. 4-21.
21. Townsend, C.: Old age, the last segregation, New York, 1971, Bantam Books, Inc.
22. Mendelson, M. A.: Tender loving greed, New York, 1974, Vintage Books.
23. Subcommittee on Long-term Care of the Special Committee on Aging, United States Senate: Nursing home care in the United States: failure in public policy, Supporting Papers No. 1-9, Washington, D.C., 1974-1975, U.S. Government Printing Office.
24. Subcommittee on Long-term Care of the Special Committee on Aging, United States Senate: Nursing home care in the United States: failure in public policy, Supporting Paper No. 4, Washington, D.C., 1975, U.S. Government Printing Office, p. xiv.
25. Davis, B. A.: Gerontological nursing comes of age, J. Gerontol. Nurs. **1:**6-7, 1975.
26. American Nurses Association: Standards of gerontological nursing practice, Kansas City, 1976, The Association.
27. Stone, V.: Personal communication, May, 1977.
28. Subcommittee on Long-term Care of the Special Committee on Aging, p. 367.
29. Burnside, I.: Nursing and the aged, New York, 1976, McGraw-Hill Book Co.
30. Andre, B. C.: Geriatric nursing programs in schools of nursing, J. Gerontol. **8:**90-93, 1953.
31. Moses, D. V., and Lake, C. S.: Geriatrics in the baccalaureate nursing curriculum, Nurs. Outlook, **16:**41-43, 1968.
32. American Nurses Association: Gerontological nursing concepts as presented in basic nursing programs as of June, 1976, Unpublished paper, Kansas City, 1977.
33. Subcommittee on Long-term care, 1975.
34. Gunter, L.: Students' attitudes toward geriatric nursing, Nurs. Outlook, **19:**466-69, 1971.
35. Kayser, J. S., and Minnigerode, F. A.: Increasing nursing students' interest in working with aged patients, Nurs. Res. **24:**23-26, 1975.
36. Heller, B., and Walsh, F.: Changing nursing students' attitudes toward the aged: an experimental study, J. Nurs. Ed. **15:**9-17, 1976.
37. DeLora, J. R., and Moses, D. V.: Specialty preferences and characteristics of nursing students in baccalaureate programs, Nurs. Res. **18:**137-144, 1969.
38. Regional Office for Europe, World Health Organization: Education and training in long-term and geriatric care, Copenhagen, 1973, World Health Organization.
39. American Nurses Association: Final report, training of registered nurses providing patient care in nursing homes, Kansas City, 1974, The Association.
40. Buseck, S. A.: Who is the nursing home nurse?—staff development for nursing home nurses, American Nurse Association clinical sessions (San Francisco, 1974), New York, 1975, Appleton-Century-Crofts, pp. 198-205.
41. Lysaught, J. P.: From abstract into action, New York, 1973, McGraw-Hill Book Co., p. 174.
42. Buseck, p. 204.
43. American Nurses Association: The scope of nursing practice, Kansas City, 1976, The Association.
44. American Nurses Association: Guidelines for short-term continuing education programs preparing the geriatric nurse practitioner, Kansas City, 1974, The Association.
45. American Nurses Association: Preparing registered nurses for expanded roles (1974-1975), Kansas City, 1975, The Association.
46. Joint Board of Clinical Nursing Studies: First report, London, 1972.
47. Lysaught, p. 174.
48. U.S. Department of Health, Education, and Welfare: Long-term care facility improvement study, Washington, D.C., July, 1975, U.S. Government Printing Office.
49. American Nurses Association, Task Force on Nursing Manpower and Training, Committee on Skilled Nursing Care: Report and recommendations. In Subcommittee on Long-term Care of the Special Committee on Aging, United States Senate: Nursing home care in the United States: failure in public policy, Supporting Paper No. 4, Washington, D.C., 1975, U.S. Government Printing Office, pp. 441-444.
50. American Nurses Association: Preparing registered nurses.
51. U.S. Department of Health, Education, and Welfare: Future directions of doctoral education for nurses, Bethesda, Md., 1971, U.S. Government Printing Office, p. 6.
52. American Nurses Association: Facts about nursing 74-75, Kansas City, 1976, The Association, p. 4.
53. Robinson, p. 593.

15 The gerontological nurse specialist

CHARLOTTE ELIOPOULOS

Although nurses have a long history of caring for the aged, it was not until 1961 that the American Nurses Association recognized geriatric nursing as a bona fide specialty. Since that time, increasing numbers of professional nurses have entered this specialty and have grown to realize that caring for the aged requires a sophisticated blend of cognitive and technical skills plus a broad and varied knowledge base, for example, gerontology, medicine, surgery, physiology, pharmacology, community health, thanatology, health education, family therapy, psychology, sociology, nutrition, and rehabilitation. Nursing's recognition of the complexities and challenges of caring for the aged has paralleled marked expansion of gerontology; impressive research activities, educational programs, and services have germinated in this field within a decade. This increased knowledge of gerontology must be translated to the nursing profession so that separate nursing technologies may be developed and implemented.

ROLE CATEGORIES OF THE GERONTOLOGICAL NURSE SPECIALIST

Gerontological nursing is now in an early developmental phase, in need of circumscription, clarification, and cultivation. Many competent nurses are working diligently in an effort to fulfill these needs. To maximize their efforts, however, nursing leadership with advanced cognitive abilities and clinical competence must exist. One such necessary leader is the advanced nursing practitioner, the gerontological nurse specialist.

The gerontological nurse specialist is a registered nurse with a minimum educational preparation of a master's degree in nursing or a related field. Although it is preferable for this nurse to have completed a graduate program for clinical specialization in gerontological nursing, it must be remembered that until recently these advanced programs were either nonexistent or inaccessible to a majority of nurses. It is useful for the gerontological nurse specialist to have several years of clinical experience prior to assuming this role for increased clinical competence and insight into the dynamics of organizations. The nurse's experience is valuable to consider since maturity promotes a fuller appreciation of the problems aged persons can experience, for example, death, retirement, role changes, and increased physical limitations.

The gerontological nurse specialist suffers the same role ambiguity as persons in other new positions. Frequently the needs of the employing agency will determine the place and function of this individual in the organization. Consequently the primary role of each gerontological nurse specialist may differ markedly. With acknowledgement of the variety of roles that this specialist can assume, four general role categories can be discussed: implementor, educator, advocate, and innovator.

Implementor

As an implementor, the gerontological nurse specialist facilitates the integration of gerontological knowledge into nursing practice, and translates gerontological concepts into operational language. Some examples of this may include:

Knowledge	*Nursing application*
Cardiac reserve is lower in older persons.[5]	1. Assist individuals in planning a schedule that paces activities. 2. Ensure that coughs are controlled to reduce cardiac stress.
Tactile sensation is decreased in older persons.[3]	1. Reposition immobile individuals at frequent intervals to prevent decubiti. 2. Encourage older persons to measure temperature of bath water before sitting in tub, avoid tight-fitting shoes, correct poor-fitting dentures, and use heating appliances with caution. 3. Examine the skin for evidence of burns and pressure sores.
Renal blood flow and glomerular filtration rate are decreased with age.[2]	1. Graph the older diabetic's blood glucose level and the results of urine testing for glucose to determine the degree of correlation. 2. Observe for signs and symptoms of adverse drug reactions caused by accumulation of toxic levels.
There is a high mortality rate among widowers.[4,6-9]	1. Forward the name of a deceased client's spouse to a resource who will contact him or her at defined times. 2. Inform the widower of local ''widow's coping groups'' or similar organizations. 3. Stimulate the development of groups to assist widowers if none exist in a given community.

The gerontological nurse specialist may disseminate gerontological principles and practices by using several strategies, one of which is nursing rounds. During these rounds, the specialist reviews with the nursing staff the nursing care of selected older individuals. It is essential that the focus of the rounds be nursing and not reiteration of medical plans. Although the content of the nursing rounds may vary among agencies, some components useful to review are as follows:

1. The individual's functional capacity to meet the regular self-care requirements of daily living such as the ability to supply and utilize nutrition, have unrestricted respirations, engage in hygienic practices, eliminate waste materials, and obtain opportunities for socialization and solitude
2. Specific assistive techniques to compensate for limitations in self-care capacity, such as supporting the right side during ambulation, applying a condom catheter during the night, providing a soft diet, keeping a written schedule of activities at the bedside, and assisting in cleansing the feet, legs, and back
3. The individual's capacity to meet the therapeutic requirements imposed by illness, such as the ability to administer medications, prepare a special diet, change a dressing, and perform catheter care
4. Specific assistive techniques to compensate for limitations in capacity to meet therapeutic demands, such as having the visiting nurse change the dressing in the

client's home every morning, devising a medication chart for home use, and teaching a neighbor how to give the injection

5. Updating and evaluating effectiveness of nursing care plan: Does the client still require assistance with exercises or can he now be instructed to do this procedure independently? Is walking to the bathroom every 2 hours too tiring for him? Is the decubitus ulcer becoming smaller in diameter? Is the individual able to answer correctly more or less of the questions on the mental status evaluation form?
6. Long-range plans
7. Referrals

As these items are reviewed, the specialist can introduce the staff to new knowledge and skills that are relevant for the client at hand. The specialist may demonstrate a particular skill, showing the staff how it can be adjusted and implemented for a specific individual. It is surprising that ideas that seemed unrealistic and idealistic in a classroom or conference setting become quite practical and acceptable when applied to an actual situation.

These rounds also can provide an opportunity for the specialist to oversee and coordinate the care of caseload of older clients. The specialist should determine that comprehensive, correct nursing plans have been made, that nursing actions are appropriate and therapeutic, that the older individual is actively involved in the planning and carrying out of his care, and that a wide range of resources are being considered in the discharge plans. Regular feedback is essential to sustain positive practices and correct any real or potential problems in the older person's care. Rather than demanding changes in gerontological nursing practice because he or she knows "what is right," the specialist must collaborate and compromise with others to be an innovator and to cause valid gerontological practices to be implemented. The gerontological nurse specialist is effective by functioning in concert with, not isolated from, other health team members.

Being a role model for gerontological nursing practice through direct clinical involvement can facilitate the specialist's implementation of desirable principles and practices. The specialist can demonstrate how gerontological knowledge can be intertwined with the nursing process to achieve effective care for older adults. The staff can observe how the specialist incorporates reminiscence into group work with older persons, the voice level the specialist uses when communicating with an individual who has a high frequency hearing loss, or how the specialist interprets data using age-related norms. Opportunities for clinical involvement may consist of either assisting other nurses in caring for older persons and identifying ways to incorporate gerontological knowledge and skills in their practice or of directly caring for a patient group and communicating plans and actions to the nursing staff. In addition to specific actions, the gerontological nurse specialist should demonstrate an attitude of respect, enthusiasm, and positivism in his or her practice that the staff can model. When nurses who enjoy working with the aged are questioned as to what stimulated their interest in this field, they frequently reveal that there was an instructor, a staff nurse or some other role model who made a lasting impression.

Client-centered conferences are also a means by which the gerontological nurse specialist can serve as an implementor. The specialist may identify a particular aged individual's nursing care problem and design a conference to assist the staff in improving their management of that person. For example, the specialist may review the care of a hospitalized aged person and discover that he has arrhythmias, especially between the hours of 8:00 A.M. and 12:00 P.M. By reading the nurses' notes, the specialist may learn that the client is bathed, eats breakfast, uses the bedside commode, goes to physical therapy, and has diagnostic tests during those morning hours. It may be appropriate for the specialist to present a conference on cardiovascular changes in aging that emphasizes pacing activities to reduce cardiac stress.

Specific concepts can be introduced in conferences with the specialist serving as a resource to assist the staff in translating the concepts into relevant actions for practice. Sensory deprivation is an example of a concept that may be discussed. The nursing staff may comprehend this concept intellectually but may need the guidance of the specialist in identifying specific behaviors to enhance their patients' sensory stimulation.

The implementor role of the gerontological nurse specialist is a vital one. The actions of the gerontological specialist who deliberately functions to apply new concepts in the care of aged persons can make new gerontological knowledge interesting, impressive, and effective in improving care for the elderly.

Educator

The gerontological nurse specialist must be prepared to take advantage of formal and informal opportunities to share knowledge and skills related to the care of the elderly. The specialist's role as educator is important in communicating new knowledge to nurses and in introducing nurses to basic gerontology. Most nurses in current practice have had no or minimal exposure to gerontology as part of their professional education. They may lack an understanding of the theories of aging, demographic characteristics of the aged population, physiological changes with age, adjustments to role changes, and other knowledge at the core of gerontological practice. The specialist should take advantage of all opportunities to increase his or her colleagues' awareness of gerontology.

In addition to increasing nurses' knowledge of the normal aging process, the specialist should teach nurses the unique factors related to pathophysiology in the aged. Nurses in all settings need to understand the principles of geriatric pharmacology, differences in symptomatology and reactions to therapy, age-related gradients used in interpretation of diagnostic tests, and specific complications for which the ill aged are at high risk. This type of information is extremely important so that nurses may be taught to eliminate the erroneous assumption that all adults can be cared for similarly. "You must not treat a young child as you would a grown person, nor must you treat an old person as you would one in the prime of life."[1] This principle was advocated in an American Journal of Nursing article in 1904; it is the challenge of the specialist to assist nurses in gaining the knowledge that can make this principle meaningful to the effective care of today's aged population.

As an educator the specialist can help gerontological nurses in one setting learn more about the mission and practice of gerontological nurses in other settings. Often acute care nurses are critical of nursing homes for providing an inadequate amount of individualized care; nurses in long-term care facilities are annoyed at obtaining an insufficient data base on patients transferred from acute hospitals; and community health nurses are outraged that a facility will discharge a debilitated individual without planning for necessary home assistance. The acute care nurse might be less critical if he or she knew the reimbursement and staffing problems of nursing homes and perhaps could promote continuity of care by learning the information important in sending a discharge summary to a nursing home.

Nurses working in institutional settings may need to be taught the problems aged persons face in the community and the resources that can be utilized to assist them. Learning about gerontological care in other settings can enhance continuity of care, promote the utilization of a wider range of alternatives to care for the aged, and foster a supportive relationship among nurses working in various gerontological care settings.

There are several strategies that the specialist can use in his or her educator role. In-service classes, seminars, and workshops can effectively communicate gerontological knowledge in a formal, structured manner. Patient care conferences and nursing rounds described earlier may present rich opportunities for learning. Directing nurses to gerontological literature and circulating selected books and articles among the nursing staff can expose them to knowledge that may stimulate further interest. Also the gerontological nurse specialist should feel a responsibility to publish in an effort to communicate knowledge to a larger nursing population.

The specialist's educator role extends beyond professionals to the general public. This can comprise two facets: (1) teaching persons of all ages about the normal aging process and (2) teaching aged persons the realities of old age and effective ways to manage age-related changes and problems. An understanding of the aging process offers persons a better chance of growing old with comfort and without fear and ignorance. Financial planning, development of leisure pursuits, and other preparations for old age may be encouraged early in life through ''education for aging.'' Misconceptions regarding the older person's sexuality, senility, and incidence of institutionalization can be clarified. Learning the realities of aging can help persons of all ages appreciate the strengths and value of the elderly.

The gerontological nurse specialist will discover that the aged are quite receptive to learning about health care and management of health problems. They are interested in understanding why their blood pressure is higher than their middle-aged children's; why ejaculation may not result with each intercourse; the importance of using medications correctly; and the rationale behind purchasing eyeglasses and hearing aides with a physician's prescription. Often aged persons are labelled ''noncompliant'' or are accused of demonstrating poor judgment when they lack an adequate knowledge base. The gerontological nurse specialist can affect the health status of aged persons by teaching promotion of health and measures to manage health problems if they should develop.

The assumption that to be an effective, dynamic teacher one must be a constant, active learner underlies the specialist's role as an educator. The gerontological nurse specialist utilizes multiple sources of learning: new literature, conferences, courses, other health care providers, and aged persons themselves. One is not only a specialist because of his or her level of expertise and educational achievement, but because of a commitment and continuous effort to update knowledge, maintain clinical competency, and grow.

Advocate

Unlike today's children who are taught to challenge and assert, the aged are of a generation who were taught to conform and accept. Unfamiliar jargon and the mystique of organizational function prevent many older persons from being heard and obtaining their rights. They are in need of advocates who can competently and eloquently support their positions and causes; the gerontological nurse specialist is one such advocate.

There are several ways in which the specialist can fulfill an advocacy role. The specialist may identify a problem that affects an individual or group of older persons and may act to seek a solution. Examples of this type of advocacy may include (1) an individual who is not receiving all the benefits for which he is entitled and a specialist who contacts the appropriate agencies to ensure that the benefits are obtained, (2) a community that lacks accessible health care facilities for the elderly and a specialist who explores with local health officials the development of a clinic for the elderly, and (3) architectural features of a geriatric facility that do not meet the needs of the residents and a specialist who recommends specific alterations. In these examples the aged may not be aware that a problem exists; that is, they may not know they are entitled to certain benefits or that specific environmental features can aid them. The specialist should accompany the problem solving activities with measures to increase the client's awareness of such activities.

Situations in which older persons identify a problem can be resolved with the assistance of the specialist. The specialist's advocacy function in this type of situation can be demonstrated by the following examples: (1) an older person who perceives that a funeral director is taking advantage of his vulnerable state and desires an alternative and a specialist who supplies him with the name of a local memorial society, (2) an individual who has concern about the therapies prescribed for him and a specialist who uses a role-playing activity to help him gain the ability and confidence to confront his physician, and (3) a local senior citizen group that would like to have more convenient transportation services and a specialist who outlines for them the procedure to follow to effect a change. In these examples the client recognizes the problem and has the capacity to solve it with the assistance of the specialist. Rather than "doing for" the aged, the specialist serves as a catalyst to increase the ageds' ability to act for themselves.

Another form of advocacy may involve the specialist's acting as an agent to solve a problem that the aged identify but that they lack the capacity to solve independently. For example, a hospitalized older person may have decided rationally that he would prefer to go home and die slowly rather than agree to the surgery his physician has advised. This individual may not have the energy level or knowledge of medical jargon to compete with his physician's convincing arguments. The specialist may need to confront the physician on the patient's behalf and defend this individual's right to refuse surgery. Likewise a group of nursing home residents may be annoyed at the lack of privacy they are afforded but may not have access to the administrator who has the authority to change this situation. The specialist may need to recommend and gain administrative support for policy changes that respect the residents' needs for privacy.

In addition to being an advocate for the aged, the gerontological nurse specialist is an advocate for gerontological nursing. The specialist may need to inform others of the complexities of gerontological nursing practice and the need to have qualified personnel in this specialty. To ensure an adequate quality and quantity of professional nurses to meet the many demands of the aged population, the specialist may need to stimulate nursing schools to include gerontological nursing in their curriculum and work with legislators to achieve policy and funding. Research may be conducted by the specialist to demonstrate that competent professionals do make a difference to gerontological care and, therefore, justify the need for greater reimbursement policies. Peer review should be encouraged by the specialist to ensure that gerontological nurses meet a minimum standard of practice.

The specialist may advocate gerontological nursing practice by being an "icebreaker" in new territories. The misconception that gerontological nursing is practiced only in long-term care facilities must be erased by gerontological nursing specialists who are compensated for their services and who demonstrate their value in acute and community care settings. The specialist can work with industries to develop preretirement education programs and health maintenance clinics for aging employees. The specialist can advise architects regarding environmental planning to meet the needs of older persons and can serve as a consultant to legislators regarding the impact of decisions on the aged. The range of opportunities for nurses to improve the health and well-being of older persons is unlimited. The specialist must be willing to join the leaders who risk entering nontraditional settings to open horizons for gerontological nursing practice.

Innovator

Through clinical practice and research the specialist strives to increase gerontological nursing knowledge and develop technologies that result in more effective care. The specialist can explore and evaluate new tools and actions and different modalities of care delivery relevant to an older population. The specialist may assume an innovative role by introducing old concepts and practices into new settings. For example, "rooming-in" has been a common practice in many obstetric and pediatric settings; why not allow family members to "room-in" occasionally with an elderly institutionalized person to maintain an intimate contact or to learn about the care of that person in preparation for discharge?

As an innovator the gerontological nurse specialist assumes an inquisitive nature, making a conscious effort to experiment for an end result of improved patient care. This requires the specialist to envision unique forms of gerontological nursing practice and to be willing to take the risks associated with transforming these visions into realities.

Nurses have had a long history of providing care to aged persons. The challenge for today's gerontological nurses is to develop and implement valid, effective technologies to use in caring for aged persons. Presently, the gerontological nurse specialist is a health team member who can assist in the discovery of creative means of providing gerontological care, facilitate the implementation of gerontological nursing concepts, and monitor the quality of gerontological nursing care. The specialist becomes a vital element in every gerontological care setting as the demand for a higher quality of gerontological care increases and the body of gerontological knowledge grows.

REFERENCES

1. Bishop, L. B.: The relation of old age to disease, with illustrative cases, Am. J. Nurs. **4:**679, 1904.
2. Davies, D. F., and Shock, N. W.: Age changes in glomerular filtration rate, effective renal plasma flow and tubular excretory capacity in adult males, Clin. Invest. **29:**496, 1950.
3. Donahue, W.: Psychologic aspects. In Cowdry, E. V., and Steinberg, F. U., editors: The care of the geriatric patient, St. Louis, 1971, The C. V. Mosby Co., p. 273.
4. Glick, I. O., Weiss, R. S., and Parkes, C. M.: The first years of bereavement, New York, 1974, John Wiley & Sons, Inc.
5. Goldman, R.: Decline in organ function with aging. In Rossman, I., editor: Clinical geriatrics, Philadelphia, 1971, J. B. Lippincott Co., p. 20.
6. Hobson, C. J.: Widows of Blackton, New Soc. Sept. 14, 1964.
7. Maddison, D., and Viola, A.: The health of widows in the year following bereavement, J. Psychosom. Res. **12:**297, 1968.
8. Parkes, C. M.: The broken heart. In Shneidman, E. S., editor: Death: current perspectives, Palo Alto, Calif., 1976, Mayfield Publishing Co., pp. 333-347.
9. Parkes, C. M., and Brown, R. J.: Health after bereavement: a controlled study of young Boston widows and widowers, Psychosom. Med. **34:**449-461, 1972.

BIBLIOGRAPHY

Lewis, E. P., editor: The clinical nurse specialist, New York, 1970, American Journal of Nursing Co.
Peplau, H. E.: Specialization in professional nursing. Nurs. Sci. **3:**268-287, August, 1965.
Riehl, J. P., and McVay, J. W., editors: The clinical nurse specialist: interpretations, New York, 1973, Appleton-Century-Crofts.

part VI

UNDERSTANDING THE LAW AND THE NURSE'S ROLE AS HEALTH ADVOCATE FOR THE ELDERLY

It is essential that all nurses, particularly those working with the elderly, recognize the growing political power of the active, involved elderly on local, county, state, and national levels. This phenomenon has occurred because an increasing number of elderly now belong to several effective national organizations. Two of the most prominent organizations are the American Association of Retired Persons/National Retired Teachers Association and the highly visible, vocal Gray Panthers. As the AARP Bulletin for March, 1978, points out:

> Probably no organization in America has experienced such phenomenal growth in size and stature over the past two decades as the AARP.
>
> Today, one in every four Americans over the age of 55 is a member of AARP and our net growth continues to exceed a million a year. With that growth has come immense influence in the nation at large as we represent the legitimate interests and needs of older citizens. No other group has had more to do with changing society's negative attitudes toward aging, ending mandatory retirement, improving the quality of life for other citizens.[1]

Indeed, particularly during the past decade, organized associations of the elderly have raised their voices in a cohesive, effective manner to further issues that will enhance the quality of life for seniors in this country.

The two chapters in this part are related in a very fundamental sense. Chapter 16, The Law and the Elderly, describes legislative changes resulting from the organized political demands of senior groups; Chapter 17 is essentially a statement of belief and philosophy of an experienced gerontological nurse that issues a challenge to nurses to serve as advocates with and for the elderly.

We believe that the nurse's informational and philosophical base for counseling and caring for the elderly will be significantly expanded through thoughtful study of these two chapters.

REFERENCE

1. American Association of Retired Persons: AARP News Bulletin **19** (3):1, March, 1978.

16 The law and the elderly

JACK L. TEDROW

For the past two decades, legalism has permeated almost every aspect of our society. This is the result of several factors: (1) the increasing complexity of our culture, with people interacting in many new ways, creating conflicts and tensions; (2) governmental expansion through the setting of standards and controls, and the resulting emphasis on individual rights in an effort to balance things out; (3) the growth of bureaucracy with its ever-increasing rules and regulations; (4) the pressure by our people on their government for special recognition and benefits; and (5) an economy that appears to demand, because of ever-present unemployment and the marked inflationary problem, changes in taxation concepts and policy. It has been said that the average person has a third, silent partner in every business transaction that takes place involving money or goods — the government, through taxes. No person escapes the impact of these controls and regulations, and most of us, in one way or another, benefit.

As people make their needs heard, and these needs because of impatience become demands, state legislatures react by passing new legislation or modifying those statutes that already exist. The Congress responds by passing, with the president's signature, public laws. The various courts may reinterpret these laws when a case in point involves issues that fall within their purview. A person challenges an aspect of the law and it may finally go on appeal to the U.S. Supreme Court, where a significant constitutional question is involved. Provisions in our federal income tax law are continually being challenged in the tax court. The first page of the Wall Street Journal usually features a column, "Tax Report," with the latest cases of interest. Each time state legislatures meet (usually once every year or once every 2 years), new laws are enacted; these appear as supplements in the statutes or codes of the particular states. (The codes are a set of books designed to keep legal professionals up to date on their state's statutes.) The various governmental agencies publish pamphlets to assist one in keeping up with developments in their departments. For instance, there are pamphlets on Social Security and Medicare to be had for the asking. Then, of course, there is a wealth of material to be found in the legal publications providing us with up-to-date court cases that bear on the problems inherent in the statute or public law. It is a completely fluid situation, and one is compelled to keep abreast of the latest changes, especially in tax law.

The federal income tax for 1977 was an attempt to simplify things for the taxpayer filling out a 1040 or 1040A (short form). In 1976, 7 million people made errors on their tax returns, and half of these overpaid by an average of $80.56! It was said that one needed a college degree to comprehend even the short form. In late 1978, President Carter signed into law a $21 billion tax cut. For those 65 or older, there was a larger exemption amounting to $4,000 exempt income, not counting deductions. Together with the increased standard deduction, a retired couple 65 years old or older has $7,400 of their ordinary income tax-free, and if their social security amounts to $6,000 a year, a total exemption of

$13,400. Annuities, pensions, and other deferred compensations are considered "earned income" and are subject to a maximum rate of 50%, the maximum tax no matter how many millions of dollars one earns each year.[1]

Another excellent example of a major change that will affect the elderly is mandatory retirement. When Bismark first proposed in 1889 the social security concept and set the age for retirement at 65, few people lived that long; those who did were glad to have the chance to take it easy. However, now people are living a lot longer and are healthier; a white man who reaches 60 years of age is now likely to live until age 77 and a white woman until age 82. Nonwhites live 1 year less. Increasing attention to diet, exercise, and nonsmoking appear to be decreasing the rate of death from heart disease.[2] This produces the problem that Bismark did not dream of — millions of people feel fine at age 65, want to remain productive, and live in a society where jobs are scarce. Young people need work opportunities, and, in the face of inflation, older people are afraid to retire on a fixed income. There had been considerable pressure on Congress to change things for the 30 million people currently covered by mandatory retirement policies.

In April, 1978, President Carter signed into law congressional action aimed at keeping employees on the payroll until age 70, provided the employer had at present 20 workers on the payroll. Also, beginning on September 30, 1978, certain federal employees were not required to retire until age 70. State and local governments could not force retirement before age 70 except in high-risk employment, such as policemen or fire fighters. Most private pension plans remained unaffected. The law was to take effect January 1, 1979, prohibiting mandatory retirement before age 70 and the labor department was asked to prepare guidelines for employers dealing with life insurance and disability benefits, pension and medicare benefits, and the required contributions of employees between ages 65 and 70.

The present Age Discrimination in Employment Act of 1967 makes it illegal to discriminate in the hiring, firing, and promoting of anyone between 40 and 65 years old, thereby permitting mandatory retirement at age 65; this is being extended to age 70 by the new legislation. This means that 150,000 to 200,000 people will remain in the labor force, hardly a dent in the 97.9 million people in the labor force as of September 1977. Of course, industry can fire elderly workers who cannot perform adequately, but the employee may not accept this appraisal of his work ability and can legally resist. There were 5,535 such complaints filed by employees in the last fiscal year, a fivefold increase since 1969. There is considerable evidence that compulsory retirement for some people leads to physical and emotional deterioration, and a great many persons believe this will happen to themselves. It appears to be a significant factor for those who do not have enough hobbies or outside interests. Those who plan to travel on retirement often give it up within 6 months. Clearly, there will be many new problems and readjustments required.

It should be clear by now that the law is society's reaction to specific problems that surface as things grow more complex and our society grows more humanistic. Indeed, the law serves to set standards, to add a degree of predictability to how things are going to work out, and to define the limits within which one may function, with sanctions imposed when one's behavior deviates substantially from those limitations, through enforcement of the law.

In an effort to "restrain" government, the Bill of Rights (the first 10 amendments) was drafted at the time the U.S. Constitution was submitted for ratification by the 13 colonies. Since that time, the public has demanded safeguards. Civil rights have been a preoccupation of our citizens since the early 1960s, and various groups of people have splintered off, demanding their rights. Recent examples of this have been the E.R.A. adherents, those for gay liberation, those who support the vote for 18-year-olds, and many others. The elderly have also had their voices raised. They are not, of course, a homogeneous group. They cut across the breadth of our population, differing in income, religion, politics, color, and ethnic background. They do not present a united front. In a recent article,[3] nine goals are set forth by the Executive Director of the American Association of Retired People:

1. Changing the image of older people
2. Ending old age discrimination by industry
3. Abolition of ceilings on earnings under Social Security
4. National health policy responsive to needs of all citizens
5. Development of a criminal justice system that protects the citizen as well as the criminal
6. Development of housing policies sensitive to needs of the elderly
7. Property tax reform
8. Election of officials who are dedicated to fighting inflation
9. Monitoring of high costs of living and taxes caused by the energy crisis

These goals cover the needs of the elderly quite well and, as will be seen, most of the legalism that involves the elderly is an attempt to deal with these particular problems.

SPECIAL LEGAL PROBLEMS OF THE ELDERLY

Do the elderly have special problems of a legal nature? The answer is yes: There is the special problem of preparation for retirement and death, dealt with, in its most sophisticated form, by the estate plan. There is the need for an income after retirement, provided for by Social Security and other benefits such as pensions derived from one's employment. It is necessary to have provisions made for medical care and hospitalization. Terminal illnesses may be prolonged. Nursing home care may be needed. The amount spent for drugs may be high. Therefore one must be familiar with Medicare; supplemental health insurance may be necessary. And there is the problem of housing, including home repairs, property taxes, and increasing utility bills. There is increasing physical and muscular weakness with aging, so older people need extra protection from hoodlums, muggers, rapists, and petty thieves. Many old people have not executed a will, many have no idea of what benefits they are entitled to under the provisions of Social Security law, and many do not know or understand the special benefits provided by the Internal Revenue Service. None of the benefits for the elderly come automatically; they must be applied for. And this comes at a time and age many people are unmotivated, bereaved, or too ill or destitute to act. Many of them need all the assistance, legal and otherwise, that they can obtain.

Retirement

Retirement itself is a difficult decision, and a surprising number of people give it little thought until a few months ahead of time. The main apprehensions appear to be what the person will do with his or her time and what kind of life can be led on a fixed income in times of inflation. A person needs to retire with dignity, knowing that his or her many years of service are truly appreciated. About three fourths of people miss the money they earned,[5] about 62% miss the work itself, and 50% sense the loss of self-esteem. This is particularly true of men with a strong "work ethic," whose entire personality is geared to work and being the breadwinner. As people age, they experience more aches and pains and may believe their health is failing when it really is not. This self-diagnosis accounts for a large number of early retirements.

One thing is certain; everyone of retirement age ought to know what to expect legally — in the way of benefits and in the way of obligations and problems.

Social Security. Let us begin with Social Security and the benefits that can be derived therefrom. It was signed into law in 1935 by President Franklin Delano Roosevelt at a time when there were county poorhouses, and just about every older person was scared to death that he or she would end up there. This was, however, a time of great family unity. The depression had forced people to stay put and many dwellings housed four generations. Youngsters married, stayed at home, and had children. The older folks were "provided for," but they were completely dependent and without dignity. Social Security was an attempt to give the older person some idea of what he would have to live on when he could no longer work. There was a great emphasis on economic security for persons of all ages in the 1930s; the depression reached its depths in 1936 and it was only with the work provided by the war industries that it ended in the 1940s. In addition to Roosevelt's many plans for economic recovery, such as the C.C.C., N.R.A., and W.P.A. (known affectionately as his alphabet soup), there was the 1934 plan of Dr. Francis Everett Townsend, originator of the old age pension plan, or Townsend Plan. This was probably the first focus on the economic problems of the aging citizen. Dr. Townsend helped write the first Social Security law.

Before looking at the recent changes in the Social Security Act, first passed in 1935 to assist the aged, the blind, and families with dependent children, let us look first at what developed as a result of social pressures on the Congress. Each month a small percentage of an employee's earnings went into a special fund along with an equal amount from his employer. Over the years, this was theoretically to provide benefits for the above-mentioned beneficiaries, beginning in 1940. But in 1950 Congress chose to provide, in addition, aid to the permanently and totally disabled regardless of age if they fulfilled the requirements as a worker. Obviously, many working people suffered chronic illnesses, such as multiple sclerosis, or cerebrovascular accidents or disabilities resulting from injuries suffered in auto accidents, industrial accidents, or other accidents that would render them incapable of earning a living and leading a productive life. Benefits have been added from time to time by Congress, since 1950, so that by 1976 the number of beneficiaries reached 31,300,000 people. With about 15% of the population receiving benefits from a program designed for less than half that number, economic problems were bound to arise. Fortunately, the number of young workers paying into the program steadily increased, especially after the "baby boom" of the mid-1940s, so that the system was able to keep functioning. However, by the mid-1970s it was obviously in trouble, and monies paid in were immediately paid out. The trust fund had become a conduit. Predictions varied, but it looked like the fund would be exhausted by 1980 or thereabouts.

The 1962 Public Welfare Amendment to the Social Security Act was designed to assist the blind, impaired, and disabled who were not receiving welfare assistance. Only 15% of people receiving Social Security benefits have had additional pension benefits. Until recently, 85 cents of every federal dollar expended for the elderly was derived from the Social Security Trust Fund. It therefore became apparent that the program must continue but somehow be made to pay its own way as originally hoped for.

Starting in 1979, the payroll taxes withheld from most paychecks and matched by employers will rise almost continuously through 1990. There are no increased benefits, but by 1982 a person 65 years old or older will be able to earn $6,000 per year in addition to his benefits without being penalized. Currently, there is a maximum of $3,000; the person is taxed $1 for every $2 earned above that amount. Lower income workers will see a tax climb of 16% or more by 1987; those who have high incomes will see an increase of 234%.[6] The average worker paid a Social Security tax of $585 in 1977. This will climb to $1,331 by 1987. The act will cost the average worker $1.20 more per week over the next 10-year period. By 1987, the tax rate, presently 5.85%, will be 7.15% and will apply to the first $42,600 earned. This will allow an average retiree a monthly benefit of about 43% of his most recent earnings (about 60% for low-income workers, and 30% for high-income workers). By 1982, the $6,000 limit on those age 70 and older will be abolished; they may earn as much as they are able. Presently, this applies at age 72. According to government actuaries, this act will keep the disability fund in the black until 2007 and the old age and survivors fund solvent until 2030.[7] The tax rate for the self-employed is presently 7.9% of earnings up to $16,500. This will rise to 10.75% by 1990. The act also repeals the monthly exception to the earnings limit, which permitted benefits to be paid for months of low earnings regardless of annual earnings. Remarriage will no longer reduce benefits to widows and widowers over 60, and a divorced spouse will receive benefits after having been married only 10 years instead of 20. Starting in 1982, a person working beyond age 65 years will increase his retirement credit by 3% each year instead of 1%. A person who retires between 62 and 65 will receive reduced cost of living increases permanently.

To obtain a copy of one's earnings record, one fills out form OAR-7004 and mails it in. To correct an error, however, the request must be made not more than 39 months after the year in which those wages were earned. A check-up every 3 years is thus a wise procedure. Nine out of ten workers in the United States are earning Social Security protection and nearly one in seven persons receives monthly Social Security checks.[8] To qualify for Social Security benefits, it is necessary to earn credits for each 3-month quarter one works and earns $50 or more and to amass enough credits to qualify. The credit stays on one's record and any return to work adds to it.[9] The amount a person receives depends on his average earnings over a period of years. Since 1972, benefits increase automatically as the cost of living rises, the increase taking effect the following July. Social Security checks are not subject to federal income tax. Maximum benefits are worked out on tables provided in booklets obtainable at Social Security offices in most communities. For example, the maximum retirement benefit for a worker who became 65 years old in 1977 was $412.70 per month. The minimum requirement for fully insured status is 1½ years; if a person has 40 quarters (120 months) of earnings, he is covered for life.

Social Security records are confidential. If a person disagrees with the decision of the Social Security Administration, a hearing may be requested before an administrative law judge of the Bureau of Hearings and Appeals. If not satisfied with that decision, one may request a review by the Appeals Council, and even go beyond that to the federal courts.

Pension plans. In the last few years, it became apparent that private pension plans were not working out for many people. These people had a certain percentage of their pay deducted and paid into a pension fund with each paycheck, often over a period of many years, only to find their jobs terminated or the employer going broke or merging with another company and the fund being lost. Many employees lost their benefits because

there had not been any vesting, that is, the employees had never been specifically designated as shareholders. In the spring of 1974, Congress enacted the Employee Retirement
Income Security Act; when a person is employed for a certain number of years, he "re-
tains" what he and his employer have invested toward his retirement, in compliance with
Part VI, sections 145 through 148 of the act. This amounts to millions of dollars that have
to be safely and satisfactorily invested and, incidentally, constitute a great power in both
the bond and stock markets.

Cost of health care

Older persons experience double the rate of illness of other age groups and are ill
about twice as long. Since 1965 the two parts of Medicare available to people 65 years old
and older provide hospital insurance and medical insurance to pay doctors and other medical items. Since July 1, 1973, Medicare coverage has been extended to those under age
65 who have been receiving disability checks for 2 or more consecutive years and to people considered to have permanent kidney failure requiring dialysis or kidney transplants.
Those who choose the medical insurance pay a quarterly premium of $106.95 (high op-
tion) or $81.75 (low option). The hospital insurance is automatic for those eligible for a
Social Security or railroad retirement check at age 65. Those applying for the hospital insurance are enrolled automatically for the medical insurance part of Medicare. The basic
hospital insurance (part A) premium is presently $55.80 a month. Premiums go up as hos-
pital costs rise; hospital costs increased 1,000% in the past decade. The medical insurance
(part B) has a $60 deductible, meaning the patient pays the first $60.00 in any calendar
year and then 20% of the remaining reasonable charges. Medicare hospital insurance
covers 90 days for each benefit period and there are an additional 60 reserve days in a lifetime that can be added for a prolonged illness.[10]

Only participating hospitals are covered, except in emergencies. For psychiatric illness, not more than 190 days of care are covered in a lifetime. After hospitalization,
treatment in a skilled nursing facility may be authorized but not for custodial care. Drugs
are not covered for outpatient visits, even though they constitute 20% of personal health
care expenses for the elderly. Dental visits, eyeglasses, and hearing aids are also omitted
from coverage even though they are problems quite common to the senior citizen. It is
thus apparent that there are many areas of limited or nonexistent coverage by Medicare.
For this reason, a great many of the elderly who can afford it have supplemental health
insurance and hospitalization policies.

The tremendous cost of medical care has been a source of great concern to Congress.
Many bills have been introduced that would provide a type of health insurance administered by the federal government. The medical profession has strongly resisted government intervention, noting the tremendous costs of "socialized medicine" in Great Britain
and Sweden. The A.M.A. has its own plan, Medi-Credit, and physicians individually
have become extremely cost conscious. However, some type of federal program appears
inevitable. No other costs of goods or services have increased as much as hospital costs
in these inflationary times.

Nursing homes

In recent years, a new industry appeared, which in some instances has proved to be
a very profitable one — the nursing home industry. At first, nursing homes were simply re-
modeled dwellings, poorly furnished, unsafe, and poorly staffed. No medical records

were kept; no charting was done. Many patients were tranquilized to the point of complete docility so that they would constitute no ''problem'' and a skeleton staff could easily operate the facility. As many as one third of the patients admitted to these nursing homes were ''forgotten'' by their families; they never received visitors, and few inquiries were made about their health. Under such circumstances, there was little incentive to improve or ''get well.'' Patients deteriorated physically and mentally. Until early 1977 there were still quite a few of these facilities in existence, but public involvement and government regulations forced many of them to close. The skilled or comprehensive nursing home gradually took over. Patients are cared for by RNs under the direction of physicians. Charts are kept up to date and staffing is done by LPNs who supervise nurses' aides.

A great deal of emphasis has been placed on safety, particularly fire protection, in nursing homes, and there are strict requirements in building codes and maintenance in keeping with federal standards. Along with public money has come public control. With 5% of the nation's elderly housed at any one time in nursing homes, it is a major concern. Medical assistance payments to nursing homes in 1971 amounted to more than a billion dollars. Through its police power, the state may direct a variety of nursing home activities, far beyond the scope of token involvement. Social Security Titles 18 and 19 (42 U.S.C. 1395 and 1396) thoroughly dominate the delivery of nursing home services. As we have seen, for nursing homes to be eligible to receive Medicare payments, there must be active treatment and the facility must be approved. These are commonly referred to as extended care facilities. They were devised to lessen the hospital load and reduce costs while providing skilled nursing services. They are a child of the 1965 congressional amendment to the Social Security Act that created Medicare. The various states may opt to cover the medically needy under Medicaid.[11] In states that do so, many people younger than age 65 years will be found in nursing homes also. Medicaid was devised to assist those of all ages with an income at or below the poverty level and for those on welfare. It is administered by the states through their social services or welfare departments.

In addition to fire protection and safety for the patients, emphasis has been on the adoption of sanitary codes, 24-hour staffing, limiting the number of admissions to the number of beds, and humane treatment of patients. The greatest needs in nursing homes are daily programs for patients including physical exercise and other forms of recreation, a mental health program that will keep patients motivated with close monitoring of sedation and tranquilizers, and a recognition of the legal rights of patients, for example, the right to share in certain significant decisions about drug administration and the right to visits from friends and family and visits to the outside world.

Taxation

Income tax. Another area in which the federal government (through congressional regulations and controls) has a major effect on the elderly is taxation. We will look first at the treatment of the elderly by the Internal Revenue Service, through the federal income tax.

Income derived from Social Security is not taxable, nor are Railroad Retirement Act benefits. A single person 65 years of age or older need not file a tax return if his or her income is $3,700 or less; for a surviving spouse 65 or older the amount is $4,700. For a married couple filing a joint return, the figure is $5,400; if one spouse is 65 or older, $5,450; if both are 65 or older, $6,200.

There is also other favored treatment. For those 55 years old and older who sell a home, there is a once in a lifetime exclusion of $100,000 in profits if it has been the principal residence for 3 of the preceding 5 years.

Money invested in an Individual Retirement Account (I.R.A.) or Keogh plan (for the self-employed) is deductable from income. In 1977, a special maximum of $1,750.00 is permitted if the I.R.A. is jointly owed by a husband and nonworking wife. The maximum one can contribute to a Keogh plan is $7,500, a provision aimed at middle-income people. The advantage of these plans is that at age 65 or older the money can be withdrawn at a tax rate commensurate with one's supposedly reduced income; it cannot be touched, of course, prior to that time, being deposited in bank accounts or special programs all labeled as such. People who hold regular jobs but do some free-lance consulting or conduct some other self-serving business on the side may enter into these programs with their extra incomes, as approved tax shelters. People using these must complete Part III of Form 5329 of the IRS material furnished them, showing how the deduction was figured.

Pensions, annuities, and deferred pay now come under the 50% limit on tax rates applied to earned income; that is if they, when added to other income, place a person within the 50% bracket, they are taxed accordingly. Stock dividends are also taxed, except that the first $100 is exempt under present law. There is no tax on the income an employment-related trust earns, when the employer invests it for the employees. Gifts in contemplation of death are taxable. That is, a person, knowing he is about to die, cannot give away property to his loved ones in an effort to escape the estate tax on his death. Qualified retirement plans are given special consideration as discussed previously. Some plans can be carried from one job to another. Such are the TIAA (Teacher's Insurance and Annuity Association) and CREF (College Retirement Equities Fund).

For those who have attained the age of 65, an additional $1,000 per year can be earned tax free. If both spouses are 65, this amounts to a $2,000 exemption if they file a joint return (section 151c, Internal Revenue code). This law also allows an additional exemption of $1,000 for the legally blind, a definition with which every ophthalmologist is familiar and which does not necessarily mean total bilateral blindness. Medical expenses, dental care, and drugs can be deducted if they exceed 3% of the taxpayer's adjusted gross income. Half the cost of medical insurance, including Medicare payments, to a maximum of $150 is deductible.

These are essentially the special benefits that the elderly are entitled to under the present Internal Revenue Code, including the 1976 and 1977 changes. The Internal Revenue Code is published by Prentice-Hall, Inc. (paperback, approximately $5); as major revisions occur, it is republished. There is also a 2-volume publication of federal regulations (Prentice-Hall, Inc.) giving detailed examples of how the code is applied to individual cases. Tax law is considered a specialty by attornies because of its fluid, ever-changing nature. No writing or chapter can be all-inclusive or completely up to date. It is hoped that this treatment of the subject will serve the purpose of acquainting the interested person with some of the highlights and complexities.

Property taxes. Another form of taxation for which the elderly often receive special treatment is property taxes. Essentially, this refers to real estate, including one's homes, as taxed by state and county governments. There are also, of course, taxes on other forms of property such as the furnishings of one's home and the tax on automobiles, but these are minor compared with those on dwellings.

It is surprising to find that 58% of elderly people own their own homes; of those, 80% are free and clear of encumbrances. This gives them borrowing power, and real estate in most places is now appreciating 10% to 20% a year. The average income is only $5,000 in this age group, so home maintenance and property taxes, ever on the increase because of inflation and the increased worth of real estate, take a big bite of that income. Sections 235 and 236 of the National Housing Act, originally enacted in 1959 and amended in 1968, attempt to provide mortgage assistance for the poor, handicapped, and elderly. These efforts have not been entirely successful as far as the elderly are concerned.

Homes, like other possessions, have a "proof of ownership," similar to a title to a car. These are called deeds and are recorded as such at the county clerk's office, usually in 2 large volumes, one under the owner's name and the other by street and city address. The usual practice is that the home is owned in joint tenancy with right of survivorship, ordinarily in the name of both husband and wife; when one spouse dies, it reverts to the other automatically. Several persons, such as children, may also be included on the deed in joint tenancy. If the house is not paid for, the deed is probably in the possession of the mortgage company or, if it is being bought on contract, in possession of the former owner. It is important that homes, once paid for, be properly recorded. A clear title means that the land or dwelling is free from encumbrances, doubts, and defects. This is determined by a title search. Such land is said to be held "in fee." With a warranty deed, the owner warrants that such is the case.

The homes of elderly people are too often in the inner or central city areas where surrounding homes are deteriorating or not worth repairing. These are often areas where crime flourishes. The rootedness of the elderly and their insufficient financial resources for relocation compel them to keep their homes. They are not inclined to make "big moves." Consequently, many live in chronic fear and apprehension in their dilapidated houses and deteriorating neighborhoods. While the average tax burden (ratio of taxes to income) in the United States in 1960 was 4%, the low-income elderly paid 10% to 36% of their income for property taxes. Many older home owners need legal assistance when they wish to challenge the tax-assessed value of such property. However, in recent years there has been a movement in many state legislatures to give elderly property owners special treatment, recognizing their economic limitations and the fact that their children are grown and that they should not be contributing to the education of children, where much tax money usually goes. Usually the cities and counties, too, would rather see money go toward paint and upkeep so that their central cities look prosperous. Such factors are included in city planning to attract new industries and tourists.

Crime

Housing location has another legal implication aside from taxes — the problem of safety and protection. In our country, crime seems rampant. Several years ago the government began to scatter the mailing days of Social Security checks so that hoodlums could not wait for a specific day to rob elderly people on their way home from the bank after cashing their checks. It is now possible to have one's Social Security check sent directly to a bank.

In a study in Nashville[12] it was found that one third of the elderly were afraid to go out alone at any time of the day, and three fourths would not go out at night. Friends and relatives, it was hoped, would stop by with what was needed. In a similar study in New York City,[13] the elderly reacted to crime, lack of personal safety, deteriorating conditions of the neighborhood, dirt and noise and the high cost of living. More than 40% report having been victims of personal crime. Those who hope to simplify their lives are attracted to condominium living; many of these provide guards and these add a safety factor. However, this has proved an economic disaster to many because maintenance that started at $50 per month may now be approaching $200 per month. Those who live in apartments often take shifts in "standing guard," providing their own security. It must be recalled that many are widows and relatively defenseless.

This defenselessness takes the form of naivete or susceptibility to fraud and quackery by both men and women, but especially women. This occurs because so often they have no one to turn to for advice and because many are so honest themselves that they cannot imagine being "taken." House repairmen of all kinds knock at their doors, from those who specialize in aluminum siding to concrete driveway experts to insulation experts (now very much in vogue). Because of their high incidence of joint and muscle pains, they are ready victims of arthritis-treatment quackery, which robs its victims of $403 million annually. Medical quacks abound, especially in the areas of cancer cures, weight reduction, "low blood sugar problems," multivitamins, and health foods as a cure for everything from the common cold to constipation. Medical quacks can be recognized by the following signs: advertising, claiming to use a "secret" or "special" cure, promising quick or easy cures, claiming to "cleanse" the body and "pep up" health, accusing the medical profession of persecuting them, and using machines and devices that are bizarre.

Consumerism has become an everyday word in the past decade. The president has seen fit to consider this a cabinet-level concern. But at the everyday local level, the only real defense against those who prey on innocent consumers, particularly the elderly, is public education. We must continually warn elderly citizens against dishonest household repairmen, dishonest automobile mechanics, and door-to-door peddlers. When older people think they have a problem, they easily become obsessed with it, and they become easy victims for those who claim to have the answer.

Driver's licenses

About 8 million of those age 65 and older hold driver's licenses. They place as much value on having their "wheels" as the teenager does in getting his, if not more. To lose one's drivers license is to lose the ability to go shopping, to visit loved ones, to go for little rides, to take vacations. It is the ticket to freedom and independence. About half of accidental deaths in the elderly result from automobile accidents, and the number dying from all accidents is more than double that of the general population, that is, 23% compared with approximately 10%. Older pedestrians and older drivers are more susceptible to fatal accidents. In a Pennsylvania study, those 65 and older made up 9% of licensed drivers and were responsible for 18% of the fatalities. In terms of property damage, they are responsible for proportionally less than those younger than 35 years.

As we have seen, the elderly often receive favored treatment by the law. The Fourteenth Amendment guarantees them, as it does all of us, equal protection of the laws and due process. However, the police powers of the state can impose certain requirements on a select group when public safety is involved. North Dakota and Washington, D.C.,[14] have special requirements for reissuing driver's licenses to those over 70 years of age. However, ability, not age, would seem to be the criterion for reissuing of licenses. Visual impairment that impedes judging distance and accommodation to light changes is a major problem; half those 65 and older need glasses when driving. There is also the problem of impaired conditioned reflexes that blunt responses, impaired judgment through an altered sense of values, increased fatigability, and lessening of neuromuscular efficiency. There are also some interesting psychological factors involved: Some elderly drivers are more likely to select their own speed rather than conform to the flow of traffic, rigidly adhere to a traffic lane and refuse to yield, assign blame to other drivers, make last minute decisions, hesitate at junctions, and conform too rigidly to the vehicle code in spite of altered conditions and even if it is unsafe to do so. All of this causes a stir and is leading to a consideration of special, more comprehensive examinations for those 65 and older seeking reissuing of their driver's licenses. The states have the power to require this if it is not blatently discriminatory.

Competency and wills

Competency is based on one's ability to care for oneself or one's affairs, this referring mainly to handling money, assets, and liabilities (debts). If a person becomes sufficiently disabled that he cannot properly provide for himself in one or both of these categories then the next of kin or a responsible party can solicit the aid of the court to have the person declared mentally incompetent and have a guardian appointed. In some states, the guardian takes care of both these aspects of the problem; in other states there is a guardian of the person (whose concern is the health, education, and care of the person) and a guardian of the estate (to handle all financial affairs). An incompetent person is not bound by contracts or business dealings except for contracts for "necessaries" such as legal, medical, and nursing services.

If a person knows that he will be incapacitated for a certain length of time, such as for major surgery or a recurrent mental illness, he may execute a revocable trust, with a trustee to administer it while he is incapacitated; he can revoke it after recovering.

It is important that every person have a will. Even though a person may feel that he has insufficient assets to "leave to anybody," his death may be accidentally caused by the negligence of another, bringing a huge sum of money, or settlement, into his estate. When a person has not made a will, his estate is divided up among the beneficiaries under the doctrine of intestate succession according to the laws of the state in which he resided at the time of his death. Wills have to go through probate, which is a determination by a court having competent jurisdiction that a will is valid.

Of course, a new will can be made and the older one destroyed, as circumstances change. Also, wills may be modified, added to, and subtracted from by a codicil. It usually does not supersede or revoke the entire will, but it is part of the will. This must conform to requirements of state law, being properly dated, signed, and witnessed. Often, handwritten (holographic) wills are admitted to probate; they must be dated and signed. Calvin Coolidge wrote his own will in a single sentence, leaving everything to his wife.

A person has sufficient mental capacity to make a will if, at the time it is executed, the person (1) is capable of understanding the nature and extent of his property, (2) appreciates the nature of the claims on him, and (3) is able to formulate an orderly scheme of disposition.[15] Aberrations that are not relevant to the issues involved are not considered significant. However, a delusion that one is poverty stricken would obviously affect testamentary capacity. Strange religious beliefs are held not to affect it. Dislike for certain family members is common, acceptable, and not delusional. All wills name an executor of the estate; if one is not provided for, the court will name one. Later, those "left out" of a will may contend that the testator was mentally incompetent at the time of the execution of the will or that he was under duress or undue influence by a certain person, such as a nurse of 20 years or a new sweetheart. They may also cite the influence of drugs. The legal burden to prove this is on the plaintiff trying to break the will. Some extraordinary family quarrels can result, and in court, with one faction sitting on one side of the aisle and the other faction sitting on the other side, one is reminded of certain weddings and funerals.

Veterans are entitled to special monetary benefits for burial expenses, currently no more than $400. The claim must be filed within 2 years after the veteran's permanent burial or cremation.[16] The Veterans Administration will also provide, free of charge, a name plaque for the grave.

There has been a considerable interest in recent years, because of the donation of and use of anatomical parts, in the question of when death legally occurs. Various states have attempted to define death. A group at the Harvard Medical School pioneered in this area and came up with the following criteria: a lack of spontaneous movement, including breathing; a complete lack of response to stimuli; absence of reflexes; and a flat EEG. Kansas and Maryland have adopted similar criteria, but generally death is pronounced by the physician in attendance, without a statutory definition.

A terminal illness may go on for a long while, and if life-saving instrumentation and gadgetry are used, life may be prolonged for additional days or weeks at considerable cost to the patient's family. Some hospitals have established committees to work with the family in determining if and when to "pull the plug" and thus avoid liability. In the past few years, many people have requested that they not be subjected to such prolongation of life once death is certain. A "living will" is a document that is not, of course, an actual will and is not considered legally binding. However, it is a form of contract that the person makes with his physician or responsible members of his family. He ordinarily places it in their hands as a written document, and they either agree verbally or sign it in agreement. As in all contracts, it is the expectations of the parties involved or the meeting of the minds that is important. All of this makes good sense and provides people with a great sense of relief.

ESTATE PLANNING

Many people prepare for their later years long in advance, through life insurance policies that will mature by then and provide a monthly income; through other investments such as stocks, bonds, or real estate; and by estate planning. A great many courses are being given and books and pamphlets prepared on the subject. These deal mainly with an effort to ease the estate taxes paid at one's death, so that more remains for one's beneficiaries. The Tax Reform Act of 1976 made great changes in the old rules turning estate planning upside down.[17] By 1981, when the law becomes fully effective, 98% of estates will escape taxation. One half of one's estate or $250,000, whichever is greater, can be left to a spouse tax free (the marital deduction). There is a new unified tax schedule for transfers of property by an individual (gifts) during his lifetime with rates, as high as 70% (gift tax). Since January 1, 1977, heirs must pay income taxes on any gains realized after 1976 inherited assets that appreciated from the value on December 31, 1976. An inventory of stocks and bonds as of that date should be on file.

A person can still give away $3,000 per year to as many people as he wishes without a gift tax; if the spouse concurs, the gift can be $6,000. There is no tax liability during their lifetime or at death. Also the first $100,000 given by one spouse to another during their lifetime is tax free. For example, a couple can give away a house worth $54,000 to a son by conveying it to him for nine notes signed by the son for $6,000 each and forgiving one of the notes each year. In 9 years, the home is his and no gift taxes have been paid. Of course, none of the notes bears interest, and there has been no appreciation that was taxed.

State death or inheritance taxes are, of course, an additional burden. Estates should be liquid enough to pay all death taxes without the need to sell property. This is often done by sufficient life insurance coverage. Estate planners often recommend trusts for transferring assets and minimizing estate problems. A trust is a right of property held by one party for the benefit of another. The confidence reposes in the trustee, often the trust officer of a bank. The trust is drawn up much like a will and may take one of several forms. A testamentary trust is created by provisions of a will and takes effect on the death of the testator. A living trust is drafted in one's lifetime; such trusts can be amended or revoked as circumstances change. Trusts have to have a body (a res), that is, contain something, be it stocks, bonds, a life insurance policy, etc. An irrevocable trust is one in which the trust passes beyond control of the one who creates it. The will may contain a ''pourover'' provision so that certain assets pour over into the living trust. The entire idea is to make sure that one's assets are not taxed unnecessarily when the first spouse dies. They will be taxed again when the surviving spouse dies, however. For instance, with a $500,000 estate, if the first spouse died in 1977, the tax would be $40,800. If the surviving spouse died in 1981, the tax would be $108,800. As can be seen, these are large amounts. This accounts for the popularity of estate planning.

Statistics show that women usually survive husbands and often they are uninformed in business matters. This is all the more reason to consider a trust, with a trustee's managing abilities. A net estate of $400,000 might result in death taxes in 1981 as high as $15,800 or as low as $800, depending on how the estate plan is drawn.[18] It is not a good idea for tax purposes to leave everything owned jointly, especially if the value is more than $100,000. The estate tax would then be 1½ times what it would be otherwise. For instance, if a man and his wife hold their house in joint tenancy, one half the value would be taxed when the second spouse dies. The state inheritance tax would probably operate in the same way. An attorney who is an expert in estate planning and knowledgeable about the tax laws in one's particular state is essential in advising one regarding estate planning. In addition to providing security for retirement years and reducing taxes, an estate plan may be able to maintain a family business or keep a farm intact. It may be used to reorganize a business enterprise and designate pension and profit sharing. Estates of persons who died in 1977 were eligible for a $30,000 credit against total estate and gift taxes, and this will gradually rise until 1981; thereafter, it will equal $47,000, or an estate of $175,000 will escape estate taxes. After December 31, 1976, every taxable gift made within 3 years of a person's death is added back into the estate.

With inflation, many older people are surprised to find out what their older home is presently worth, and the value of farmland may exceed their wildest dreams. Many people who would not have considered an estate plan a decade ago are very interested now.

POLITICAL ACTIVITIES

Senior citizens have considerable political clout. The elderly constitute more than 17% of the electorate in the United States, and more than two thirds vote regularly. Politicians cannot afford to ignore them or their demands, and they scramble to get their names in the Council Newsletter of the National Council of Senior Citizens (N.C.S.C.) in Washington, D.C., the headquarters for 3,000 affiliated organizations and branches. Current interests, in addition to those mentioned earlier, include reduced fares on public transit systems; 50 cities have responded. More than two dozen states have reduced property taxes. Older people also seek reductions in costs of drugs, reduced premiums on health and auto insurance, and special rates in the cost of travel. Many members of Congress and state legislatures are in their 60s and 70s, and this gives the elderly well-respected, powerful spokesmen. A thousand older people outside a state capitol, some in wheelchairs, can have a pronounced impact on those who govern.

SUMMARY

The law as it applies to the elderly, or any aspect of the law for that matter, is not something that can be carried around in one's head. It is too fluid, too detailed for that. But a kind of organized outline can be remembered. One needs to become familiar with the language of the law and, knowing that, where to look it up. Lawyers live essentially in their libraries, and just keeping current is a difficult task. It is hoped that this chapter provides somewhat of an outline, and although not greatly detailed, will assist the reader in grasping an overview of the ramifications of the law as it applies to the elderly and their specific problems. If a great deal of the presentation appears to involve dollars and cents, that is because it does. The economic health of the elderly person depends on his knowledge of the matters discussed in this chapter and, of course, much more.

REFERENCES

1. U.S. News and World Report, p. 73, Feb. 6, 1978.
2. U.S. News and World Report, p. 70, Nov. 7, 1977.
3. Ross, I.: Breaking the 65 barrier, Reader's Digest, p. 42, Jan., 1978.
4. Brickfield, C. F.: Count us in! Modern Maturity, Dec.-Jan., 1977-1978.
5. Miller, H.: Must people retire at 65? U.S. News and World Report, p. 37, Aug. 22, 1977.
6. Salt Lake Tribune, p. 1, Dec. 16, 1977.
7. Pierson, J.: Wall Street Journal, p. 2, Dec. 16, 1977.
8. Social security brings benefits, Salt Lake Tribune, p. 10B, June 26, 1977.
9. Your Social Security, U.S. Department of Health Education and Welfare Publication No. (SSA) 77-10035, 1977, p. 11.
10. Your Medicare handbook. U.S. Department of Health, Education and Welfare, Publication No. (SSA) 77-100050, 1977, p. 14.
11. 42 U.S.C., Sect. 139 6a(a) (10) (B) 1970.
12. Bourg, C. J.: Elderly in a southern metropolitan area, Gerontologist **15:**15-22, Feb., 1975.
13. Cantor, M. H.: Life space and the social support system of the inner city elderly of New York, Gerontologist **15:**23-27, Feb., 1975.
14. Freeman, J. T.: Elder drivers: growing numbers and growing problems, Geriatrics **27:**46-56, July, 1972.
15. Testamentary capacity, J.A.M.A. **215:**2029-2030, 1971.
16. Encyclopedia of U.S. government benefits, p. 893, Union City, N.J., 1968, Wm. H. Wise & Co., Inc.
17. For your family's future, U.S. News and World Report, pp. 47-48, May 30, 1977.
18. Clay, W. C.: The law and your will, U.S. News and World Report, pp. 49-50, May 30, 1977.

17 The nurse's role as advocate with the elderly

DOROTHY V. MOSES

ADVOCACY

Advocacy is an old term that has been around for many years and has a variety of meanings and usages. Throughout history there have always been advocates because there have always been individuals or groups who were powerless or helpless. Any student of the Bible will recognize some of the earliest examples of advocacy for the poor and sick. In our own country history is rich with recorded examples of advocacy, from the first Pilgrims who established our Thanksgiving Day and acted as spokesmen for the native Americans, to the suffragettes who advocated in their own behalf, and to the current active presence of the Gray Panthers. Most of the social reforms in history were instigated and carried through by advocates. Much knowledge and awareness of the advocacy process is needed to be a successful advocate.

Traditionally the term "nursing" has meant giving care, helping the sick, and following the doctor's orders. Unfortunately this limited perception of the nursing role has been accepted by too many members of today's society. If we as nurses continue to maintain the traditional role and authority patterns we are doomed to oblivion as a profession. Before we can function successfully as advocates for our elderly clients we must first become advocates for ourselves and actively participate in individual and group action to change our public image. As a group, nurses constitute the largest number of health care providers in this country and with a little organized effort could have an enormous impact on changing the health care system that everyone is currently criticizing.

According to Arnold Kisch,[1] one of the major obstacles to achieving change in the health care system is the role of the physician in this system. The disproportionate power granted to the physician in relation to all other health professionals is a combination of traditional mystique and the law. These sources grant the physician justified recognition of his technical eminence and seek to safeguard his power from usurpation and abuse by untrained persons.[1] The problem, however, is that the physician's preeminence has been allowed to extend far beyond the sphere of technological knowledge to encompass all aspects of health care services. There is a vast difference between medical care and health care. Medical care is just one small facet of the entire health care system, and currently the situation is a case of the "tail wagging the dog." Physicians are an expensive commodity and utilizing them in all health-related efforts further inflates health care costs that in turn limit access to health care for many people. This power granted to physicians discourages meaningful delegation of authority that hampers other health professionals from realizing their full potential.

One definition of advocacy particularly applicable to nursing is Mark Berger's in which he describes advocacy as an activity through which people closely identified with

221

the needs of some socially, politically, or economically deprived subgroup can promote changes in the nature of the power structure to improve the situation for their clients.[2] This definition implies knowledge of the power structure and knowledge of the process of creating change. The key word in this definition is "activities," which means action. With action there may also be risks. Recognizing the risks involved, the American Nurses Association at their 1976 convention in Atlantic City passed the following resolution:

Protection of the nurse who acts as an advocate for the aged

Whereas, The American Nurses Association believes that nurses must be advocates for the people they serve, and *whereas,* in this advocacy role, the nurse assumes responsibility for the elderly person who may not be able to defend himself against any abuse, and *whereas,* the nurse, by assuming this role, may jeopardize her employment and her livelihood; therefore be it *resolved,* that the American Nurses Association actively support the advocacy role of the nurse and explore ways to defend nurses whose positions are jeopardized because of such activity.

The American Nurses Association has been in a leadership role for some time in attempting to improve the health care services for the elderly, with specific emphasis on improving nursing care. This was attested to by Claire Townsend in her report for Ralph Nader's study group on nursing homes. She states that "The nurses and the American Nurses Association are not the villains of this study" and goes on to implicate Congress, the Social Security Administration, and nursing home owners. She further states, "nurses have shown more responsibility than physicians and nursing home operators and for this the aged and the nation can be grateful."[3]

In 1961 the American Nurses Association established a group devoted to the interest of geriatric nursing and in 1968 when the Divisions of Practice in the American Nurses Association were established, the geriatric division had 15,570 members. By 1970 this number had more than doubled to 37,811 members. The Division on Geriatric Nursing Practice was the first division to publish their Standards of Nursing Practice in 1973. In 1976 these standards were revised and the name of the division was changed to Gerontological Nursing Practice. This division has also been the most active division in certifying nurses for excellence in practice. The National League for Nursing has been interested and active in attempting to improve the teaching of geriatric nursing in schools of nursing as well as in producing many papers and bibliographies on the care of the aged in all settings.

Despite the activities of national nursing organizations, the current situation in long-term care for the aged is still critical and much more needs to be done. Why does the nation's largest organization of health care professionals, the American Nurses Association, have little or no voice in the decision making processes by which hospitals, nursing homes, and other long-term care facilities are accredited? The American Nurses Association has been trying for 25 years to find an answer. The four-member Accreditation Council for Long-Term Care Facilities of the Joint Commission of Hospitals has consistently voted against American Nurses Association membership on this council and has provided no rationale for such action.

The March-April, 1977, issue of the Journal of Gerontological Nursing contains reports of the Illinois League for Nursing Conference, "Toward Quality Health Care for the Aged," and is highly recommended for further reading. The national offices of both the American Nurses Association and National League for Nursing are pleased to furnish further information regarding their programs on behalf of improving nursing care for the elderly.

WHY THE NEED FOR ADVOCACY

When health care of the aging is mentioned, one usually thinks of nursing homes. Presently nursing home beds in this country outnumber acute hospital beds. Between 1960 and 1970 the number of nursing home facilities increased by 140% and the number of beds increased by 232%, with a current capacity of more than 1 million beds. However, of the 815,000 employed registered nurses in the nation, less than one-tenth are employed in long-term care facilities. As a result, 80% to 90% of the nursing care in these long-term facilities is provided by individuals whose educational preparation is not consistent with the diverse and complex needs of the elderly. To meet the complex, interrelated physical, social, and psychological needs of the elderly requires a high level of sophistication and knowledge. As we grow older the interdependence of these factors becomes more critical. This fact has profound significance for the delivery of health care services to the elderly.

A great deal of national attention has recently been focused on the abuses in nursing home care. Newspapers, magazines, and books have documented these situations well. A great deal of emphasis is currently placed on alternatives to institutionalization. This is worthwhile and long overdue; however we must not forget that there will always be a necessary role for institutions. Perhaps too much criticism has been raised and not enough suggestions offered for creative solutions. The bibliography following this chapter includes books that not only document the abuses and miserable situations but that also offer some suggested solutions for improvement. Whenever an article criticising long-term care appears in nursing publications, an amazing number of nurses write to the editors complaining about such criticism. It seems that the writers of such letters feel as though they have been personally attacked. It is a well-documented fact that many institutions for the aged provide an excellent, high level of care and they are to be commended. However no nurse should be satisfied as long as there is one institution left in which abuse and neglect are tolerated.

Many critics blame inadequate funding as the major cause of the poor level of care. Again, if some nursing homes can provide good care with this funding, why cannot the others? While focusing on the situation in nursing homes, it is also necessary to concentrate constantly on preventive services and ways of keeping elderly clients well and functioning in the community with necessary supportive services. There has been much controversy lately as to whether or not there is a shortage of nurses. If there is not a shortage, there is surely maldistribution. Efforts to attract high quality nurses to nursing homes have been most difficult. Many reasons have been advanced encompassing financial compensation and the type of duties involved to the lack of educational programs in stressing this phase of nursing. Unfortunately too much of the nurse's time is involved with paperwork and administrative duties. More research and study are needed on how this area of nursing can provide positive incentives and attract more nurses. At the same time the entire nursing profession needs to commend, recognize, and support the nurses who are dedicated and devoted to the care of the aged. These nurses are struggling against almost insurmountable odds and rightly deserve much appreciation and support.

PREPARING FOR ADVOCACY

Successful advocacy involves a great deal of stamina and just plain hard work. But perhaps motivation is more important. It really comes down to a moral and ethical question that involves our sense of feeling and caring about the sick aged. If there is any group in our society that is powerless and helpless it is the sick aged, particularly those in institutions. We must continually remind ourselves of the great contributions these people have made in achieving our present state of civilization. We must accord them the dignity and respect that they have so richly earned. Each one of us must do a great deal of soul searching and consciousness raising to effectively function as advocates. Throughout our lifetimes we all belong to many subgroups and generally have freedom of choice as to which group we will belong to. However one subgroup that none of us can avoid, barring premature death, is the subculture of the aged. It has been postulated that this fear of becoming old may be one of the barriers that keeps us away from working with the elderly. A sense of moral indignation at the neglect and warehousing of the sick aged may be the best motivation to become an advocate. We must see that the care of the aged is humanized by caring individuals.

Many elderly are fearful of complaining about neglect and poor care in nursing homes because of their fear of retaliation if it is discovered that they have complained. To counteract this dilemma, the federal government has established an ombudsman program throughout the country. Many states have state offices for this function, and the movement has spread to many local areas. Investigation of state and local activities and programs in these areas is essential for nurses. All nurses should be familiar with the national bill of rights for patients in long-term care. Nurses need to be active in seeing that it is enforced. California had such a bill of rights established before the federal bill was enacted. In addition the state attorney general in California has published a pamphlet called ''Understanding the New California Nursing Home Law.'' This pamphlet explains how clients, friends, or relatives can go about filing complaints.

My own moral indignation was recently reactivated while I was sitting in my own physician's waiting room. I started talking to an elderly lady sitting next to me. She explained to me that she had fallen and injured her knee and was waiting for an x-ray report. She showed me her knee, which was badly bruised and swollen, and she had a cane because she could hardly bear weight on the knee. In a few minutes the nurse came to the door, called the lady by name, and told her that her x-ray was negative and she could go home. My newly found friend looked toward me and her face fell. She weakly commented, ''But my knee still hurts!'' My immediate tendency was to jump up and chastise that nurse. However, using the principle of attempting to assist people in helping themselves, I told the lady she should ask to see the physician again. Her reply was, ''Oh no, he is too busy. I don't want to bother him,'' and she started to get up to leave. I kept insisting that she had a right to receive some treatment for her discomfort and that I would tell the nurse that she needed to see the doctor. However she kept protesting that she did not want to cause any trouble and she would just go home. She limped out of the office.

How many times does such a scene take place in other physicians' offices across the country? I was extremely angry at the nurse as well as at the doctor. When I finally was called in to see my doctor I told him the story and also told him what I thought about the entire incident. I was personally reassured to find out that the physician involved was not mine but another member of the group who practiced together. However I did extort a promise from my physician that he would report the incident to the involved nurse and physician. The elderly themselves need a great deal of conscienceness raising about their worth and their rights to demand attention and care.

In addition to the moral motivation, knowledge and research are necessary. Nurses need knowledge about the normal aging process as well as knowledge about disabilities and diseases to which the aged are more vulnerable. We need to be familiar with and understand the current programs and financing structures available for programming. For example, Medicare is probably the cruelest hoax perpetrated on the aged. Medicare is primarily crisis oriented and meets only about one third of the health care needs of the aged. They are spending far more money out of their own pockets for medical care today than they ever did before the advent of Medicare.

We need to carefully examine and look at the implications for long-term care of all the currently proposed national health care plans. Why are the Gray Panthers so strongly advocating passage of the Dellums bill (HR 694)? This is a piece of legislation that has been given very little attention by the national press. Support of this bill was the number one priority of the Gray Panthers in 1978. It is not a health insurance proposal but is a true health services act, which eliminates all deductibles and provides a range of services from preventive to long-term care. This bill is based on the concept of locally controlled health maintenance organizations, which would be responsive to consumers as participants in governing the programs. There is increasing dissatisfaction among health consumers and unless nurses stay tuned in, they may miss many golden opportunities to assist in changing the system. Another opportunity for nurses is participation in a local health systems agency, established under Public Law 93-641. This provides an opportunity to get involved in the planning process.

Understanding the political process and the resistance to change of vested interest groups is extremely important in successful advocacy. Under the Older American's Act local area agencies on aging, known as A.A.A., are charged with responsibility for planning and monitoring local programs. These groups need skilled nursing input and participation. The political process is not easy to understand, particularly in today's pluralistic system. The best learning method is probably active participation at the local level, moving up to the state and federal levels. Writing letters to legislators is important, particularly if those letters are original and sincere. Presenting testimony at hearings is also vital.

READY FOR ACTION

The simple fact is that attitudes and conditions can be changed. The aged do not have time to wait. There is no need to wait 25 years — it can happen today. The major ingredient in promoting change is an aroused citizenry that exerts continual pressures on its elected representatives. While the title of this chapter concerns advocacy *with* the elderly, much of the focus has been on advocacy *for* the elderly because the sick aged, as a group, are least able to take action on their own behalf. However there are many active, alert, and capable elderly who will be more than ready to join in the action.

The Gray Panthers are a coalition of both old and young people who are drawn together by deeply felt common concerns. This movement has spread rapidly across the country until now most major cities have an active group. Margaret E. Kuhn, known as ''Maggie,'' was one of a small group that started the movement in the early 1970s because they were outraged at the injustice and dehumanization accorded the elderly in our society. She wrote a chapter in Kirschner's book *Advocacy and Age* in which she described vividly the goals and activities of the Gray Panther movement. Maggie is such a vibrant example of true advocacy that anyone meeting and listening to her inevitably has his social conscience stirred. In her chapter she outlines ten steps for successful advocacy. Whereas these steps are directed primarily at the aged themselves, they certainly apply to any age group. These steps include concepts such as personal liberation from the agism of society, awareness and analysis of one's assets, and an inventory of one's skills. Next one must update his knowledge and acquire a thorough understanding of society, including the power structure and political process. Learning to overcome frustrations and resisting efforts and pressures to be pushed aside are also important steps in successful advocacy.

All of the writings on advocacy stress the importance of being informed, or doing one's homework. It is basic and essential to start with research and have documentation of the facts. One needs to identify an area in which one has a degree of expertise to offer. Then one must carefully evaluate and be willing to take the risks involved. Nurses must be advocates for each and every patient with whom they are involved. This means that nurses function individually as advocates as well as in groups. Groups with common goals may frequently band together on certain issues, but this can be difficult at times since many groups are fearful of losing their individual identification. However if the ultimate goal is valuable enough there must be a certain amount of risk and of give and take. Good press relations are imperative and if the story is valuable, the press is usually interested.

Advocacy can be a complicated process requiring much skill, experience, sensitivity, persistence, frustration tolerance, and plain hard work. The rewards of success can well be worth all the effort involved. Poorly planned campaigns may serve to alienate potential supporters and end in frustration and failure. It is better to start small with clearly identified objectives that can be readily achieved. Creative leadership and organization based on carefully planned strategies will usually succeed if the cause is of true social significance. Whereas every nurse cannot be expected to seek employment in long-term care facilities, all nurses should be concerned about the care of the aged because it is a group to which we will all belong some day and we may well be consumers of such care. Above all we should show our respect, appreciation, and support of those nurses actively engaged in the care of the aged.

REFERENCES

1. Kisch, A.: The health care system and health, Nurs. Dig. **4**:41, Fall, 1976.
2. Berger, M.: An orienting perspective on advocacy. In Kerscher, P., editor: Advocacy and age, Los Angeles, 1976, University of Southern California Press, p. 2.
3. Townsend, C.: Old age: the last segregation, New York, 1971, Grossman Publishers, p. 107.

BIBLIOGRAPHY

Burnside, I.: Nursing and the aged, New York, 1976, McGraw-Hill Book Co.
Butler, R. N.: Why survive? being old in America, New York, 1975, Harper & Row, Publishers.
Horn, L., and Griesel, E.: Nursing homes: a citizen's action guide, Boston, 1977, Beacon Press.
J. Gerontol. Nurs. **3**(2): entire issue, March-April, 1977.
Kerschner, P. A., editor: Advocacy and age, Los Angeles, 1976, University of Southern California Press.
Moss, F. E., and Halamandaris, V. J.: Too old, too sick, too bad, Germantown, Md., 1977, Aspen Systems Corp.
Storlie, F.: Nursing and the social conscience, unit 5, the aged poor, New York, 1970, Appleton-Century-Crofts.
Townsend, C.: Old age: the last segregation, New York, 1971, Grossman Publications.

part VII
LOOKING TO THE FUTURE

The youth orientation of our society and other western cultures has tended to distort our concept of the aging as productive, contributing citizens. These attitudes as well as our commitment in the health care disciplines necessitate more serious study of physiological, psychosocial, and cultural needs of the elderly.

Looking ahead, we anticipate a significant growth in gerontological content of nursing programs at all levels because the nursing profession has always attempted to respond to the nursing needs of society. Growing government concern for the needs of the aging, prompted by the effective lobbying efforts of numerous national organizations of the elderly, along with the continuing growth of the elderly population, indicates increased commitment and educational activity in geriatric and gerontological nursing fields.

The final chapter of the text is a summary dealing with issues and trends in gerontology in this country. Contributed by Paul A. L. Haber, who has been active and involved in the field of health care for the elderly for many years, this chapter covers in a succinct manner the numerous issues and trends taking shape in this country concerning the provision of health care for the elderly. He notes that the plight of the aged has at long last reached the public ear and eye.

Haber also points to the need for gerontological nursing to address itself to the field of research in aging and notes that nursing can make some significant contributions to the knowledge base in gerontology in several unique areas. This chapter is rich with suggestions for the future of gerontological nursing and we recommend close scrutiny of its contents.

18 Issues and trends in gerontology

PAUL A. L. HABER

The fields of geriatrics and gerontology will command the attention of all of us — health care workers, planners, sociobiologists, politicians, economists, and many more — for the remainder of our lives. It is well known that the median and mean ages of our population are increasing, but what escapes detection is that the very old are also going to increase to undreamed of proportions in the next 50 years. This excess of aging populations is probably a new phenomenon. Never before in recorded human history (and most probably never before in animal history) has biology permitted a similar increase in the relative and absolute numbers of aging and aged individuals. Therefore it is necessary to reevaluate many of our national attitudes toward the aged.

SOCIETAL ATTITUDES TOWARD THE AGED

The fact that our population is going to be made up increasingly of older individuals will have a pervasive, even a decisive effect on the national goals and the national perspective. Every facet of life as we know it will be affected. We may need less primary education in favor of more continuing lifelong learning. Our buying habits will certainly be affected. Whole industries may suffer decrements, such as baby food, furniture, and clothing suppliers. Others may spring up to take their places, such as leisure industries for retirement-age people. The health care industry is certain to be affected. Although there may be more need for long-term institutional care, there will certainly be a greatly increased need for various home health services and for acute medical care services in hospitals and other institutions for treatment of chronic diseases.

What will be needed is some rational explication of current controversies concerning the provisions of health care. Can these controversial health care provisions and policies be adjusted to an increasingly complex and therefore specific technology without at the same time undergoing infinite fragmentations? Can they be brought to bear with efficiency and cost effectiveness as a separate system that parallels the mainstream of American medical and health care systems, or must they be integrated with all other health care? These and other considerations thrust themselves on us as questions whose solutions must be promptly forthcoming.

Probably the most central of all the issues of aging is the basic one of the role and perception of the aged person in our society. Innumerable authors have discoursed at length on this subject, but none more eloquently and convincingly than Simone de Beauvoir.[1] She points out that there is a general degradation of the aged in society commensurate with a loss of functioning and earning power but that this is not necessarily true in all societies. In some primitive societies the aged are viewed as repositories of wisdom and coping skills. What is of added interest is that since they are closer to death, they may be viewed in the role of intercessor between the generally younger population of the tribe and death.

Bernice Neugarten has spent much of her career grappling with the issues of the

229

aged's role in society. One device she has employed to help resolve that issue has been her convenient division of the elderly into two groups—the young-old (those between ages 55 and 75 years old) and the old-old (those over 75 years old).[2] She has dealt with a number of economic, political, social, and behavioral dimensions of the problem on the basis of her divisions and, if one accepts her premise that the young-old are relatively more healthy, productive, and independent than the old-old, her solutions flow with logic and coherence. Neugarten has an optimistic view of what the future has to hold for both groups and she buttresses this view with a number of surprising and comforting facts. One such fact is that despite popular opinion to the contrary, there will be more children per older family in the future than at present. For example, there will be 2.85 children per aged woman of 75 years in 2010 as opposed to 2.0 children per 75-year-old woman at the present time.

America has often been cited as the prime example of the "youth-oriented" society and much has been made of the fact that we discriminate economically, legally, and politically against the aging. But it is also true that the plight of the aged has reached the public ear and eye and it cannot be truthfully held that the aged are ignored and pushed aside. There are now a number of well-funded and surprisingly potent organizations within and without the federal government whose function it is to promote the welfare of the aged and aging communities. Among these are the National Council on Aging, the National Association of Retired Persons, the Gerontological Society, and various ethnic groups that have developed specific bodies to deal with minority and ethnic problems of the aged. In the government both houses of Congress have committees that deal with problems of the aged. In the scientific community the National Institute on Aging, the American Geriatric Society (dealing with the medical aspects of aging), and various other medical and scientific bodies are concerned with aging. Of a more embracing nature is the Administration on Aging, which administers a number of programs brought about as a result of legislation, chiefly under the Older Americans Acts of the preceding few years.

The net result of the work of all the previously mentioned organizations is an increase in public consciousness of the problems associated with the process of aging. And it is clear that much progress has been made. The institution of the Social Security System testifies to our growing preoccupation with aging. Medicare's concentration on the aged as beneficiaries and the growth of budgetary allotments for the Older Americans Act also indicates that the problems of the aged are not being swept under the rug.

Growing awareness of the aged as consumers is part of the American scene and the news media are increasingly sensitive to the fact that they literally cannot afford to continue to stereotype the aged. In the autumn and early winter of 1977 to 1978 an ongoing series of television programs aimed at entertaining and informing the aged and those concerned about the status of the aged was aired by station KQED, San Francisco, under the title of "Over Easy."

In short, what we have witnessed in the past 2 or 3 decades in this country is a spontaneous and gratifying shift against "agism." This movement has been shared by the government, scientific bodies, consumer groups, and the general public. The attitudes of the aged themselves have also undergone profound changes during that time. What is most heartening about this trend is that whereas it has some sound economic roots (as in the enactment of Social Security and the improvement of pension fund plans), it is not confined alone to finances, but spreads into concerns about health, housing, consumerism, legal rights, and political activity.

One area to which I should like to call specific attention is the field of education.

Whereas there have been some encouraging although tentative efforts, what is needed is a greater commitment on the part of educators and the aged themselves to the process and structure of lifelong learning. As sources of funding begin to dry up in higher education, there may be increased attention paid to the educational needs of the elderly. It is hoped that this movement will be spurred by newer observations regarding the learning and memory retention abilities of the aged, both of which have been found to be greater than previously supposed.[3]

THE NURSE'S ROLE IN GERONTOLOGY

One of the major issues in the whole field of geriatric nursing is the role of the nurse. From my perspective as physician-administrator of a large comprehensive care system, I perceive that the nurse's role covers several areas.

Institutional situations

The traditional role of the nurse in an institutional setting is an area that must be dealt with forthrightly. It has become fashionable to deprecate the role of the institution in dealing with the problems of the elderly. Such attitudes are pernicious. A great many ills have been attributed to the institution — the institution is dehumanizing, it is impersonal, it creates dependency, it robs the patient of the will to live, and so forth. Institutions can be all of those things, but these things are not intrinsic characteristics of institutions. An enlightened and motivated management and staff team may and can avoid all of the previously mentioned pitfalls. What happens all too often, however, is that the staff tends to disengage from the patients, and that management ignores the inevitable consequences in the name of efficiency. What is needed is a rededication on the part of nursing as a profession toward improving conditions in the institutional caring for elderly long-term patients. The institution itself is neither malevolent nor benevolent. It is neutral, but thoughtless regimentation and eradication of personal life-style can make it dehumanizing. Nursing has an opportunity and obligation to reinvest itself in the traditional institution, but in a way that is new and innovative.

One role increasingly filled by nursing is that of administrator of long-term care institutions. Education needs to recognize this role and structure programs specifically for the nurse-administrator of the long-term care health facility. A premium should be placed on acquisition and retention of nurses in this role on the basis that nursing brings a different but vitally needed perspective to the role of administrator. I favor many states' increasing trends toward formal licensure of nursing home administrators. However, I suggest something more: addition of the discipline of nursing administrator.

Home health care situations

Comments on the role of the nurse in home health care situations are found throughout this book. Nursing has a vital role to play in the coordination, management, and delivery of health services to the aged in their own homes. The role of the institution as a health care provider for the elderly should be played only when other noninstitutional resources have been exhausted. Again, the nursing perspective and nursing skills are essential in the provision of services to the homebound elderly patient.

Outpatient situations

There remains something to be said about the role of the nurse in the outpatient clinic. Here specially trained nurses can act in several fashions. They can perform the role of

triage coordinator, separating the truly sick from the worried well, and can make decisions as to the appropriate disposition of patients not requiring hospitalization or immediate institutionalization. The geriatric nurse can help provide primary care for the aged
patient. The nurse practitioner and the clinical nurse specialist have already demonstrated their effectiveness and this has been commented on in a recent publication of the
Public Health Service.[4]

Planning health care services

One area in which nursing must play a larger role is in the planning and mobilization
of resources for the aged. A specific area of concern is in the planning and operation of
senior centers and other senior group programs.[5] A publication of the National Council
on Aging points out that although either full- or part-time nurses are on the staffs of senior
citizen centers, health services are still inadequate. In any event the challenge to nursing is
clear. Nursing must increase its effort to contribute services and views in planning the
gamut of services for the health care of the elderly. Health planners everywhere should
seek out nursing assistance and consultation in preparing health care disciplines. Nursing
educators should be aware of the increased training requirements implicit in the fulfillment of these roles.

COST OF HEALTH CARE

One major issue affecting the health care of the elderly is cost. It is estimated that the
total cost of health care for all Americans will be $180 billion by 1980. The average cost
of any single hospital stay of 7 to 8 days was $996.20 in 1974[6]; it now exceeds $1,000.
The elderly use more hospital days and the incidence of acute care goes up very rapidly
with advancing age. Consequently the total cost of health care for the elderly is disproportionately greater than it is for younger populations, and the burden is increased because
the elderly as a group are least able to afford such care. The role of government then becomes much greater in providing the resources for such health care. Of course the role of
third party payers in the form of insurance is a considerable one. In 1974 private health
insurers paid $27.8 billion in benefits to the American people to help cover health care
expenses.[7]

It is clear that the cost of health care is going to continue to escalate for three reasons.
First, the cost of everything goes up with inflation. Second, for a long time the health care
industry has paid less than minimum wages for certain categories of workers; as minimum
wage laws cover more persons, the health care industry will have to meet this increased
cost. Third and most important, the rise of expensive, new technology carries with it
escalating costs. Only the government can provide the prodigious resources necessary to
defray these costs.

Everyone, or almost everyone, is prepared to let the government bear these health care
costs. At a session of the 1971 White House Conference on Aging there was a fair degree
of concensus on the subject of who should bear the cost of health services to the elderly,
but there was also a simultaneous proscription against government "interference." However, government regulation is a necessary consequence of government funding. The taxpayer footing the bill has a right to know how and where his money is spent and this can
be accounted for only if the appropriate controls are established.

In the health care industry there is a more profound need for regulation because of the
standards of performance. At the same 1971 White House conference the same proscrip-

tion against government regulations for insuring quality control was exhibited by some of the participants. Everyone agreed that the government had to impose uniform national standards of care with respect to quality, but only a few seemed to realize that such a requirement projects even more federal involvement in the care of the elderly.

In short, if increased quality and quantity of health care for the elderly are to be provided, there appears to be no alternative to a commensurate increase in government involvement and regulation. This should not cause dismay among those who are interested in the issue of providing health services for the elderly. It does summon them to greater vigilance and responsibility as it does all workers involved in health care for the elderly, both in and outside government.

RESEARCH IN AGING

Another issue of paramount importance deals with the direction that research efforts in the field of aging should take. There are a number of dimensions involved, but the debate comes down to the need for a decision about whether it is more important to add years to the life expectancy of the individual or to concentrate on research that deals with attempts to add vigor and mobility to the life span already achieved. Popularly phrased, it is whether to "add years to life or life to years." One dimension of the debate pits biomedical against psychosocial research. Both forms of research are needed.

The newly created National Institute on Aging of the National Institutes of Health solved the issue well by creating three task forces to develop the plan for the future direction of the Institute. One task force dealt with biomedical research, another with psychosocial research, and a third with delivery systems for human services, including health delivery systems. The last task force was created to exploit the basic research issues of the first two task forces and to convert them into usable gains for addressing the problems of the aged.

Biomedical research

The field of biomedical research seems ripe for several important gains soon, if not immediately. New knowledge about the nature of cellular aging focuses on the nature and action of DNA. The whole field of genetic control of aging is now open for further exploration and exploitation. Furthermore we are now able to identify many diseases whose causes are traceable to specific genetic defects, often to the malformation of a single enzyme. Such diseases can upset the normal metabolic pathways and may permit us to take remedial action in pathologic states such as diabetes. The immunology of the normal and aged human being is coming under increased investigation and is yielding some secrets to geriatric scientists. Studies of membrane activity and the function of the hitherto unknown organelles of the cell promise increased knowledge of the inner workings of the cell.

Basic biochemical knowledge of the cell as the key to understanding the aging process is accompanied increasingly by studies dealing with the functioning of organ systems and whole organisms. Clinical studies on the aging are multiplying in number, in sophistication, and in payoffs. The cardiovascular, respiratory, skeletal, endocrine, and special sense organ systems, to name just a few, are undergoing intensive investigation through clinical studies in various academic and clinical settings throughout the world and particularly in the United States. What is most gratifying about the nature of this trend is that the quality, as well as the quantity, of research seems to be improving. Not long ago, the most talented and reputable scientists did not consider aging a field worthy of their energies. This is no longer the case and the best brains in biology, biochemistry, physiology, physics, and medicine are now engaged in expanding knowledge about aging.

Psychosocial research

Basic knowledge is being sought and found in the psychosocial aspects of aging. Macro- and microsystems are being analyzed to determine the best patterns of adaptation for the aging. The disciplines of sociology, economics, psychology, and anthropology are being engaged in this effort. Institutes of gerontology have sprung up in a number of academic settings and tend to be in the forefront of psychosocial investigation. Out of such research will come better information about how to cope with the problems of housing, work, retirement careers, and life-style that the aging experience.

Research in both biomedical aspects and psychosocial aspects of aging is needed. Biomedical research may add to the life expectancy as well as to the maximum functioning of the aged individual. And certainly the psychosocial knowledge gained from research may improve the lot of the individuals whose life span has been extended. Results are counterproductive when the two camps compete for resources.

Nurses in research

Nursing as a profession must commit itself to contributions to the field of research in aging. Nursing can offer skills in at least three areas. The first area is in the classical biomedical research area. Nurses with basic scientific skills should be encouraged to seek research fellowships and to prepare themselves for careers in basic scientific research. Nursing is in a pivotal position to carry on studies dealing with improving efficiency in health care delivery. Nursing has already been involved in studies dealing with different types of ward and clinic administration with a view toward increasing delegation of authority. The final area of research should be in what is properly called "nursing arts." This field has long been neglected.

The sad fact is that not enough money is being spent on research in aging. The total federal budget, including that spent by the National Institute on Aging and the Veterans Administration, is probably less than $50 million. Undoubtedly the total figure spent by other academic institutions and private foundations may be several times greater, but those funds are still not adequate to do the job.

DEALING WITH DEATH

Much of the public attitude about the problem of the aged is characterized by feelings concerning the problem of death and the process of dying. It is highly probable that much of the public and societal attitudes toward the aged are conditioned, not determined, by the attitude toward death itself. Since the aged are more susceptible to death and dying, and institutions such as nursing homes tend to include large numbers of these patients, it follows that attitudes toward death—fears, phobias, and prejudices—will generalize to include the institutions also. Thus if physicians have unresolved conflicts (as many do) in dealing with death, they will detach themselves from nursing homes and other long-term care institutions for the elderly in which death is a commonplace experience.

The problem remains how best to deal with the issue of death. This problem has many ramifications, all of them fraught with highly charged emotional issues. The central theme revolves around whether we should preserve life at all costs or whether it is more humane, moral, and economic to permit and even to abet the termination of life when there seems to be no hope of recovery. It has become possible through the use of heroic measures to preserve and prolong life far beyond the point that our ancestors thought of as the end. Artificial heart pacemakers, artificial respirators, and artificial kidneys can assume many of the patient's vegetative functions. In the struggle against death, the dedicated health care worker — physician, nurse, or therapist — has a duty to preserve and prolong life. The patient can have no other skilled ally in the fight against death. It is true that often the patient wishes surcease and that is a factor that must be weighed in the balance, but many times it is impossible to know what the patient really wants. The enormity of making an irrevocable mistake makes the prudent physician shrink from taking that awesome responsibility on his shoulders. It appears that the best mechanism for determining whether and when to "pull the plug" must be through recourse to our legal mechanisms and the courts, for it must be a societal decision arrived at in ways that society can adjust to and control.

Dealing with the dying patient

There are other dimensions to the problem of dealing with death. The vexing question of how to deal with the dying patient in his terminal state is still a matter of controversy. For some patients the answer lies in being permitted to die at home among relatives and friends. For others the nursing home may be the best solution since it can provide a guilt-free trained corps of workers who can minister to the dying patients' needs. The concept of the hospice is an interesting approach and one that merits further trial and study. In recent usage, the hospice is a place where the dying go to die. All hope of recovery is abandoned and the total effort is to make the process of dying as painless and peaceful as possible. The patient is not burdened with difficult, often painful diagnostic or therapeutic efforts but instead is kept free of pain by judicious and frequent administration of appropriate anodynes and analgesics. The patient is encouraged to come to terms with the prospect of death. The hospice had to be created to see if such a regimen could help the dying patient; in a hospital the intervention of massive diagnostic and therapeutic maneuvers makes this approach impossible.

Staff attitudes

Another parameter of the issue of dealing with death and dying concerns working with the staff of any health care institution. This is done in the hopes of revealing to the staff their own anxieties and fears about dealing with the process of dying. Working through with the staff their ingrained difficulties in dealing with death should not be confined to long-term care institutions alone but should also take place in acute care institutions in which death is always regarded as an unexpected intruder. Lectures, courses, and demonstrations involving the entire health care team must take place on an increased scale if this goal is to be met. Again, the nursing profession has a unique leadership role in molding staff attitudes toward dealing with this problem. Nursing is probably more heavily involved in caring for the dying patient on a day-to-day basis than any other of the health care professions. The nurse can be a tremendous source of solace, not only to the dying patient but to the other staff members as well.

THE ELDERLY AND PUBLIC CONCERN
Housing

A major issue for the elderly is the problem of where to live — their own dwellings, apartments, or homes or in congregate housing that serves the elderly and thus minimizes cost, problems of maintenance, loneliness, and abandonment. It is impossible to generalize about what the elderly want for themselves. The best solution to the problem is to maximize the possibilities of choices for the elderly. It is far better for the elderly to continue to live in their habitual abode, but this often imposes financial and physical burdens that are difficult for the aged to bear. A greater array of home services should be available. Home-care programs are a major step in this direction but much more needs to be done. Meals-on-Wheels can help, as can congregate feeding programs, such as those inaugurated and operated by the Administration on Aging using funds supplied by the Older Americans Act. Too often the difficulty of procuring and preparing meals for the elderly is so great that the individual gives up and resorts to the ubiquitous "tea and toast" routine that leads inevitably to malnutrition. Indeed, one large home for the elderly in Philadelphia has reported that the commonest disability on admission of elderly patients from their own homes was, not surprisingly, that associated with malnutrition.

Here again nursing can play many roles. Nursing needs to bring its insights to the home health care programs and to the various surrogates for institutional care. Nursing also needs to be active in the role of decision making for housing for the elderly. One important aspect of the problem is whether to make the housing contain all the elements of shopping, entertainment, and health care on the thesis that convenience makes access easier for all those services. But at least one prominent architect experienced in providing housing for the aged disagrees and states that having the services nearby, but not in the housing envelope, will motivate the elderly inhabitants to get out and immerse themselves in the neighborhood, thus neatly avoiding the pitfalls of isolation and abandonment.

Energy

Still another set of issues concerns the special vulnerability of the aged in certain areas of public concern, particularly energy. Whereas it is true that the elderly as a class are probably lower consumers of energy than other groups, the fact remains that they are more energy dependent than any other group. As we age our energy derived from physiological internal sources fades and our dependence on other external forms of energy becomes greater. This applies to heat, light, mobility, and other forms of energy consumption. During the recent gasoline cutback, it became clear that many of the elderly suffered disproportionately because those who cared for them frequently had to bring services to the home of the aged citizen by automobile. Those who are concerned with the plight of the aged American will have to be vigilant to prevent incursions on the life-style of the elderly brought about by straight across-the-board energy consumption restrictions.

GERONTOLOGY FOR HEALTH CARE PROFESSIONALS

A final issue to be considered deals more with the problem of physicians than it does with nursing, but it needs to be considered for many of the health care professions. The question simply is whether to train specialists in aging or whether to try to train all members of the profession in the rudiments of caring for the aged. In medicine the problem is whether it is more economic and efficient to train a sufficient member of geriatricians or to try to incorporate some geriatric training into every medical student's curriculum. The problem is far from solved. Meetings have been held under the auspices of the American Geriatrics Society and the National Institute on Aging that brought together leading figures in medical academia and the fields of geriatrics and gerontology. It now appears that it is easier to add to the ranks of geriatricians by seeking recruits from the fields of internal medicine, general practice, and psychiatry than it is to train an entire corps of geriatricians. It may be possible in the future to attract bright, energetic, young physicians who are willing to dedicate their professional futures to the field of geriatrics. However, it is probably not possible now to attract enough physicians of that type to help solve the present problem of insufficiently trained physicians in geriatrics. It is heartening to note, however, that more and more schools of medicine are beginning to be aware of the problem. Nursing has not yet experienced this particular dilemma, but it is clear that it will soon.

Lack of gerontological training for some reason does not seem to plague the allied health professionals, particularly the behavioral science professions, to the same degree. Thus it is possible to have social workers, sociologists, and psychologists who specialize in the field of aging and who seem to be able to acquire enough competence to conduct themselves with distinction.

SUMMARY

I have reflected on some of the issues and trends that characterize our approach to the problem of aging. The future is promising for those interested in working with the aged. To be sure, there is a keenly felt need for more of everything — funds, trained health care workers, facilities, equipment, and, above all, understanding and the will to solve difficult problems. There are signs that help is on the way. There is remarkable growth in the interest and energy expended on studying and attending to the problems of the aged, and it appears that this growth will continue at an accelerated pace. Particularly for nurses, a career in geriatrics seems to hold much promise. Undoubtedly the role of the nurse will be expanded, and it is my fervent hope that it will be sooner rather than later.

REFERENCES

1. de Beauvoir, S.: The coming of age, New York, 1973, Warner Books, Inc.
2. Neugarten, B., and Havighurst, R. J.: Social policy, social ethics and the aging society, (report prepared for National Science Foundation), Chicago, 1976, U.S. Government Printing Office, pp. 5-7.
3. Eisdorfer, C., and Fann, W.: Psychopharmacology and aging, New York, 1973, The Plenum Press, p. 130.
4. Cheyovitch, T. K., Lewis, C. E., and Gortner, S. R.: The nurse practitioner in an adult outpatient clinic, Bethesda, Md., 1976, U.S. Department of Health, Education and Welfare, Public Health Service, Health Resources Administration.
5. Leanse, J., and Wagner, S. B.: Senior centers, report of senior groups programs in America, Washington, D.C., 1975, the National Institute for Senior Citizens, National Council on the Aging.
6. Source book of health insurance data 1975-76, New York, 1976, Health Insurance Institute, p. 56.
7. Ibid, p. 13.